Hematopoietic Stem Cell Protocols

METHODS IN MOLECULAR MEDICINE™

John M. Walker, Series Editor

METHODS IN MOLECULAR MEDICINE™

Hematopoietic Stem Cell Protocols

Edited by

Christopher A. Klug, PhD

*University of Alabama-Birmingham,
Birmingham, AL*

and

Craig T. Jordan, PhD

*University of Kentucky,
Lexington, KY*

Humana Press ✳ Totowa, New Jersey

© 2002 Humana Press Inc.
999 Riverview Drive, Suite 208
Totowa, New Jersey 07512

humanapress.com

This publication is printed on acid-free paper. ∞
ANSI Z39.48-1984 (American Standards Institute) Permanence of Paper for Printed Library Materials.

Cover design by: Patricia Cleary

Cover photograph: Scanning electron microscope image of a long-term stroma-supported culture of mouse bone marrow cells. The spherical cells are clustered in so-called 'cobblestone areas', and their association with stromal cells can be seen in some places.

Photo: Julian D. Down and Rob E. Ploemacher.

Production Editor: Kim Hoather-Potter

For additional copies, pricing for bulk purchases, and/or information about other Humana titles, contact Humana at the above address or at any of the following numbers: Tel: 973-256-1699; Fax: 973-256-8341; E-mail: humana@humanapr.com; Website: humanapress.com

Printed in the United States of America. 10 9 8 7 6 5 4 3 2 1

Library of Congress Cataloging in Publication Data

Main entry under title: Methods in molecular medicine™.

Hematopoietic stem cell protocols / edited by Christopher A. Klug and Craig T. Jordan.
        p. ; cm. — (Methods in molecular medicine; 63)
    Includes bibliographical references and index.
    ISBN 0-89603-812-2 (alk. paper)
    1. Hematopoietic stem cells—Laboratory manuals. I. Klug, Christopher A. II. Jordan, Craig T. III. Series.
    [DNLM: 1. Hematopoietic Stem Cells—cytology. 2. Cytological Techniques—methods. 3. Hematopoietic Stem Cells—physiology. WH 380 H48693 2001]
    QP92.H4534 2001
    611'.41—dc21   2001016559

Preface

The ability to highly purify and characterize hematopoietic stem cells (HSC) from mice and humans has opened up an exceedingly rich field of basic science research with enormous clinical potential. Many of the techniques used in studies of HSC biology have become more standardized over the last several years, which makes it possible to compile a set of methods that can be used by both seasoned investigators and novices in the stem cell field. We have attempted to be as comprehensive as possible and yet focus on what we perceive to be the most widely used approaches for studies of murine and human HSC.

This first edition of *Hematopoietic Stem Cell Protocols* will therefore have some obvious omissions that were dictated by contemporary circumstances. It is our hope that readers will feel free to contribute their personal suggestions for further chapters as well as on how existing chapters can be improved for future editions. We certainly expect that old approaches will be refined, new assays will be developed, and other animal model and vector systems will be described that will become the new gold standards for future work. Our sincere thanks goes out to all of the contributors and to those in the stem cell field that have enlarged our thinking and provided new tools to further understand this fascinating cell type.

Christopher A. Klug, PhD
Craig T. Jordan, PhD

Contents

Contributors

SARA J. ABRAHAM • *British Columbia Cancer Research Centre, Vancouver, British Columbia, Canada*

JENNIFER ANTONCHUK • *Terry Fox Laboratory, British Columbia Cancer Agency, Vancouver, British Columbia, Canada*

JULIE AUDET • *Terry Fox Laboratory, Departments of Chemical and Bio-Resource Engineering, University of British Columbia, Vancouver, British Columbia, Canada*

ALEXANDER V. BELYAVSKY • *New York Blood Center, New York, NY, Engelhardt Institute of Molecular Biology, Moscow, Russia*

IVAN BERTONCELLO • *Peter MacCallum Cancer Institute, Melbourne, Victoria, Australia*

GILLIAN B. BRADFORD • *Howard Hughes Medical Institute, Herman B. Wells Center for Pediatric Research, Indiana University School of Medicine, Indianapolis, IN*

CLAUDIU V. COTTA • *Department of Pathology, University of Alabama at Birmingham, Birmingham, AL*

MO A. DAO • *Division of Research Immunology/Bone Marrow Transplantation, Children's Hospital; Departments of Pediatrics and Craniofacial Developmental Biology, Los Angeles, CA*

MARELLA DE BRUIJN • *Department of Cell Biology and Genetics, Erasmus University, Rotterdam, the Netherlands*

GERALD DE HAAN • *Department of Stem Cell Biology, University of Gröningen, Gröningen, the Netherlands*

ELAINE DZIERZAK • *Department of Cell Biology and Genetics, Erasmus University, Rotterdam, the Netherlands*

CONNIE J. EAVES • *Terry Fox Laboratory, British Columbia Cancer Agency, StemCell Technologies Inc., Vancouver, British Columbia, Canada*

R. KEITH HUMPHRIES • *Terry Fox Laboratory, British Columbia Cancer Agency, Vancouver, British Columbia, Canada*

LIBUSE JERABEK • *Stanford University School of Medicine, Stanford, CA*

CRAIG T. JORDAN • *Markey Cancer Center, University of Kentucky, Lexington, KY*

CHRISTIAN P. KALBERER • *Terry Fox Laboratory, British Columbia Cancer Agency, Vancouver, British Columbia, Canada*

GORDON M. KELLER • *Department of Medicine, National Jewish Medical and Research Center, Denver, CO*

MARION KENNEDY • *Department of Medicine, National Jewish Medical and Research Center, Denver, CO*

CHRISTOPHER A. KLUG • *Comprehensive Cancer Center, University of Alabama-Birmingham, Birmingham, AB*

PETER M. LANSDORP • *Terry Fox Laboratory, British Columbia Cancer Agency, Vancouver, British Columbia, Canada*

BRENDA R. LEE • *SyStemix, Inc., Palo Alto, CA*

ANNE G. LIVINGSTON • *Ralph H. Johnson VA Medical Center, Medical University of South Carolina, Charleston, SC*

ERNEST A. MCCULLOCH • *The Ontario Cancer Institute, Princess Margaret Hospital, Toronto, Ontario, Canada*

CINDY L. MILLER • *StemCell Technologies Inc., Vancouver, British Columbia, Canada*

SEAN J. MORRISON • *Departments of Internal Medicine and Cell and Developmental Biology, Howard Hughes Medical Institute and University of Michigan, Ann Arbor, MI*

FRANCK E. NICOLINI • *Terry Fox Laboratory, Vancouver, British Columbia, Canada*

JAN A. NOLTA • *Division of Research Immunology/Bone Marrow Transplantation, Children's Hospital, Departments of Pediatrics and Craniofacial Developmental Biology, Los Angeles, CA*

MAKIO OGAWA • *Ralph H. Johnson VA Medical Center, the Medical University of South Carolina, Charleston, SC*

DONALD ORLIC • *Hematopoiesis Section, Genetics and Molecular Biology Branch, National Human Genome Research Institute, National Institute of Health, Bethesda, MD*

ROB PLOEMACHER • *Institute of Hematology, Erasmus University, Rotterdam, the Netherlands*

MICHAEL J. REITSMA • *StemCells Inc., Sunnyvale, CA*

SERGEY V. SHMELKOV • *New York Blood Center, New York, NY, Engelhardt Institute of Molecular Biology, Moscow, Russia*

EDWARD F. SROUR • *Indiana Cancer Research Institute, Indiana University School of Medicine, Indianapolis, IN*

RICHARD E. SUTTON • *Center for Cell and Gene Therapy, Baylor College of Medicine, Houston, TX*

C. SCOTT SWINDLE • *Department of Pathology, University of Alabama at Birmingham, Birmingham, AL*

STEPHEN J. SZILVASSY • *Lucille P. Markey Cancer Center, University of Kentucky, Lexington, KY*

TERRY E. THOMAS • *StemCell Technologies Inc., Vancouver, British Columbia, Canada*
NOBUKO UCHIDA • *StemCells Inc., Sunnyvale, CA*
JAN W. M. VISSER • *New York Blood Center, New York, NY*
SAIPHONE WEBB • *Department of Medicine, National Jewish Medical and Research Center, Denver, CO*
IRVING L. WEISSMAN • *Stanford University School of Medicine, Stanford, CA*

1

Isolation and Analysis of Hematopoietic Stem Cells from Mouse Embryos

Elaine Dzierzak and Marella de Bruijn

1. Introduction

Recently, there has been much interest in the embryonic origins of the adult hematopoietic system in mammals *(1)*. The controversy surrounding the potency and function of hematopoietic cells produced by the yolk sac compared to those produced by the intrabody portion of the mouse embryo has prompted much new research in the field of developmental hematopoiesis *(2–8)*. While the yolk sac is the first tissue in the mammalian conceptus to visibly exhibit hematopoietic cells, the intrabody region—which at different stages of development includes the splanchnopleural mesoderm, para-aortic splanchnopleura (PAS) and the aorta-gonad-mesonephros (AGM) region— clearly contains more potent undifferentiated hematopoietic progenitors and stem cells before the yolk sac. Furthermore, the most interesting dichotomy revealed by these studies is that terminally differentiated hematopoietic cells can be produced in the mouse embryo before the appearance of cells with adult repopulating capacity. Thus, the accepted view of the adult hematopoietic hierarchy with the hematopoietic stem cell (HSC) at its foundation does not reflect the hematopoietic hierarchy in the developing mouse embryo *(9)*. Because this field offers many questions concerning the types of hematopoietic cells present in the embryo, the lineage relationships between these cells, and the molecular programs necessary for the development of the embryonic and adult hematopoietic systems, this section presents the approaches taken and the materials and methods necessary to explore the mouse embryo for the presence of the first adult repopulating HSCs.

From: *Methods in Molecular Medicine, vol. 63: Hematopoietic Stem Cell Protocols*
Edited by: C. A. Klug and C. T. Jordan © Humana Press Inc., Totowa, NJ

2. Materials

2.1. Isolation and Dissection of Embryonic Tissues

1. Dissection needles: sharpened tungsten wire of 0.375-mm diameter (Agar Scientific Ltd.) attached to metal holders typically used for bacterial culture inoculation.
2. Dissection microscope: any suitable dissection microscope with magnification range from ×7–40 with a black background stage and cold light source.
3. Culture plates: 60 × 15 mm plastic tissue culture dishes.
4. Medium: phosphate-buffered saline (PBS) with 10% fetal calf serum (FCS), penicillin (100 U/mL) and streptomycin (100 μg/mL).

2.2. Organ Explant Culture

1. Millipore 0.65 μm DV Durapore membrane filters: Before use, filters are washed and sterilized in several changes of boiling tissue-culture water (Sigma, cat. #W-3500) and dried in a tissue-culture hood.
2. Stainless-steel mesh supports: Supports were custom-made in our workshop by bending a 22 mm × 12 mm rectangular piece of stainless-steel wire mesh so that it stands 5 mm high with a 12 mm × 12 mm supportive platform. Supports are washed in nitric acid (HNO$_3$) for 2–24 h, then rinsed five times in sterile milliQ water. Subsequently, they are sterilized in 70% ethanol and rinsed two times in tissue-culture water (Sigma). Then, the supports are dried in a tissue-culture hood.
3. 6-Well tissue culture plates.
4. Curved fine point forceps.
5. Medium: Myeloid long-term culture (LTC) media (M5300, StemCell Technologies). Supplemented with hydrocortisone succinate (Sigma), 10^{-5} *M* final concentration.
6. Scalpel blade.

2.3.1. Preparation of a Single-Cell Suspension from Dissected Embryonic Tissues

1. Collagenase Type I (Sigma): Make a 2.5% stock solution in PBS and freeze aliquots at –20°C. For use, make a 1:20 dilution of stock collagenase in PBS-10% FCS-Pen-Strep. One mL of 0.12% collagenase will disperse approx 10 embryonic tissues when incubated at 37°C for 1 h.

2.4.1. PREPARATION AND STAINING OF SINGLE-CELL SUSPENSION

1. Propidium iodide (Sigma).
2. Heat-inactivated FCS.
3. Hematopoietic-specific antibodies, available from sources such as Pharmingen.

2.5.1. Colony-Forming Unit-Spleen (CFU-S) Assay

1. Tellyesniczky's solution: for 100 mL, mix 90 mL of 70% ethanol, 5 mL of glacial acetic acid, and 5 mL of 37% formaldehyde (100% formalin).

2.5.2.1. PERIPHERAL BLOOD DNA PREPARATION AND PCR ANALYSIS

1. Blood Mix: 0.05 M Tris-HCl pH 7.8, 0.1 M EDTA, 0.1 M NaCl, 1% SDS, 0.3 mg/mL Proteinase K.
2. RNase A: 10 mg/mL stock solution.
3. Phenol-Chloroform-Isoamyl alcohol.
4. 2 M sodium acetate (pH 5.6).
5. Isopropanol.
6. 70% ethanol.
7. LacZ PCR primers: lacz1 5'GCGACTTCCAGTTCAACATC3'
                                    lacz2 5'GATGAGTTTGGACAAACCAC3'
8. YMT2 PCR primers: ymt1 5'CTGGAGCTCTACAGTGATGA3'
                                    ymt2 5'CAGTTACCAATCAACACATCAC3'
9. Myogenin PCR primers: myo1 5'TTACGTCCATCGTGGACAGC3'
                                    myo2 5'TGGGCTGGGTGTTAGTCTTA3'
10. Deoxynucleotide 5' triphosphate (dNTP) mix: stock solution of 10 mM each of deoxyadenosine 5' triphosphate (dATP), deoxythymidine 5' triphosphate (dTTP), deoxyguanosine 5' triphosphate (dGTP), deoxycytidine 5' triphosphate (dCTP).
11. PCR (10X) mix: 100 mM Tris-HCl, pH 9.0, 15 mM MgCl$_2$, 500 mM KCl, 1% Triton-X-100, 0.1% w/v stabilizer.
12. *Taq* polymerase.

2.5.2.2. MULTILINEAGE ANALYSIS

1. Complete medium: RPMI-1640, 5% FCS, 2 mM L-glutamine, 10 mM HEPES, 100 U/mL penicillin, 100 µg/mL streptomycin, and 100 µM 2-mercaptoethanol.
2. Lipopolysaccharide (Sigma).
3. Murine interleukin 2 (IL-2)(Biosource)
4. Concanavalin A (Sigma).
5. L-cell conditioned medium.
6. Lineage-specific antibodies are routinely used (available from sources such as Pharmingen).

3. Methods

3.1. Isolation and Dissection of Embryonic Tissues

1. To obtain embryonic tissues for the analysis of HSCs and progenitors, adult male mice are mated with two females in the late afternoon. Females are checked for the presence of a vaginal plug the following morning. If a plug is found, this is considered embryonic d 0 (E0) (*see* **Note 1**).

Dzierzak and de Bruijn

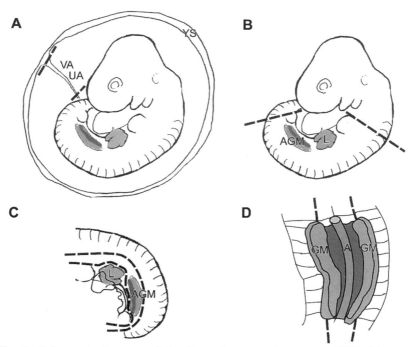

Fig. 1. Schematic diagram of the dissection procedure on an E10/E11 mouse embryo. Dark broken lines show the regions in which a series of cuts are performed on the mouse embryo. **(A)** The yolk sac (YS) is removed by cutting the vitelline artery (VA) and umbilical artery (UA) the site where they join the yolk sac. A second cut adjacent to the embryo body frees the arteries. **(B)** The dissection needles cut the head and tail regions from the trunk of the embryo which contains the AGM and liver (L). **(C)** The internal organs (gastrointestinal tract, heart, and liver) are dissected away first, and then the dorsal tissues (the neural tube and somites) are removed. **(D)** After turning the remaining trunkal region of the embryo so that the ventral side is facing upwards, the dissection needles are inserted under the AGM region, and the remaining somitic tissue is dissected away.

2. Pregnant females at the chosen day of gestation are sacrificed, and uteri removed into a 60 × 15 mm tissue-culture dish containing PBS-FCS (PBS with 10% FCS, penicillin 100 U/mL and streptomycin 100 µg/mL).
3. Using a dissection microscope (×7–8 magnification) and fine forceps or scissors, remove the muscular wall of uterus from the individual decidua. Then with small grasps of the forceps, remove Reichert's membrane, which is the thin tissue layer surrounding the yolk sac *(13)*. During these manipulations, the embryos are transferred to other culture dishes containing PBS-FCS to wash away maternal blood contamination.

4. The yolk sac is isolated by grasping with the fine-tipped forceps and tearing open this tissue which surrounds the embryo. The yolk sac is torn off at the blood vessels (vitelline and umbilical vessels) which connect it to the embryo proper (**Fig. 1A**). The embryo is now covered only by a very thin amnionic sac that may have been broken during the dissection. The vitelline and umbilical arteries may now be obtained with fine scissors by cutting them off at the connection to the embryo body proper (for staging of embryos, *see* **Note 2**).
5. For the dissection of fetal liver and the AGM region from the embryo proper, we switch to the use of dissection needles and a slightly higher magnification. Dissection needles are made from small pieces of sharpened tungsten wire attached to metal holders, which are typically used for bacterial culture inoculation. A sharpening stone, normally used to sharpen knives, is used to produce a fine point at the tip of the tungsten wire. One needle is generally used to hold the embryo in the area where cutting is desired. The other needle is slowly moved alongside the holding needle in a cutting action. Only small precise areas are dissected with each needle placement.
6. Briefly, to dissect an E10/E11 embryo as it is lying on its side, the dissection needles are used to cut the trunk of the embryo from the tail and head (*see* **Fig. 1B**). The needles are then used to remove the lung buds, heart, liver and gastrointestinal (GI) tract from the embryo. The liver can then be dissected cleanly from the heart, GI tract, and remaining connective tissue (**Fig. 1C**).
7. Next the somites and neural tube, running along the dorsal side of the embryo, are removed with care to maintain the integrity of the dorsal aorta (**Fig. 1C**). The trunk of the embryo is now adjusted so the ventral side is facing upwards. The AGM region is now clearly visible. The remaining somites can be cut away by inserting the needles under the AGM (**Fig. 1D**).

3.2. Organ Explant Culture

An organ explant culture has been developed to examine the growth of colony-forming units-spleen (CFU-S) and long-term repopulating hematopoietic stem cells (LTR-HSC) in individual embryonic tissues *(5)*. Beginning at E8.5 (9 somite-pair stage), the circulation between the mouse embryo body and the yolk sac is established *(6)*. Thus, in vitro culture of explanted tissues allows for the analysis of these tissues in an isolated manner, preventing cellular exchange. The culture method was optimized for the maintenance/production of CFU-S and LTR-HSC by placing the dissected tissues at the air/medium interface in the culture rather than submerging them in medium. No exogenous hematopoietic growth factors are added; thus the CFU-S and HSC rely only on the endogenous signals provided by the embryonic tissue.

3.2.1. Culture Procedure

1. One wire mesh support is placed into each well of a 6-well culture plate, and the wells are filled with 5 mL of medium.

2. With forceps, a filter is placed onto the mesh support and allowed to become permeated with medium. The medium level should be adjusted so that the filter is at the air-medium interface.

3. Individual dissected embryonic tissues are placed on the filters, using curved forceps. Up to six individual tissues can be cultured per filter. Empty wells of the culture plate are filled with PBS or sterile water (to maintain humidity), and the culture plate is carefully placed in a 37°, 5% CO_2 incubator. Tissue explants are cultured for 2–3 d.

3.2.2. Harvest of Cultured Tissues

1. Using forceps and gloved hands, the filter holding explanted tissues is removed from the culture plate. The filter is held in one hand, while a scalpel blade is used to scrape each tissue individually from the surface of the filter.

3.3. Transplantation of Embryonic Hematopoietic Cells into Adult Recipients

In vivo transplantation assays have long been established for the purpose of examining cell populations for the presence of HSCs or progenitors *(16)*. In measuring the hematopoietic capacity of embryonic tissues, we have used both the short-term CFU-S assay (3,5,17) and the LTR-HSC assay *(5,10,11)*. While the frequency of CFU-S and LTR-HSCs is a useful measurement for adult bone-marrow populations, since these cells are in limited numbers within an individual embryo, pools of embryo-derived cells are typically used in transplantation assays. Thus, after staging mouse embryos from the available litters by counting somite pairs, only embryos within a desired developmental window are used (for example, from late E10, we would pool embryos of 36–40 somite pairs [sp]). The embryos are dissected and a single-cell suspension is prepared from the pooled tissues, noting the number of tissue embryo equivalents. It is thus possible to determine the absolute numbers of CFU-S and repopulating units in an individual embryo within a temporal context at the earliest stages of development.

3.3.1. Cell Preparation

1. Collagenase treatment is performed to obtain a single-cell suspension from dissected embryonic tissues or from explant cultures of embryonic tissues. Tissues are placed into 1.0 mL of 0.12% collagenase in PBS-FCS-Pen-Strep and incubated at 37°C for 1 h. During the incubation, the tube is occasionally tapped to aid the dispersion of the tissue.

2. After incubation, the tube is placed on ice. Five mL of PBS-10% FCS is added to the cells and using a blunt-ended pipet held against the bottom of the test tube, the tissue suspension is pipetted back and forth up to 20 times to disperse the cells. Cells are centrifuged at 250g and washed two times.

Table 1
Number of Viable Cells Obtained from Mouse Embryonic Tissues after Collagenase Treatment

Embryonic day	Somite pairs	Cell number ($\times 10^4$) per tissue	
		PAS/AGM	Yolk sac
E9	20–29	8.4 +/– 3.8	12.5 +/– 4.8
E10	30–39	12.0 +/–3.5	20.1 +/– 6.9
E11	>40	21.2 +/– 6.2	47.1 +/– 3.8

3. Viable cell counts are performed using Trypan blue dye exclusion. After collagenase treatment, it is expected that only approx 50–75% of the embryonic cells will be viable. **Table 1** provides a summary of the expected number of viable cells that can be obtained from the PAS/AGM and yolk sac from E9, E10, and E11 embryos after collagenase treatment.

4. For immediate in vivo injection, the desired number of cells or known embryo equivalents of cells are suspended in PBS (0.2 mL–0.5 mL per recipient). If some time will elapse before injection, cells are suspended in PBS with 10% FCS, and later washed and resuspended in PBS alone. All cell suspensions are kept on ice.

5. To promote the survival of the irradiated recipient mice so that the engraftment properties of hematopoietic cells from embryonic tissues can be measured, we typically cotransplant a small number of normal unmarked (recipient-type) adult spleen cells (2×10^5) into each recipient along with the marked test cells *(10,11)*. These cells are included in the volume (0.2–0.5 mL) to be injected intravenously into the lateral tail vein. Also, competitive transplantation strategies with unmarked HSCs *(18)* can be used to test for the quality of the donor-marked hematopoietic cells.

3.3.2. Transplantation Protocol

Male or female (nontransgenic) 2–3-mo-old mice can be used as recipients for donor embryonic cells in CFU-S or LTR-HSC assays. When using the Y chromosome as the genetic marker for donor embryonic cells, female recipients of the same strain are required. As in all transplantation protocols, the use of a transgene marker in donor embryonic cells requires the use of either male or female nontransgenic recipients of the same strain as the donor transgenic. We have used inbred strains (C57BL/6, C57BL/10) and F1 strain combinations ([CBA × C57BL/10]F1, [129 × C57BL/6]F1) as recipients in our transplantation experiments.

1. The mice designated for transplantation experiments are housed in filter-top microisolator cages which eliminate the possibility of viral infection within the colony. Before transplantation, recipients are maintained on 0.037% HCl water (3.7% stock diluted 1:100) for at least 2 wk.

2. On the day of transplantation, recipients are irradiated with a split dose of 9 gy for LTR-HSC and 10 gy for CFU-S from a gamma radiation source. The first dose of 4.5–5 gy is given 3 h before the second dose of 4.5–5 gy. The dose of irradiation should be tested within each facility, because variation in the lethal dose of gamma sources and in the strains of mice have been observed.
3. Prior to injection, adult mice are warmed briefly under a heating lamp to dilate the blood vessels and restrained in a holder through which the tail can be threaded. The tail is cleaned with 70% ethanol to make visible the veins lateral to the dorsal-lateral tail artery.
4. Injection of 0.2–0.5 mL (per recipient) into the lateral tail vein is performed using a 1-mL tuberculin syringe and 25–26-gauge needle. Thereafter, mice are maintained on antibiotic water containing 0.16% neomycin sulfate (Sigma) for at least 4 wk.

3.4. Flow Cytometric Analysis/Sorting of Cells from Embryonic Tissues

The cell-surface marker characterization of functional HSCs and the progenitors within the developing mouse conceptus pose special problems in isolation, viability, and analysis. As discussed in previous sections, the numbers of cells isolated from the hematopoietic tissues of early-stage embryos are limited. For phenotypic analysis only, without any functional transplantation, only a few embryos are required. However, several litters of embryos must be isolated and dissected on the same day when functional cells are to be sorted fluorescence-activated cell-sorting (FACS). For example, a good cell-sorting experiment using two different antibodies for the isolation of cells to be transplanted in limiting dilution into adult recipients requires approx 20–40 AGM regions from marked E11 embryos *(11)*. Studies such as these require teamwork, allowing the rapid dissection of embryos by several researchers simultaneously.

3.4.1. Preparation, and Staining of Single-Cell Suspension

1. Embryonic tissues are collagenase-treated as described in **subheading 3.3.1, steps 1–3**. After washing, the cells are suspended in PBS with 10% heat-inactivated FCS.
2. Incubation with CD16/CD32 (2.4G2) monoclonal antibody (MAb) (anti-FcRII and III, Pharmingen) is performed for 20 min on ice to lower nonspecific staining.
3. This is followed by incubation with antibodies of interest (for example, CD34-biotin and c-kit-Fluorescein-5 isothiocyanate (FITC), Pharmingen) for 20–30 min on ice. Cells are then washed twice in PBS with 10% FCS and Pen-Strep and subsequently incubated with fluorochrome-conjugated streptavidin when required.

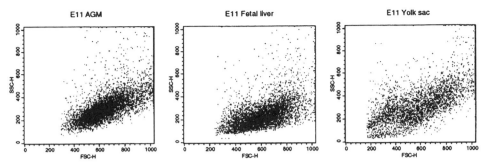

Fig. 2. FACScan plots for forward-scatter and side-scatter of AGM, yolk sac, and fetal liver cells from E11 mouse embryos. Debris and dead cells (based on PI staining) are gated out. The number of cells analyzed per sample is 1.5×10^4.

4. Again, labeled cells are washed twice and filtered through a 40-μm nylon mesh screen (Falcon) to remove cell clumps. After washing, cells are resuspended in PBS with 10% FCS containing 0.5 μg/mL propidium iodide (PI, Sigma) *(11)*.

3.4.2. Sorting

1. Viable cells are defined by exclusion of PI-positive and high obtuse scatter or low forward scatter on a FACStar Plus or Vantage cell sorter (Becton-Dickinson) or any other appropriate cell sorter. **Fig. 2** shows forward-scatter and side-scatter FACScan plots of AGM, fetal liver and yolk sac cells from E11 embryos. Varying distributions of the cells from each of these tissues on the basis of size and granularity are observed after gating out dead cells (PI positive) and debris.
2. Collection gates for marker-positive cells are set by comparison to cells stained with fluorochrome-conjugated immunoglobin isotype controls *(11)*. Viable fluorescent positive cells are collected and reanalyzed for purity and counted.
3. For functional transplantation assays, sorted cells are suspended in PBS at the desired cell number or embryo equivalent for injection as described in **Subheading 3.3.1., step 4**. We have obtained the best results on cells transplanted as soon as possible after the sorting procedure (this is about 8 h after starting the dissection of the embryos).

3.5. Analysis of Transplanted Adult Mice

3.5.1. CFU-S Assay

1. To determine the CFU-S$_{11}$ content of embryonic tissues, tissues are collagenase-treated as described in **Subheading 3.3.1., step 1** and cells are injected into the tail vein of lethally irradiated (10 gy) mice *(3,5,17)*. Control irradiated mice that do not receive cells should be included in each experiment, to check for residual endogenous spleen-colony formation.

2. Eleven days after transfer, the spleens are excised and fixed in Tellyesniczky's solution, and the macroscopic surface colonies are counted. Up to 10–12 colonies per spleen can easily be counted. Thus, the cell dose chosen for injection should be determined to ensure that no more than this number is obtained per spleen. A typical dose of cells for injection is in the range of 2–4 embryo equivalents ($4–8 \times 10^5$) of E11 AGM cells per recipient adult mouse.

3. To exclude contribution in CFU-S activity by either maternally derived cells or residual endogenous CFU-S, genetically marked donor cells can be used to check for the origin of the CFU-S (*see* **Note 3**).

4. After isolation of spleens from the recipient mice, the tissue is not fixed, but placed in PBS in a small tissue-culture plate. Individual spleen colonies are dissected using cataract scissors under a dissection microscope *(3)*. DNA is isolated from each individual colony, and a donor-marker-specific polymerase chain reaction (PCR) is performed to determine the genetic origin of the colonies.

3.5.2. LTR-HSC Assay

To test for long-term hematopoietic repopulation in the transplanted animals, the peripheral blood of recipients is analyzed two times for the presence of donor-derived cells: once at 1–2 mo posttransplantation as a preliminary screening for engraftment, and once at 4–6 mo posttransplantation for true HSC-derived contribution *(19)*. To assay for multilineage reconstitution, donor-positive mice are sacrificed 4–6 mo posttransplantation, hematopoietic organs are taken, and donor contribution to the various hematopoietic lineages is determined as described in **Subheading 3.5.2.1., steps 1–6.**

3.5.2.1. PERIPHERAL BLOOD DNA PREPARATION AND PCR ANALYSIS

1. Peripheral blood (100–200 µL) is collected from the retro-orbital plexus or via the tail vein from recipient mice (in the absence of any anticoagulants) and placed directly into an eppendorf tube containing 500 mL of "blood mix." Samples are shaken and placed in a 55°C water bath for 4–24 h.

2. After a quick spin in the microfuge to remove any of the sample condensed on the top of the Eppendorf tube, 20 µL of RNase A (10 µg/mL) is added, and the sample is incubated in a 37°C water bath for 1 h.

3. This is followed by phenol-chloroform extraction (500 µL) in an Eppendorf shaker for 15 min. After a 15 min spin in a microfuge at 16,000*g*, the aqueous phase (550 µL) is transferred to a clean Eppendorf tube and DNA is precipitated after addition of 50 µL of 2 *M* sodium acetate (pH 5.6) and 400 µL isopropanol.

4. The samples are spun again at 16,000*g* for 15 min, the isopropanol is removed, and the DNA is washed with 700 µL of 70% ethanol. After another spin for 15 min at 16,000*g*, the ethanol is decanted, and the DNA is dried and resuspended in 50 µL of water. Samples are stored at –20°C until use.

5. Analysis of blood DNA for the donor genetic marker is done by PCR. We have routinely used a LacZ transgene or a Y-chromosome marker as the genetic

marker. Simultaneously, a PCR for DNA normalization is performed using myogenin primers. One mL of DNA is added to 1 mL of deoxynucleotide 5' triphosphate (dNTP) mix, 5 µL of 10X PCR buffer, 1 µL of each primer (100 ng each), 1 ml *Taq* polymerase plus water to a total volume of 50 µL. The conditions for the LacZ-myogenin PCR are: 92 °C for 5 min, followed by 30 cycles at 92 °C for 1 min, 55°C for 2 min, 72°C for 2 min, and a final single cycle at 72 °C for 7 min. The sizes of the amplified products are 670 base pairs (bp) for LacZ and 245 bp for myogenin. The conditions for the YMT-2 male marker-myogenin PCR are: 92°C for 5 min, followed by 30 cycles at 92°C for 1 min, 60°C for 2 min, and 72°C for 2 min, and a final single cycle at 72°C for 7 min. The sizes of the amplified products are 342 bp for YMT-2 and 245 bp for myogenin. These conditions may vary, depending on the instrument used for PCR.

6. After the PCR, the amplified products are run on a 1.5–2% agarose gel with appropriate donor-marker contribution controls (100%, 10%, 1%, and 0%, which are made by mixed transgenic or male DNA with nontransgenic or female DNA). Gels are blotted according to standard Southern blotting procedures and [^{32}P]-labeled probes are used for hybridization. Percentage engraftment by donor cells is determined by quantitation of radioactive bands on a phosphorimager.

3.5.2.2. MULTILINEAGE ANALYSIS

To test for long-term multilineage hematopoietic reconstitution, the peripheral blood, bone marrow, thymus, lymph nodes, and spleen are isolated from reconstituted mice at least 4 months after transfer. When a cell-surface marker can be used to detect donor-cell repopulation (as with the Ly-5.1/Ly-5.2 congenics) multilineage repopulation can be tested through FACS analysis of the different tissues, using a donor-specific MAb in combination with hematopoietic lineage-specific antibodies. When a genetic marker is used to detect donor-type reconstitution, cells of the different hematopoietic lineages are purified and DNA is isolated from them. This can be done by growing cells in the presence of lineage-specific stimuli/growth factors—in order to obtain relatively pure populations of B, T, and myeloid cells—or alternatively, by sorting cells to high purity by FACS using antibodies that recognize the different hematopoietic lineages.

1. For culture of B or T cells, spleen cells are grown for 3–4 d in "complete medium" supplemented with either 10 µg/mL lipopolysaccharide or 10–40 U/mL murine interleukin 2 (IL-2) together with 5 µg/mL concanavalin A, respectively.

2. Macrophages can be obtained by growing peritoneal, spleen, or bone-marrow cells for 4–10 d in complete medium in the presence of 10% L-cell-conditioned medium as a source of M-CSF. After culture, the purity of the cells can be determined through FACS analysis using B, T, and macrophage-specific antibodies, and DNA is isolated.

3. To sort B, T, myeloid, and erythroid cells from spleen and bone-marrow cell

suspensions, the following lineage-specific antibodies are routinely used (available from sources such as Pharmingen). For B cells, these are RA3–6B2 (anti-CD45R, B220) and 1D3 (anti-CD19). For T cells, the combination of 53–6.7 (anti-CD8a, Ly-2) and H129.19 (anti-CD4, L3T4)) MAb is a good option, as the CD4 and CD8 antigens are expressed at a higher level on T cells than the pan-T cell marker CD3, thereby facilitating their detection. Myeloid cells can be purified using M1/70 (anti-CD11b, Mac-1), which recognizes complement receptor 3, expressed on both macrophages and granulocytes. As CD11b is also expressed by a subset of B cells (the CD5-positive B cells) present in the peritoneal cavity and spleen, it is advised to use this marker in combination with a B cell-marker when sorting myeloid cells from these tissues. To purify for erythroid cells, TER-119 is generally used.

4. After sorting, the purity of the isolated populations is checked, and usually exceeds 95%. DNA is isolated from at least 10^4 sorted cells and donor-type reconstitution tested by PCR using donor-specific primers as described in **Subheading 3.5.2.1., steps 5** and **6.**

4. Notes

1. We have routinely used a transgene as the genetic marker of the donor embryonic cells *(10,11)*. Other markers available are the Y chromosome marker (if embryos are typed for sex) *(5)* and the Ly5.1/5.2 congenic system *(12)*. When using transgenes as markers, the use of homozygous transgenic males mated to normal females will eliminate any detectable contribution of the maternal blood cells which can be a source of contamination during the dissection of embryos.

2. The embryos within a litter are staged by counting somite pairs (sp) *(14)* and examining eye pigmentation and the shape of the limb buds *(15)*. Since embryos within a single litter can vary by as much as 0.5 d in gestation, this assures that embryonic tissues used for experiments will be developmentally similar. For better contrast, a dissection microscope with a black background stage and a cold light source is used to illuminate the embryos from the side (at 10–15× magnification). E8–8.5 embryos have 1–7 sp; E8.5–9 embryos have 8–14 sp; E9–9.5 embryos have 13–20 sp, and E9.5–10 embryos have 21–30 sp. Embryos of 30–35 sp are considered early E10, 36–37 sp mid-E10, and 38–40 late E10. At E11, sp are greater than 40, the eye pigmentation ring is closing, and the limb buds are rounded with the beginning of internal digital segmentation.

3. It is rare to find maternal contribution to CFU-S activity, because embryos and tissues are washed throughout the dissection procedure. However, when very low CFU-S numbers per spleen are obtained or endogenous CFU-S activity is found in the control spleens, use of the donor genetic marker may be necessary to clearly prove the donor-origin of the CFU-S.

Acknowledgments

The authors thank all members of the laboratory, past and present, especially Dr. Alexander Medvinsky, Dr. Maria-Jose Sanchez and Dr. Albrecht Muller for contributing to the development of the protocols and procedures described in this chapter. Also, we thank Drs. Marian Peeters and Robert Oostendorp for critical comments on the manuscript. Our research is supported by the Netherlands Scientific Organization (901–08–090), the Leukemia Society of America (1034–94), the KWF (EUR 99–1965), and the National Institutes of Health (DK54077–02).

References

1. Dzierzak, E., Medvinsky, A., and de Bruijn, M. (1998) Qualitative and quantitative aspects of haemopoietic cell development in the mammalian embryo. *Immunology Today* **19(5),** 228–236.
2. Moore, M. A. and Metcalf, D. (1970) Ontogeny of the haemopoietic system: yolk sac origin of in vivo and in vitro colony forming cells in the developing mouse embryo *Br. J. Haematol.* **18(3),** 279–296.
3. Medvinsky, A. L., Samoylina, N. L., Muller, A. M., and Dzierzak, E. A. (1993) An early pre-liver intraembryonic source of CFU-S in the developing mouse. *Nature* **364(6432),** 64–67.
4. Godin, I. E., Garcia-Porrero, J. A., Coutinho, A., Dieterlen-Lievre, F., and Marcos, M. A. (1993) Para-aortic splanchnopleura from early mouse embryos contains B1a cell progenitors. *Nature* **364(6432),** 67–70.
5. Medvinsky, A. and Dzierzak, E. (1996) Definitive hematopoiesis is autonomously initiated by the AGM region. *Cell* **86(6),** 897–906.
6. Cumano, A., Dieterlen-Lievre, F., and Godin, I. (1996) Lymphoid potential, probed before circulation in mouse, is restricted to caudal intraembryonic splanchnopleura. *Cell* **86(6),** 907–916.
7. Yoder, M. C., Hiatt, K., Dutt, P., Mukherjee, P., Bodine, D. M., and Orlic, D. (1997) Characterization of definitive lymphohematopoietic stem cells in the day 9 murine yolk sac. *Immunity* **7(3),** 335–344.
8. Godin, I., Garcia-Porrero, J. A., Dieterlen-Lievre, F., and Cumano, A. (1999) Stem cell emergence and hemopoietic activity are incompatible in mouse intraembryonic sites. *J. Exp. Med.* **190,** 43–52.
9. Dzierzak, E. and Medvinsky, A. (1995) Mouse embryonic hematopoiesis. *Trends Genet.* **11(9),** 359–366.
10. Muller, A. M., Medvinsky, A., Strouboulis, J., Grosveld, F., and Dzierzak, E. (1994) Development of hematopoietic stem cell activity in the mouse embryo. *Immunity* **1(4),** 291–301.
11. Sanchez, M. J., Holmes, A., Miles, C., and Dzierzak, E. (1996) Characterization of the first definitive hematopoietic stem cells in the AGM and liver of the mouse embryo. *Immunity* **5(6),** 513–525.
12. Spangrude, G. J., Heimfeld, S., and Weissman, I. L. (1988) Purification and characterization of mouse hematopoietic stem cells. *Science* **241(4861),** 58–62.

13. Hogan, B., Costantini, F., and Lacy, E. (1986) Manipulating the Mouse Embryo: A Laboratory Manual, Cold Spring Harbor Laboratory, Cold Spring Harbor, NY.
14. Kaufman, M. (1992) *The Atlas of Mouse Development*, Academic Press Limited, London, pp. 5–8.
15. Samoylina, N. L., Gan, O. I., and Medvinsky, A. L. (1990) Development of the hemopoietic system: Splenic colony forming units in mouse embryogenesis. *Sov. J. Dev. Biol.* **21**, 127–133.
16. Lemischka, I. R. (1991) Clonal, in vivo behavior of the totipotent hematopoietic stem cell. *Seminars in Immunology* **3**, 349–355.
17. Medvinsky, A. L., Gan, O. I., Semenova, M. L., and Samoylina, N. L. (1996) Development of day-8 colony-forming unit-spleen hematopoietic progenitors during early murine embryogenesis: spatial and temporal mapping. *Blood* **87(2)**, 557–566.
18. Harrison, D. E., Jordan, C. T., Zhong, R. K., and Astle, C. M. (1993) Primitive hemopoietic stem cells: Direct assay of most productive populations by competitive repopulation with simple binomial, correlation and covariance calculations. *Exp. Hematol.* **21(2)**, 206–219.
19. Jordan, C. T. and Lemischka, I. R. (1990) Clonal and systemic analysis of long-term hematopoiesis in the mouse. *Genes Dev.* **4(2)**, 220–232.

2

The Purification of Mouse Hematopoietic Stem Cells at Sequential Stages of Maturation

Sean J. Morrison

1. Introduction

Hematopoietic stem cells (HSCs) are rare, self-renewing progenitors that give rise to all lineages of blood cells. HSCs can be found in all hematopoietic organs, from the para-aortic mesoderm *(1,2)* and yolk sac *(3,4)* in fetuses to the bone marrow (reviewed in **ref. 5**), blood and spleens of adults.

HSCs can be isolated by flow-cytometry, based on surface-marker expression. Multipotent hematopoietic progenitors have been purified as $Thy-1^{lo}Sca-1^{+}Lineage^{-/lo}$ bone-marrow cells *(9)*. Although this population contained all multipotent progenitors in C57BL/Ka-Thy-1.1 mice *(10)*, it was heterogeneous, containing transiently reconstituting multipotent progenitors in addition to long-term reconstituting HSCs *(11,12)*. We found cell-intrinsic differences between long-term self-renewing HSCs and transiently reconstituting multipotent progenitors that permit the independent isolation of these progenitor populations *(13)*. Three distinct multipotent progenitor populations were isolated from the bone marrow of C57BL/Ka-Thy-1.1 mice *(13–15)*: the $Thy-1^{lo}Sca-1^{+}Lineage^{-}Mac-1^{-}CD4^{-}c-kit^{+}$ population contained mainly long-term self-renewing HSCs (*see* **Note 1**), the $Thy-1^{lo}Sca-1^{+}Lineage^{-}Mac-1^{lo}CD4^{-}$ population contained mainly transiently self-renewing multipotent progenitors (*see* **Note 2**), and the $Thy-1^{lo}Sca-1^{+}Mac-1^{lo}CD4^{lo}$ population contained mainly non-self-renewing multipotent progenitors (*see* **Note 3**). These populations form a lineage in which frequency *(13)*, self-renewal potential *(14)*, cell-cycle status *(13,16)*, and gene expression *(17,18)* vary with each stage in the progression toward lineage commitment *(14)*. The ability to isolate HSCs at sequential

From: *Methods in Molecular Medicine, vol. 63: Hematopoietic Stem Cell Protocols*
Edited by: C. A. Klug and C. T. Jordan © Humana Press Inc., Totowa, NJ

stages of development permits direct analyses of their properties and the properties of their immediate progeny.

The properties of HSCs also change during ontogeny *(19,20)*. For example, fetal liver HSCs give rise to bone-marrow HSCs *(21,22)*, but HSCs in the bone marrow and fetal liver are phenotypically and functionally distinct *(23,24)*. HSCs can be purified from fetal liver as Thy-1^{lo}Sca-1$^+$Lineage$^-$Mac-1$^+$CD4$^-$ cells (*23, see* **Note 4**). This population contains all of the multipotent progenitors from the fetal liver of C57BL/Ka-Thy-1.1 mice. Overall, HSCs can be isolated at four sequential stages of development in the fetal liver and bone marrow.

Other markers have also been identified that permit the purification of long-term self-renewing HSCs from mouse bone marrow. Rhodamine 123^{lo}Hoechst^{lo} cells *(25)*, or rhodamine 123^{lo}Sca-1$^+$Lin$^-$ cells that are Thy-1^{lo} *(26)* or c-kit$^+$ *(27)* are pure or nearly pure populations of long-term reconstituting HSCs. Although rhodamine$^{med-high}$ cells are enriched for transiently reconstituting multipotent progenitors *(27–29)*, no evidence has established that it is possible to purify transiently reconstituting multipotent progenitors based on elevated levels of rhodamine staining. Long-term self-renewing HSCs can also be purified as CD34$^-$Sca-1$^+$c-kit$^+$Lin$^-$ cells *(30)*. Although transiently reconstituting multipotent progenitors are enriched in the CD34$^+$ fraction, no evidence indicates that they can be purified based on CD34 expression. Finally, AA4.1-Lin$^-$Aldehyde dehydrogenase$^+$ cells have also been found to be highly enriched for long-term HSCs, but the phenotype of transiently reconstituting multipotent progenitors with respect to these markers has not been addressed *(31)*. Thus other markers permit the purification of HSCs, but they have not been shown to permit the simultaneous purification of transiently reconstituting multipotent progenitors

2. Materials

2.1. Isolation of Bone Marrow

1. Adult Thy-1.1$^+$, Ly-6.2 (Ly-6^b) mice such as C57BL/Ka-Thy-1.1 or AKR/J. Typically, 6–10-wk-old mice are used, but older mice can also be used for the isolation of HSCs.
2. Staining medium: Hank's Balanced Salt Solution (HBSS) with 2% heat-inactivated calf serum.
3. Nylon screen to filter the bone-marrow cells after isolation (for example, the cell strainer with 70 μm nylon mesh from Falcon, product #2350 is suitable).
4. 3-mL syringes with 25-gauge needles to flush marrow out of femurs and tibias.
5. Use 6-mL or 15-mL tubes to stain bone-marrow cells. Note that cells must be transferred to 6-mL Falcon 2058 tubes for fluorescence-activated cell-sorting

(FACS) on Becton Dickinson machines or Falcon 2005 tubes for FACS on Cytomation machines.

2.2. Staining of Bone Marrow

Most of the antibodies described in this protocol are available from Pharmingen (San Diego, CA), and hybridomas are readily available from a number of laboratories.

1. Lineage-marker antibodies: KT31.1 (anti-CD3), GK1.5 (anti-CD4), 53–7.3 (anti-CD5), 53–6.7 (anti-CD8), M1/70 (anti-CD11b; Mac-1), Ter119 (anti-erythrocyte-progenitor antigen; Ly76), 6B2 (anti-B220; CD45R), and 8C5 (anti-Gr-1; Ly-6G). Note that all antibodies should be titrated before use, and used at dilutions that brightly stain antigen-positive cells without nonspecifically staining antigen-negative cells.
2. Fluorescein-5-isothiocyanate (FITC)-conjugated 19XE5 antibody (anti-Thy-1.1; CD90.1).
3. Biotinylated E13, anti-Sca-1 (Ly6A/E) antibody.
4. Allophycocyanin (APC)-conjugated anti-c-kit (CD117) antibody, such as 2B8. Note that some anti-c-kit antibodies, like 2B8, give brighter staining than others, like 3C11, and are preferable.
5. APC-conjugated M1/70 (anti-Mac-1 antibody). This must provide bright staining without nonspecific background in order to cleanly distinguish Mac-1^{lo} cells (*see* **ref. 32**).
6. Phycoerythrin-conjugated GK1.5 (anti-CD4 antibody). This must give bright staining without nonspecific background in order to cleanly distinguish CD4^{lo} cells.
7. Streptavidin conjugated to Texas Red or PharRed (APC-Cy7), depending on the configuration of the FACS machine (lasers and filters). The dye conjugated to streptavidin must be compatible with simultaneous analysis of FITC, phycoerythrin, and APC.
8. A viability dye such as propidium iodide (PI) or 7-aminoactinomycin D (7-AAD). Depending on FACS machine configuration, 7-AAD may be superior because it has a more narrow emission spectrum and therefore causes fewer compensation problems with other dyes.

2.3. Pre-Enrichment of Progenitors with Magnetic Beads

1. A MACS cell separation unit from Miltenyi Biotec (Auburn, CA).
2. MiniMACS (MS$^+$) columns (designed to hold 10^7 cells) or midiMACS (LS$^+$) columns (designed to hold 10^8 cells) from Miltenyi Biotec. In bone-marrow preparations obtained from 3–6 mice, 1 or 2 miniMACS columns can be used. In preparations using larger amounts of bone-marrow midiMACS columns are preferred.
3. Streptavidin-conjugated paramagnetic beads from Miltenyi Biotec.

2.4. FACS

1. A FACS machine with at least four-color capability, such as a Becton Dickinson FACS Vantage (San Jose, CA), or a Cytomation MoFlo (Fort Collins, CO).

2.5. Isolation of Fetal Liver HSCs

Reagents for the isolation of fetal liver HSCs are the same as described in **Subheadings 2.1.** and **2.2.**, except that fetal livers are obtained from E12 to E15 timed pregnant mice. To maximize the yield of HSCs, E14.5 livers are preferred.

3. Methods

3.1. Isolation of Bone Marrow

Obtain bone marrow from a 6–12-wk-old mouse of appropriate genotype (Ly-6.2, Thy-1.1)

1. Sacrifice the mouse by cervical dislocation and dissect the femurs and tibias.
2. Cut the ends off the bones to facilitate access to the marrow cavity.
3. Flush the marrow out of each bone using a 25-gauge needle to force staining medium through the marrow cavities. Collect the marrow and staining medium in a Petri dish.
4. Prepare a single-cell suspension by drawing the marrow and staining medium through the needle into the syringe. Expel the marrow back out of the syringe into a 6-mL or 15-mL tube, depending on the amount of marrow to be stained. The marrow will tend to dissociate as it passes through the needle, but the resulting cell suspension must still be filtered as it is expelled into the tube, by placing a nylon screen over the mouth of the 6-mL or 15-mL tube.

3.2. Staining of Bone Marrow

The bone marrow contains three different multipotent progenitor populations: long-term self-renewing Thy-1^{lo}Sca-1^{+}Lineage^{-}Mac-1^{-}CD4^{-}c-kit^{+} cells, transiently self-renewing Thy-1^{lo}Sca-1^{+}Lineage^{-}Mac-1^{lo}CD4^{-} cells, and non-self-renewing Thy-1^{lo}Sca-1^{+}Mac-1^{lo}CD4^{lo} cells. Because of differences in Mac-1 and CD4 staining, the bone marrow must be divided into three aliquots to stain for each population separately.

3.2.1. Staining for Long-Term Self-Renewing Thy-1^{lo}Sca-1^{+}Lineage^{-} Mac-1^{-}CD4^{-}c-kit^{+} Cells

1. Suspend bone-marrow cells in antibodies at a density of 10^8 cells per mL. Cells are stained first with unlabeled antibodies against lineage markers. The lineage cocktail is a mixture of antibodies against CD3 (KT31.1), CD4 (GK1.5), CD5

(53–7.3), CD8 (53–6.7), B220 (6B2), and Gr-1 (8C5), erythrocyte-progenitor antigen (Ter119), and Mac-1 (M1/70). In order to maximize the enrichment of long-term self-renewing HSCs, it is necessary to eliminate Mac-1^{lo} and CD4^{lo} transiently reconstituting multipotent progenitors. Thus, it is critical to use antibodies against Mac-1 and CD4 that stain brightly (*see* **Figs. 2–4**). In some cases it is preferable to use directly conjugated antibodies against Mac-1 and CD4. If directly conjugated antibodies are used, they should not be included in the lineage cocktail, but should be included with other directly conjugated antibodies in **step 4**. Always incubate in antibodies for 20–25 min on ice. After this incubation period, dilute the cells in at least 10 vol of staining medium, then centrifuge for 6 min at 600g.

2. Aspirate the supernatant, then resuspend the cell pellet in anti-rat immunoglobulin (IgG) second-stage antibody conjugated to phycoerythrin. For example, suitable second stage antibodies are available from Jackson Immunoresearch (West Grove, Pennsylvania). After incubating for 20 min on ice, wash off unbound antibody by diluting in staining medium and centrifuging.

3. Resuspend the cell pellet in 0.1 mg/mL rat IgG to block unbound sites on the second-stage antibody. Incubate for 10 min on ice.

4. Without washing or centrifuging, add all directly conjugated antibodies to the cell suspension including biotinylated anti-Sca-1, and APC-conjugated anti-c-kit (2B8), FITC-conjugated anti-Thy-1.1, as well as phycoerythrin-conjugated antibodies against CD4 and Mac-1 if these were not included in the lineage cocktail. After incubating for 20 min, wash the cells twice by diluting in staining medium followed by centrifugation.

5. The cells can now either be pre-enriched using magnetic beads (*see* **Subheading 3.3.**), or prepared for FACS of unenriched cells. If FACS will be performed on unenriched cells, complete the staining by incubating in streptavidin conjugated to Texas Red or PharRed for 20 min on ice. After washing, resuspend the cells in staining medium containing a viability dye (PI at 1 μg/mL or 7-AAD at 2 μg/ mL), and leave on ice pending FACS (*see* **Subheading 3.4.**). If cells are to be pre-enriched using magnetic beads, *see* **Subheading 3.3.**

3.2.2. Staining for Transiently Self-Renewing Thy-1^{lo}Sca-1$^+$Lineage$^-$ Mac-1^{lo}CD4$^-$ Cells

1. Stain for 20 min in a cocktail of antibodies against all lineage markers except Mac-1. Directly conjugated Mac-1 antibody will be used later in the protocol. Dilute in staining medium, and centrifuge.

2. Resuspend the cell pellet in phycoerythrin-conjugated anti-rat IgG. After incubating for 20 min, dilute and centrifuge.

3. Resuspend the cell pellet in 0.1 mg/mL rat IgG to block unbound sites on the second-stage antibody. Incubate for 10 min on ice.

4. Without washing or centrifuging, add all directly conjugated antibodies to the cell suspension, including biotinylated anti-Sca-1, APC-conjugated anti-Mac-1 (M1/70), FITC-conjugated anti-Thy-1.1, and phycoerythrin-conjugated anti-CD4

when it is not included in the lineage cocktail. After incubating for 20 min, wash the cells twice by diluting in staining medium followed by centrifugation.

5. The cells are now ready for pre-enrichment with magnetic beads (*see* **Subheading 3.3.**), or the staining can be completed by incubating in streptavidin conjugated to Texas Red or PharRed for 15–20 min on ice. The cells should then be resuspended in staining medium containing a viability dye (PI at 1μg/mL or 7-AAD at 2 μg/mL) pending FACS (*see* **Subheading 3.4.**).

3.2.3. Staining for Isolation of Non-Self-Renewing Thy-1^{lo}Sca-1$^+$Mac-1^{lo}CD4^{lo} Cells

1. Stain in directly conjugated antibodies: biotinylated anti-Sca-1, FITC-conjugated anti-Thy-1.1, phycoerythrin-conjugated anti-CD4, and APC-conjugated anti-Mac-1.

2. Pre-enrich with magnetic beads by proceeding to **Subheadings 3.3**, or stain in streptavidin-Texas Red, and then resuspend in PI or 7-AAD pending FACS (*see* **Subheading 3.4.**). Note that Thy-1^{lo}Sca-1$^+$Mac-1^{lo}CD4^{lo} cells appear to be negative for other lineage markers.

3.3. Pre-Enrichment of Progenitors with Magnetic Beads

Since the populations described in **Subheadings 3.2.1.–3.2.3.** represent only 0.01–0.03% of normal adult bone-marrow cells, FACS can be very time-consuming without pre-enrichment. Progenitors can be pre-enriched by selecting Sca-1$^+$ cells using streptavidin-conjugated paramagnetic beads, such as those provided by Miltenyi Biotec.

1. Resuspend the cell pellet in degassed staining medium plus streptavidin-conjugated paramagnetic beads. Staining medium can be degassed by incubating it under vacuum for 20 min. For 10^8 cells, use 0.4 mL staining medium plus 0.1 mL magnetic beads. Exercise care not to introduce air bubbles while resuspending cells. Incubate for 15 min at 4°C.

2. During this incubation period, prepare a miniMACS column (capacity 10^7 cells in the magnetic fraction) by running degassed staining medium through it. This column size is appropriate for enriching progenitors from up to 2.5 × 10^8 bone-marrow cells (~3 mice). If larger amounts of bone marrow are being processed, then midiMACS columns with a capacity of 10^8 cells in the magnetic fraction can be used.

3. Without washing or centrifuging, add Texas Red or PharRed-conjugated streptavidin to the cell suspension (depending on FACS configuration). Incubate for an additional 15 min at 4°C. Dilute in staining medium, then centrifuge.

4. Resuspend the cell pellet in 0.2 mL of medium per 10^8 cells. Add the resuspended cells to a MACS column and place the column in the magnet. After the liquid phase has passed through the magnet, return the cell suspension to the top of the magnet twice, allowing the cells to pass through the column a total of three

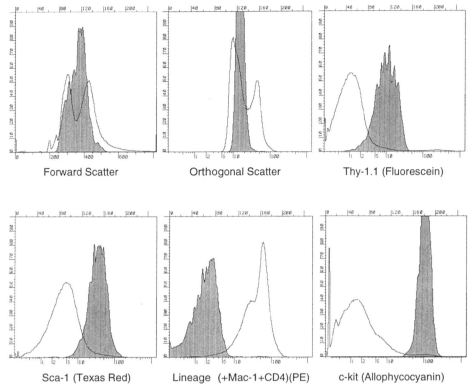

Fig. 1 A reanalysis of long-term self-renewing HSCs isolated by FACS from the bone marrow of C57BL/Ka-Thy-1.1 mice. The shaded histograms represent Thy-1^{lo}Sca-1^+Lineage$^-$Mac-1^-CD4$^-$c-kit$^+$ cells, and the unshaded histograms represent whole bone-marrow cells.

times. Unbound cells in the fluid phase within the column must be washed out by running staining medium through the column (typically 1 mL for miniMACS and 5 mL for midiMACS) . The magnetic fraction (retained within the column) should be enriched in Sca-1^+ cells. It can be eluted from the column by removing the column from the magnet, and forcing approx 0.5 mL of staining medium through the column with a plunger provided by the manufacturer.

5. Pellet the magnetic fraction by centrifugation, then resuspend in staining medium containing a viability dye such as PI (1 μg/mL) or 7-AAD (2 μg/mL).

3.4. FACS

In order to purify the multipotent progenitor populations, two consecutive rounds of sorting should be performed. In each round, sort the cells into staining medium. Containing a viability dye (PI or 7AAD) to mark any cells that die after the first round of sorting.

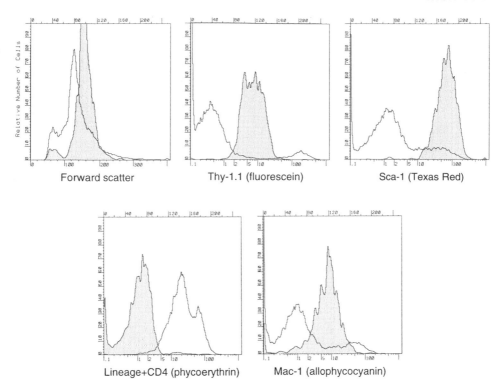

Fig. 2. A reanalysis of transiently self-renewing multipotent progenitors isolated by FACS from the spleens of cyclophosphamide/G-CSF treated mice *(15)*. The shaded histograms represent Thy-1^{lo}Sca-1^{+}Lineage^{-}Mac-1^{lo}CD4^{-} cells, and the unshaded histograms represent unseparated splenocytes. Although these cells were isolated from the spleens of mobilized mice, the fluorescence profile of Thy-1^{lo}Sca-1^{+}Lineage^{-}Mac-1^{lo}CD4^{-} cells isolated from bone marrow is very similar *(13)*. Note that although c-kit was not used as a marker to isolate these cells, all cells in this population are c-kit^{+} *(13,15)*.

1. The fluorescence profiles of Thy-1^{lo}Sca-1^{+}Lineage^{-}Mac-1^{-}CD4^{-}c-kit^{+} cells relative to whole bone-marrow cells are shown in **Fig. 1**. Cells considered negative for a marker have fluorescence levels consistent with autofluorescence (unstained) background. Cells are Thy-1^{lo} if they have fluorescence greater than autofluorescence, but less than that exhibited by T cells.

2. The fluorescence profiles of Thy-1^{lo}Sca-1^{+}Lineage^{-}Mac-1^{lo}CD4^{-} cells are shown in **Fig. 2**. Although **Fig. 2** shows cells isolated from the spleens of cyclophosphamide/granulocyte colony stimulating factor (G-CSF)-mobilized mice, the fluorescence profiles are very similar to that observed in bone marrow. Mac-1^{lo} cells have fluorescence greater than autofluorescence background, but less than most mature myeloid cells.

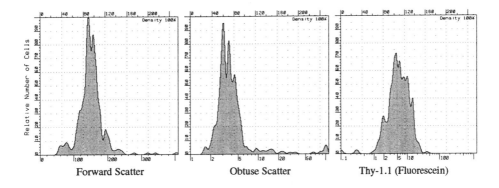

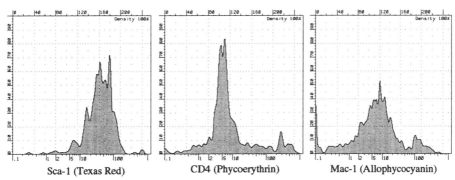

Fig. 3. A reanalysis of non-self-renewing multipotent progenitors isolated by FACS from the bone marrow of C57BL/Ka-Thy-1.1 mice. The shaded histograms represent Thy-1^{lo}Sca-1$^+$Mac-1^{lo}CD4^{lo} cells. The fluorescence profile of the whole bone-marrow cells from which the Thy-1^{lo}Sca-1$^+$Mac-1^{lo}CD4^{lo} cells were isolated is not shown. Although c-kit was not used as a marker to isolate these cells, all cells in this population are c-kit$^+$ *(13)*. Note the increased frequency of contaminating CD4^{hi} and Mac-1^{hi} cells in this population. Because no negative markers are used in the isolation of this population, it is more difficult to isolate cleanly. Two consecutive rounds of sorting are required to eliminate contaminants.

3. The fluorescence profiles of Thy-1^{lo}Sca-1$^+$Mac-1^{lo}CD4^{lo} cells are shown in **Fig. 3**. CD4^{lo} cells have fluorescence greater than autofluorescence background but less than CD4$^+$ T cells. Bright CD4 and Mac-1 staining are required to distinguish CD4^{lo} and Mac-1^{lo} cells from background.

3.5. Purification of Fetal-Liver HSCs

1. Prepare a single-cell suspension from E12 to E15 fetal liver. Remove the fetal livers and make a single-cell suspension by drawing the cells into a syringe through a 25-gauge needle and then expelling the cells into a tube through a nylon screen.

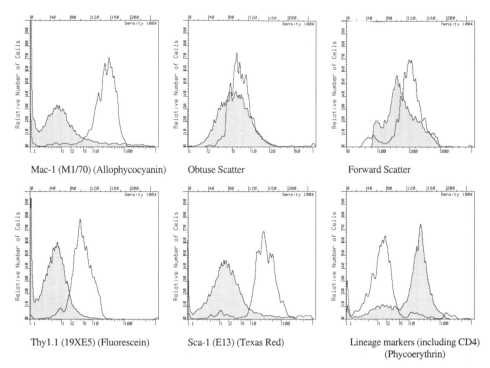

Mac-1 (M1/70) (Allophycocyanin)   Obtuse Scatter   Forward Scatter

Thy1.1 (19XE5) (Fluorescein)   Sca-1 (E13) (Texas Red)   Lineage markers (including CD4)
                                                                          (Phycoerythrin)

Fig. 4. A reanalysis of HSCs isolated by FACS from the livers of C57BL/Ka-Thy-1.1 fetuses. The unshaded histograms represent Thy-1^{lo}Sca-1$^+$Lineage$^-$Mac-1$^+$CD4$^-$ cells, and the shaded histograms represent unseparated fetal liver cells. Note that the bulk of lineage marker staining on unseparated fetal liver cells derives from Ter119$^+$ erythroid precursors.

2. Stain the fetal liver cells with a cocktail of antibodies against lineage markers including CD3 (KT31.1), CD4 (GK1.5), CD5 (53–7.3), CD8 (53–6.7), B220 (6B2), Gr-1 (8C5), and erythrocyte-progenitor antigen (Ter119). Of these markers, Ter119 is most important, because most fetal liver cells are Ter119$^+$. After 20 min incubation on ice, dilute and centrifuge.

3. Resuspend the cell pellet in anti-rat IgG second-stage antibody conjugated to phycoerythrin. After incubating for 20 min on ice, wash by diluting in staining medium and centrifuging.

4. Resuspend the cell pellet in 0.1 mg/mL rat IgG to block unbound sites on the second-stage antibody. Incubate for 10 min on ice.

5. Without washing or centrifuging, add all directly conjugated antibodies to the cell suspension, including biotinylated anti-Sca-1, APC-conjugated anti-Mac-1, and FITC-conjugated anti-Thy-1.1. After incubating for 20 min, wash the cells twice by diluting in staining medium, followed by centrifugation.

6. The cells can now either be pre-enriched using magnetic beads (*see* **Subheading**

3.3.), or prepared for FACS without enrichment. If unenriched cells will be sorted, complete the staining by incubating in streptavidin conjugated to Texas Red or PharRed for 15–20 min on ice. After washing, resuspend the cells in staining medium containing a viability dye (PI at 1 µg/mL or 7-AAD at 2 µg/mL) and leave on ice pending FACS.

7. Isolate Thy-1^{lo}Sca-1$^+$Lineage$^-$Mac-1$^+$CD4$^-$ cells by sorting and then resorting to ensure purity. The fluorescence profile of fetal liver HSCs relative to unseparated fetal liver cells is shown in **Fig. 4**.

4. Notes

1. Long-term self-renewing Thy-1^{lo}Sca-1$^+$Lineage$^-$Mac-1$^-$CD4$^-$c-kit$^+$ cells represent approx 0.01% of normal young adult C57BL/Ka-Thy-1.1 bone marrow *(13)*. Approximately 3% of these cells are in S/G$_2$/M phase of the cell cycle, 24% are in G$_1$ phase, and the balance are in G$_0$ *(16)*. When used to competitively reconstitute lethally irradiated histocompatible mice, 1 out of every 10 intravenously injected cells is able to home to bone marrow and detectably reconstitute *(13)*. More than 70% of clones give long-term multilineage reconstitution. Sixty-seven percent to 83% of single cells (depending on the nature of the donor) form primitive colonies in methylcellulose supplemented by steel factor, IL-3, and IL-6, but few cells form colonies when stimulated by IL-3 or granulocyte-macrophage colony-stimulating factor (GM-CSF) alone *(15,20)*. Although these cells have been most thoroughly characterized from young adult bone marrow, they can also be isolated from the bone marrow of older mice *(20)*, cyclophosphamide/G-CSF-mobilized peripheral blood/spleen *(15)*, and reconstituted mice *(14)*. The frequency and cell-cycle status of HSCs is strain specific *(33,34)*. Thy-1^{lo}Sca-1$^+$Lineage$^-$Mac-1$^-$CD4$^-$ c-kit$^+$ cells isolated from AKR/J mice represent more than 0.03% of young adult bone-marrow cells (unpublished data). Although more frequent in AKR/J mice, these cells are similarly enriched for long-term reconstituting activity, with one out of every 11 cells homing to bone marrow and giving long-term multilineage reconstitution (unpublished data).

2. Transiently self-renewing Thy-1^{lo}Sca-1$^+$Lineage$^-$Mac-1^{lo}CD4$^-$ multipotent progenitors represent approx 0.01% of young adult C57BL/Ka-Thy-1.1 bone marrow *(13)*. Approximately 7% of these cells are in S/G$_2$/M phase of the cell cycle. When used to competitively reconstitute lethally irradiated histocompatible mice, one out of every 10 intravenously injected cells is able to home to bone marrow and detectably reconstitute *(13)*. Most clones give transient multilineage reconstitution, and only 15% of clones give long-term reconstitution. Fifty-three percent to 71% of single cells (depending on the nature of the donor) form primitive colonies in methylcellulose supplemented by steel factor, IL-3, and IL-6, but no more than 10% of cells form colonies when stimulated by IL-3 or GM-CSF alone *(14,15,20)*. Although these cells have been most thoroughly characterized from young adult bone marrow, they can also be isolated from the bone marrow of older mice *(20)*, cyclophosphamide/G-CSF-mobilized peripheral blood/spleen *(15)*, and reconstituted mice *(14)*.

3. Thy-1^{lo}Sca-1$^+$Mac-1^{lo}CD4^{lo} cells represent approx 0.03% of young adult C57BL/
   Ka-Thy-1.1 bone marrow *(13)*. Approximately 18% of these cells are in S/G$_2$/M
   phase of the cell cycle. When used to competitively reconstitute lethally irradiated histocompatible mice, one out of every 10 intravenously injected cells is able
   to home to bone marrow and detectably reconstitute *(13)*. Only 7% of clones give
   long-term reconstitution. Of the remaining clones, around half give transient
   multilineage reconstitution, and half transiently reconstitute the B-lineage only
   (13). The clones that only detectably reconstitute the B-lineage may be lymphoid-
   committed, since in contrast to the Thy-1^{lo}Sca-1$^+$Lineage$^-$Mac-1$^-$CD4$^-$c-kit$^+$ and
   Thy-1^{lo}Sca-1$^+$Lineage$^-$Mac-1^{lo}CD4$^-$ populations, only 26% of Thy-1^{lo}Sca-1
   $^+$Mac-1^{lo}CD4^{lo} cells are able to form myeloerythroid colonies in methylcellulose
   (14). This population cannot be detected in the bone marrow of old mice *(20)*,
   mice that have been reconstituted for more than 6 wk *(14)*, or from the blood or
   spleens of cyclophosphamide/G-CSF-mobilized mice *(15)*.
4. Thy-1^{lo}Sca-1$^+$Lineage$^-$Mac-1$^+$CD4$^-$ cells represent approx 0.04% of fetal liver
   cells from E12.5 to E14.5, but only approx 0.015% of cells at E15.5 *(23)*. At least
   25% of these cells are in S/G$_2$/M phases of the cell cycle at any one time, and the
   number of fetal liver HSCs doubles with each day of development, suggesting
   that all cells undergo a daily self-renewing division. When used to competitively
   reconstitute lethally irradiated histocompatible mice, one out of every six intravenously injected cells is able to home to bone marrow and detectably reconstitute
   (13). Approximately 70% of clones give long-term multilineage reconstitution.

References

1. Muller, A. M., Medvinsky, A., Strouboulis, J., Grosveld, F., and Dzierzak, E.
   (1994) Development of hematopoietic stem cell activity in the mouse embryo.
   Immunity **1,** 291–301.
2. Godin, I., Dieterlen-Lievre, F., and Cumano, A. (1995) Emergence of multipotent
   hematopoietic cells in the yolk sac and paraaortic splanchnopleura in mouse embryos, beginning at 8.5 days postcoitus. *Proc. Natl. Acad. Sci.* USA **92,** 773–777.
3. Huang, H. and Auerbach, R. (1993) Identification and characterization of hematopoietic stem cells from the yolk sac of the early mouse embryo. *Proc. Natl. Acad.
   Sci.* USA **90,** 10,110–10,114.
4. Yoder, M. C., Hiatt, K., and Mukherjee, P. (1997) In vivo repopulating hematopoietic stem cells are present in the murine yolk sac at day 9.0 postcoitus. *Proc.
   Natl. Acad. Sci. USA* **94,** 6776–6780.
5. Morrison, S. J., Uchida, N., and Weissman, I. L. (1995) The biology of hematopoietic stem cells. *Annu. Rev. Cell Dev. Biol.* **11,** 35–71.
6. Molineux, G., Pojda, Z., Hampson, I. N., Lord, B. I., and Dexter, T. M. (1990)
   Transplantation potential of peripheral blood stem cells induced by granulocyte
   colony-stimulating factor. *Blood* **76,** 2153–2158.
7. Bodine, D. M., Seidel, N. E., Zsebo, K. M., and Orlic, D. (1993) In vivo administration of stem cell factor to mice increases the absolute number of pluripotent
   hematopoietic stem cells. *Blood* **82,** 445–455.

8. Fleming, W. H., Alpern, E. J., Uchida, N., Ikuta, K., and Weissman, I. L. (1993) Steel factor influences the distribution and activity of murine hematopoietic stem cells in vivo. *Proc. Natl. Acad. Sci. USA* **90,** 3760–3764.

9. Spangrude, G. J., Heimfeld, S., and Weissman, I. L. (1988) Purification and characterization of mouse hematopoietic stem cells. *Science* **241,** 58–62.

10. Uchida, N. and Weissman, I. L. (1992) Searching for hematopoietic stem cells: evidence that Thy-1.11o Lin- Sca-1+ cells are the only stem cells in C57BL/Ka-Thy-1.1 bone marrow. J. Exp. *Med.* **175,** 175–184.

11. Harrison, D. E., and Zhong, R.-K. (1992) The same exhaustible multilineage precursor produces both myeloid and lymphoid cells as early as 3–4 weeks after marrow transplantation. *Proc. Natl. Acad. Sci. USA* **89,** 10,134–10,138.

12. Uchida, N., Fleming, W. H., Alpern, E. J., and Weissman, I. L. (1993) Heterogeneity of hematopoietic stem cells. *Curr. Opin. Immunol.* **5,** 177–184.

13. Morrison, S. J. and Weissman, I. L. (1994) The long-term repopulating subset of hematopoietic stem cells is deterministic and isolatable by phenotype. *Immunity* **1,** 661–673.

14. Morrison, S. J., Wandycz, A. M., Hemmati, H. D., Wright, D. E., and Weissman, I. L. (1997) Identification of a lineage of multipotent hematopoietic progenitors. *Development* **124,** 1929–1939.

15. Morrison, S. J., Wright, D., and Weissman, I. L. (1997) Cyclophosphamide/granulocyte -colony-stimulating factor induces cells to proliferate prior to mobilization. *Proc. Natl. Acad. Sci. USA* **94,** 1908–1913.

16. Cheshier, S., Morrison, S. J., Liao, X., and Weissman, I. L. (1999) In vivo proliferation and cell cycle kinetics of isolated long-term self-renewing hematopoietic stem cells. *Proc. Natl. Acad. Sci. USA* **96,** 3120–3125

17. Morrison, S. J., Prowse, K. R., Ho, P., and Weissman, I. L. (1996) Telomerase activity of hematopoietic cells is associated with self-renewal potential. *Immunity* **5,** 207–216.

18. Klug, C. A., Morrison, S. J., Masek, M., Hahm, K., Smale, S. T., and Weissman, I. L. (1998) Hematopoietic stem cells and lymphoid progenitors express different Ikaros isoforms and Ikaros is localized to heterochromatin in immature lymphocytes. Proc. *Natl. Acad. Sci. USA* **95,** 657–662.

19. Lansdorp, P. M., Dragowska, W., and Mayani, H. (1993) Ontogeny-related changes in proliferative potential of human hematopoietic cells. *J. Exp. Med.* **178,** 787–791.

20. Morrison, S. J., Wandycz, A. M., Akashi, K., Globerson, A., and Weissman, I. L. (1996) The aging of hematopoietic stem cells. *Nat. Med.* **2,** 202–206.

21. Fleischman, R. A., Custer, R. P., and Mintz, B. (1982) Totipotent hematopoietic stem cells: normal self-renewal and differentiation after transplantation between mouse fetuses. *Cell* **30,** 351–359.

22. Clapp, D. W., Freie, B., Lee, W.-H., and Zhang, Y.-Y. (1995) Molecular evidence that in situ-transduced fetal liver hematopoietic stem/progenitor cells give rise to medullary hematopoiesis in adult rats. *Blood* **86,** 2113–2122.

23. Morrison, S. J., Hemmati, H. D., Wandycz, A. M., and Weissman, I. L. (1995)

The purification and characterization of fetal liver hematopoietic stem cells. *Proc. Natl. Acad. Sci. USA* **92**, 10,302–10,306.

24. Rebel, V. I., Miller, C. L., Eaves, C. J., and Lansdorp, P. M. (1996) The repopulation potential of fetal liver hematopoietic stem cells in mice exceeds that of their adult bone marrow counterparts. *Blood* **87**, 3500–3507.

25. Wolf, N. S., Kone, A., Priestley, G. V., and Bartelmez, S. H. (1993) In vivo and in vitro characterization of long-term repopulating primitive hematopoietic cells isolated by sequential Hoechst 33342–rhodamine 123 FACS selection. *Exp. Hematol.* **21**, 614–622.

26. Spangrude, G. J., Brooks, D. M., and Tumas, D. B. (1995) Long-term repopulation of irradiated mice with limiting numbers of purified hematopoietic stem cells: in vivo expansion of stem cell phenotype but not function. *Blood* **85**, 1006–1016.

27. Li, C. L. and Johnson, G. R. (1995) Murine hematopoietic stem and progenitor cells: I. Enrichment and biologic characterization. *Blood* **85**, 1472–1479.

28. Li, C. L. and Johnson, G. R. (1992) Rhodamine 123 reveals heterogeneity within murine Lin-, Sca-1+ hematopoietic stem cells. *J. Exp. Med.* **175**, 1443–1447.

29. Zijlmans, J. M., Visser, J. W. M., Kleiverda, K., Kluin, P. M., Willemze, R., and Fibbe, W. E. (1995) Modification of rhodamin staining with the use of verapamil allows identification of hematopoietic stem cells with preferential short-term or long-term bone marrow-repopulating ability. *Proc. Natl. Acad. Sci. USA* **92**, 8901–8905.

30. Osawa, M., Hanada, K.-I., Hamada, H., and Nakauchi, H. (1996) Long-term lymphohematopoietic reconstitution by a single CD34–low/negative hematopoietic stem cell. *Science* **273**, 242–245.

31. Jones, R. J., Collector, M. I., Barber, J. P., Vala, M. S., Fackler, M. J., May, W. S., et al. (1996) Characterization of mouse lymphohematopoietic stem cells lacking spleen colony-forming activity. *Blood* **88**, 487–491

32. Morrison, S. J., Lagasse, E., and Weissman, I. L. (1994) Demonstration that Thy-lo subsets of mouse bone marrow that express high levels of lineage markers are not significant hematopoietic progenitors. *Blood* **83**, 3480–3490.

33. deHaan, G., Nijhof, W., and VanZant, G. (1997) Mouse strain -dependent changes in frequency and proliferation of hematopoietic stem cells during aging: correlation between lifespan and cycling activity. *Blood* **89**, 1543–1550.

34. deHaan, G. and VanZant, G. (1997) Intrinsic and extrinsic control of hematopoietic stem cell numbers: mapping of a stem cell gene. *J. Exp. Med.* **186**, 529–536.

3

Flow Cytometry and Immunoselection of Human Stem Cells

Terry E. Thomas, Sara J. Abraham, and Peter M. Lansdorp

1. Introduction

Human hematopoietic stem cells (HSCs) can be obtained from a variety of hematopoietic tissues, including bone marrow, blood, cord blood, and fetal liver. Various techniques have been used to fractionate hematopoietic cell populations based on differences in size and density, expression of cell-surface antigens, differential dye uptake, and sensitivity to cytotoxic drugs. The very low frequency of HSCs in hematopoietic tissues presents an enormous challenge to purification strategies aimed at isolation of sufficient cells of suitable purity for further study. The most effective approaches invariably involve several cell-separation steps which differ in capacity and degree of selectivity.

Hematopoiesis is generally viewed as a hierarchical system in which undifferentiated pluripotent stem cells give rise to committed progenitors, which in turn give rise to fully differentiated mature blood cells. This involves numerous differentiation steps and extensive proliferation. The expression of certain cell-surface antigens is often characteristic of a particular differentiation stage and commitment to a specific hematopoietic lineage. Functionally distinct subpopulations of fully differentiated mature blood cells often express unique surface markers. Unfortunately, no unique markers currently exist for HSCs that are typically defined in functional transplantation assays *(1,2)* by their potential for sustained multilineage repopulation. Hematopoietic progenitor cells of various differentiation stages can be detected and quantified by other well-established assays. Mature, lineage-committed colony-forming cells (CFCs) can be distinguished from more primitive precursors detected in Long-

From: *Methods in Molecular Medicine, vol. 63: Hematopoietic Stem Cell Protocols*
Edited by: C. A. Klug and C. T. Jordan © Humana Press Inc., Totowa, NJ

Term Culture-Initiating Cell (LTC-IC) assays *(3–5)*. Systematic analysis using the LTC-IC assay of subpopulations of cells separated on the basis of their expression of certain cell-surface antigens has led to the identification of cells with a rare cell phenotype which are highly enriched both for LTC-IC and stem-cell activity *(4,6–9)*.

1.1. Rare Cell Isolation: Multi-Step Strategies

Fluorescence-Activated Cell-Sorting (FACS) has the ability to isolate individual cells based on multiple, independent parameters including light-scatter properties and the expression of several cell-surface markers. Simultaneous multi-parameter analysis and sorting of individual cells produces cell suspensions of very high purity (>99%). However, FACS is a relatively slow method of isolating cells capable of sorting $2–50 \times 10^3$ cells/s ($1.2–30 \times 10^5$ cells/min). The very low frequency (<0.01%) of stem cells in hematopoietic tissues means that a large number of cells must be processed to obtain a usable number of stem cells. For this reason, pre-enrichment steps are typically used to remove mature cells and reduce the sample size for subsequent analysis and sorting by FACS.

The degree of stem-cell enrichment offered by pre-enrichment steps varies depending on what proportion of the "non-stem cells" are removed. Antibody-mediated batch-wise immunoselection techniques offer the greatest degree of pre-enrichment, but often require an initial lysis or density separation to remove red cells. Density separations will typically also remove granulocytes, decreasing the nucleated cell count and enriching for stem cells. The procedure for isolating human HSCs described in this chapter involves three steps: a density centrifugation to remove red cells and granulocytes; an immunomagnetic lineage depletion to remove the remaining mature differentiated cells; and finally, multi-parameter FACS.

1.2. Antibody-Mediated Cell Separation: Positive vs Negative Selection

Most immunomagnetic pre-enrichment and FACS techniques separate cells based on antibody binding to cell-surface antigens. There are two basic approaches to antibody-mediated cell separation: *positive selection*, where the desired cell is labeled with an antibody and recovered, or *negative selection*, where the unwanted cells are antibody-labeled and removed. FACS can simultaneously select a cell with positive selection (the cell expresses a designated marker) and negative selection (the cell does not express a designated marker). Batch-wise techniques, like magnetic cell separation, are limited to either positive or negative selection in a given separation step. The advantage of positive selection pre-enrichment methods is that only one antibody is required. With negative selection, numerous cell types must be targeted for removal, requiring several antibodies. The disadvantages of positive selection are that the desired cells are labeled with antibody and must be recovered from the separation matrix in an additional second step. More significant than these technical considerations is the question: "Is it better to pre-enrich stem cells based on the antigen they do express (positive selection) or the lack of expression of certain antigens (negative selection)?" In order to answer this question, the potential enrichment and recovery offered by the two approaches must be evaluated.

1.2.1. Positive Selection

The most commonly used stem-cell enrichment technique is CD34-positive selection. CD34 is expressed on 1–4% of normal adult human bone marrow and on ~0.1% of the nucleated cells present in steady-state peripheral blood. Cytokine mobilization and/or myelotoxic therapies may increase the level of $CD34^+$ cells in blood to >1.0% *(10–13)*. Selection of $CD34^+$ cells from bone marrow or mobilized peripheral blood therefore typically achieves approx 25–100-fold enrichment of $CD34^+$ stem cells. Yin et al. have recently identified a marker on a more primitive subpopulation of $CD34^+$ cells *(14)*. The AC133 monoclonal antibody (MAb) binds to a cell-surface antigen present on 20–60% of $CD34^+$ cells, including those with long-term in vivo repopulating activity, but is not expressed on all CFC *(14)*. Positive selection with AC133 offers two-five fold greater enrichment of stem cells than CD34 positive selection.

1.2.2. Negative Selection

The more primitive blast cells, progenitor cells, and stem cells can be significantly enriched from blood and bone marrow by the removal of the cells which express mature lineage markers. This involves "purging" the cell suspension with several antibodies or a "cocktail of antibodies." Examples of these mature lineage markers are glycophorin A, CD2, CD3, CD4, CD8, CD14, CD16, CD19, CD20, and CD56. These antigens define mature subpopulations of cells, such as erythrocytes, T cells, B cells, NK cells, monocytes, and granulocytes. The degree of enrichment of stem cells offered by such "lineage depletion" depends on the type and number of antibodies used, but typically ranges from 50–200 fold *(15)*.

A number of cell-surface molecules are expressed early in the differentiation of the various hematopoietic lineages, but are still absent on stem cells. These markers have been used to differentiate more mature lineage-committed CFC from cells which are detected in assays for stem-cell function (Long-Term Culture-Initiating Cell (LTC-IC) assay and Competitive Repopulating Unit (CRU) assay) *(4,6–9)*. **Fig. 1** shows the progenitor potential of different subpopulations of normal human bone marrow CD34$^+$ cells sorted based on their expression of CD38, CD71, and CD45RA *(16)*.

Both CD34 positive selection and the basic lineage depletion using negative selection result in ~100-fold enrichment of HSCs. Negative selection with a extended depletion cocktail, including antibodies to markers expressed by committed progenitors but absent on stem cells (e.g., anti-CD38, CD71, CD45RA) offers an additional 10-fold enrichment. Positive selection with AC133 only offers an additional two- to fivefold enrichment. Significant advantages to negative selection are that it avoids coating the recovered cells with antibody, and that the yield of cells of interest is typically higher. Furthermore, recent studies suggest that a portion of human hematopoietic stem cells are CD34 negative, and that these Lin$^-$CD34$^-$ cells may give rise to the most primitive CD34$^+$ cells *(17,18)*. For these various reasons, immunomagnetic lineage depletion techniques as described in the this chapter appear to have significant advantages over CD34 or AC133 positive selection to enrich stem cells prior to FACS.

1.3. Primitive Cell Phenotype

FACS can be used to simultaneously select for the presence or absence of several cell-surface markers. A number of markers have proven useful in identifying a subpopulations of CD34$^+$ cells which are more highly enriched for cells with stem-cell function *(4,8,19)*. Fig. 1 illustrates how this approach has been useful in separating the most primitive CD34$^+$ CD45RA$^-$CD71$^-$ adult human marrow cells (containing all the LTC-IC) from the CD34$^+$CD45RA$^+$CD71$^\pm$ granulopoietic CFC and the CD34$^+$CD45RA$^-$CD71$^+$ erythroid CFC. Thy-1 is selectively expressed on primitive human hematopoietic progenitors and not on the majority of lineage-restricted human CFC *(19)*. Thy-1 is expressed on approx 25% of CD34$^+$ cells in human fetal liver, cord blood, and bone marrow, and on a majority of LTC-IC, whereas a majority of the CFC are in the CD34$^+$ Thy-1$^-$ fraction *(19,20)*. Very primitive phenotypes include; CD34$^+$CD45RA^{lo}CD71^{lo} *(8,21)*, CD34$^+$CD45RA^{lo}CD71^{lo}Thy-1$^+$ *(19,20)* and CD34$^+$CD38$^-$ *(6)*. Protocols for purifying these populations by FACS are given in this chapter. Exclusion of the supravital dye rhodamine-123 (Rh-123) is also indicative of a more primitive subpopulation of CD34$^+$ cells *(7)*. Recently, it has also been suggested that the fluorescence from the Hoechst 33241 DNA dye can be used to enrich HSCs *(22)*. These various promising dye exclusion cell-sorting strategies have the disadvantage that additional incubation steps are required, and are not described in detail in this chapter.

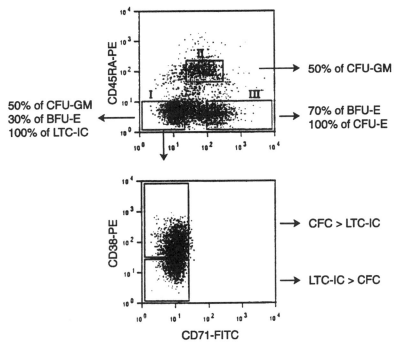

Fig. 1. The progenitor potential of different subpopulations of normal human bone marrow CD34+ cells. CD34+ cells were sorted based on their expression of CD45RA, CD71 and CD38, and the sorted cell populations were assayed for CFC and LTC-IC using recombinant growth factors and engineered feeders as described in **ref. *16***. All of the LTC-IC, one-half of the CFU-GM, and one-third of the BFU-E were found in the CD34+CD45RA−CD71− population. The CD34+CD45RA+ population contained the other half of the CFU-GM. All of the CFU-E and 70% of the BFU-E were found in the CD34+CD45RA−CD71+ population.

1.4. Capacity, Recovery, and Yield

In designing a multi-step cell purification strategy one must consider the capacity of the various methods, the degree of cell enrichment offered with each step, the loss of desired cells with each step and the compatibility of the various techniques. For example, the pre-enrichment step must not restrict the parameters which can be used in the subsequent FACS. This chapter describes a cell-separation strategy which has been successfully used to highly enrich stem cells from blood, bone marrow, and cord blood. It involves three separation steps: density separation, lineage depletion via magnetic immunoabsorption and FACS. The cell recovery and fold enrichment of stem cells with each step is discussed in **Subheading 4**. Procedures are also given for the preparation samples from a variety of cell and tissue sources prior to enrichment of specific cell types.

2. Materials

2.1. Sample Preparation

1. Media: Buffered salt solutions without Ca^{++} or Mg^{++}: Dulbecco's phosphate-buffered saline (D-PBS, StemCell Technologies Inc, Vancouver, Canada 37350) or Hank's HEPES Buffered Salt Solution (Hank's, StemCell Technologies Inc, Vancouver, Canada 37150).
2. Protein source: Fetal bovine serum (FBS, StemCell Technologies Inc, Vancouver, Canada 6100) or human serum albumin (HSA, 25% solution, Baxter, DIN 118303). Add FBS or HSA to the desired buffered salt solution with a final concentration of 2–6%. Store at 4°C for up to 1 y.
3. Density-separation medium: Ficoll-Paque, 1.077 g/cm^3 (Pharmacia Biotech 17084008). Store and use at room temperature.
4. Lysing solution: 0.8% NH_4Cl with 10 mM ethylenediaminetetraacetate (EDTA) (StemCell Technologies Inc, Vancouver, Canada 07800). Aliquot into suitable volumes for a single day's use and store at –20°C. Thaw and keep at 4°C for use. Discard unused portion at the end of each day.
5. DMSO: Dimethyl sulfoxide (Sigma D 5879). Store at room temperature. Wear proper protective clothing (gloves and gown) to avoid skin contact. DMSO is rapidly absorbed through the skin, and its solvent properties facilitate the absorption of substances which may be present on the skin surface.
6. DNase: Type II-S from bovine pancreas (Sigma D 4513). Prepare 1.0 mg/mL in PBS, without Ca^{++} or Mg^{++}. Aliquot into suitable volumes for a single day's use and store at –20°C. Thaw and keep at 4°C for use. Discard unused portion at the end of each day.
7. Anticoagulant citrate dextrose solution: Anticoagulant citrate dextrose solution, Formula A, (Baxter Health Care Corporation, DIN 788139) contains 2.45 g dextrose monohydrate, 2.2 g sodium citrate dihydrate, and 730 mg citric acid, anhydrous per 100 mL. Use at a 1/10 dilution. Ten times stock is also available.
8. Dispase II: Dispase II (Boehringer Mannheim, 165 859) stock is made by disolving 5 mg powder in 1 L sterile PBS.

2.2. Pre-Enrichment Immunomagnetic Cell Separation

1. Lineage depletion antibody cocktail: A mixture of bispecific tetrameric antibody complexes recognizing dextran and the following cell-surface antigens: glycophorin A, CD2, CD3, CD14, CD16, CD19, CD24, CD56, CD66b, and optionally CD36, CD45RA, CD38 (StemSep™ Progenitor Enrichment cocktail, StemCell Technologies Inc, Vancouver, Canada). Antibody cocktail is stable for 2 y at 4°C. Do not freeze.
2. Colloidal magnetic dextran iron particles: Supplied from StemCell Technologies Inc., Vancouver, Canada, at OD_{450} of 10.0. Use at 60 µL per mL of cells. Colloid should be stored frozen, but can be frozen and thawed several times. Shelf life is 1 y at –20°C, 6 wk at 4°C, and 3 d at 21°C.
3. High-gradient magnetic cell separation columns: Columns for StemSep™ mag-

Table 1
Optimum Number of Nucleated Cells in the Start Suspension
for Various StemSep™ Column Sizes

Column diameter (inches)	Optimum no. of cells per column	Will fit StemSep™ magnet (color-coded)
1.0	10^{10}	black
0.6	5×10^8	green, blue, black
0.5	10^8	green, blue, black
0.3	5×10^7	all magnet sizes
0.1	$10^6 - 10^7$	red, green

netic cell separation are available in five different sizes, depending on the total number of nucleated cells to be processed per column (*see* **Table 1**). Columns may be run with a peristaltic pump feed (*see* **Table 2** for flow rates and pump settings) or by gravity feed.

4. Magnet: StemSep™ high-gradient magnetic cell separation requires a magnetic field of >0.5 Tesla. Magnets should be kept away from pacemakers, other magnets, computer disks, watches and other objects that are affected by magnetic fields. StemCell Technologies supplies a variety of magnets designed to hold 1–4 columns of various sizes (*see* **Table 1**).

2.3. Fluorescence-Activated Cell-Sorting

1. Medium: Hank's HEPES-buffered salt solution (StemCell Technologies, Inc., Vancouver, Canada 37150). Fetal Bovine Serum (FBS, StemCell Technologies Inc, Vancouver, Canada 6100). For FACS, prepare Hank's containing 2% FBS (HF).
2. Fluorescence-conjugated antibodies: Refer to **Table 3** for details of the fluorescence-conjugated antibodies required for FACS.
3. Propidium iodide: Propidium iodide (PI, Sigma P 4170) is an irritant and mutagen. Wear appropriate protective equipment, and avoid inhalation and contact with eyes, skin, or clothing. To minimize exposure risk, dissolve directly in original container. In the fume hood, add 1 or 2 mL D-PBS to a 25-mg vial. Transfer the solution to a labeled 50-cc centrifuge tube. Repeat this process several times to ensure that all the powder is dissolved and the container is well rinsed. Keep track of the total volume pipeted, and bring the final volume in the tube to 25 mL for a 1.0 mg/mL stock solution. Filter-sterilize, dispense into 1 mL-aliquots, and store at 4°C. Protect from light. Stable for at least 1 y. For use, prepare a fresh 2 μg/mL working solution in HF.
4. FACS instrument: Flow cytometer/cell sorter equipped with both a 5-W argon and a 30-mW helium neon laser, as well as appropriate filters, detectors, and software. A cell sorter with an argon (488 nm) laser only may be used, but Cy5 conjugates will not be excited/detected. Cy5-PE conjugates may be substituted, but this precludes the use of propidium iodide for viable cell discrimination.

Table 2
Flow Rates and Pump Settings: StemSep™ Pre-Enrichment

Column size	Priming		Loading sample and washing	
(inches)	mL/min	Pump setting[a]	mL/min	Pump setting[a]
1.0	2.0	10.0	5.0	27.0
0.6	0.6	3.0	2.0	10.0
0.5	0.3	1.5	1.0	5.0
0.3	0.2	1.0	0.6	3.0

[a]Note: Pump setting for four-channel pump supplied by StemCell Technologies Inc. only.

3. Methods

3.1. Sample Preparation

3.1.1. Sample

The ideal sample is fresh, anticoagulated hematopoietic tissue (*see* **Note 1**). The preparation details vary, depending on the specific tissue source (*see* **Note 2**). for characteristics of whole blood, mobilized leukapheresis preparations of peripheral blood, whole bone marrow, bone-marrow buffy coat, fetal liver and cord blood, and recommended processing choices. If samples cannot be processed within 48 h, they should be frozen (*see* **Note 3**).

3.1.2. Density Separation Procedure (Ficoll)

1. Dilute samples 1:1 in D-PBS without Mg^{++} or Ca^{++}.
2. Pour 20 mL Ficoll into a 50-mL tube and slowly layer (tilting tube and running the cells down the side of the tube) 25 mL of diluted blood or marrow on top.
3. Centrifuge at room temperature $1100g$ for 20 min.
4. Remove half of the top layer, and discard.
5. Carefully pipet off "cloudy" interface layer (approx 10 mL) and transfer into a clean 50-mL tube. Wash these cells with 50 mL PBS without Mg^{++} and Ca^{++}.
6. Resuspend cells in media with serum or protein (D-PBS or Hank's with 2–6% FBS or HSA).

3.1.3. Red Cell Lysis Procedure

1. Centrifuge cells, and wash twice in D-PBS without Mg^{++} and Ca^{++}.
2. Resuspend in *cold* NH_4Cl solution at 3–4 times the original sample volume.
3. Incubate on ice for 10 min.
4. Centrifuge cells, and wash twice in D-PBS without Mg^{++} and Ca^{++}. Resuspend cells in media with serum or protein (D-PBS or Hank's with 2–6% FBS or HSA).

Table 3
Fluorescence-Conjugated Antibodies for FACS

Antibody to	Clone	Fluorochrome	Reference	Source	Amount per mL of cells (μg)
Reagents for Sorting CD34⁺CD45RA^{lo}CD71^{lo} Cells					
CD34	8G12, Qben 10, or 581	Cy5	Lansdorp et al., 1990 *J.Exp.Med.* **172**, 363	Pharmingen 34378X[a] Immunotech 1576[a]	20
CD71	OKT9	FITC	R. Sutherland et al., 1981 PNAS 78: 4515	Coulter 6604077	1
CD45RA	8D2	PE	Lansdorp et al., 1991 *Cytometry* **12**, 723	Pharmingen (clone HI100)	4
Additional Reagent for Sorting CD34⁺CD45RA^{lo}CD71^{lo}Thy-1⁺ Cells					
Thy-1[b]	5E10	PE	Craig et al., 1993 *J.Exp.Med.* **177**, 1331	Pharmingen 33085A	5
Reagents for Sorting CD34⁺CD38⁻ Cells					
CD34	8G12	FITC	Lansdorp et al., 1990 *J Exp Med.* **172**, 363	Becton Dickinson 348053	20
CD38	HB-7	PE	Craig et al., 1993 *J.Exp.Med.* **177**, 1331	Becton Dickinson 347687	1
Irrelevant Antibody Isotype Controls (Mouse IgG₁)					
		FITC		Becton Dickinson 349041	1
		PE		Becton Dickinson 349043	4
		Cy5		Pharmingen 33818X	20

[a]These reagents are conjugated to PE-Cy5 rather that Cy5 alone. This permits excitation with 488 nm, (i.e., the procedure can be done with a single laser instrument); however, PI cannot be used for sorting out nonviable cells.
[b]If cells are to be sorted for CD34⁺CD45RA^{lo}CD71^{lo}Thy-1⁺, resort CD34⁺CD45RA^{lo}CD71^{lo} cells labeled with anti-Thy-1 (5E10) PE. 5μg/mL of cells. Labeling procedure is the same as for the initial sort.

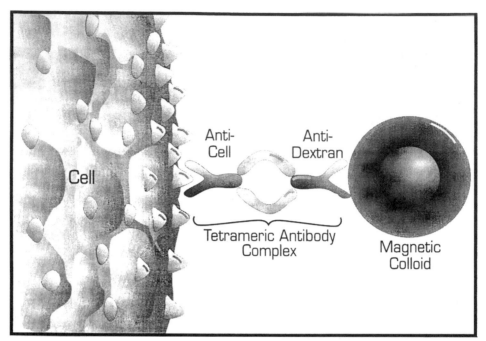

Fig. 2. Schematic drawing of StemSep™ magnetic cell labeling. Cells are crosslinked to magnetic dextran iron particles, using tetrameric antibody complexes. These complexes are comprised of two murine IgG_1 MAb molecules held in tetrameric array by two rat anti-mouse IgG_1 MAb molecules. One murine antibody recognizes the cell surface antigen and the other murine antibody recognizes dextran. Reproduced with permission from StemCell Technologies Inc., Vancouver, BC, Canada.

3.2. Pre-Enrichment-Lineage Depletion Using Immunomagnetic Cell Separation

3.2.1. StemSep™ Lineage Depletion

Colloidal magnetic dextran iron particles are selectively bound to target cells using bispecific tetrameric antibody complexes *(23,24)*. These complexes recognize both dextran and the target cell-surface antigen (**Fig. 2**). Labeled cells are passed over a column placed in a magnetic field. Cells with antibody complexes—and therefore dextran iron—on their surfaces are retained within the column. The desired cells, which have not been labeled with antibody, pass through the column and are collected. The small size of the colloidal magnetic dextran iron particles facilitates their delivery to the cells. The use of bispecific tetrameric antibody complexes avoids expensive and inefficient covalent coupling of antibodies to magnetic particles, thus ensuring reproducibility and ease of scale-up.

3.2.2. Antibody Cocktail Options

The number and type of antibodies in the lineage depletion cocktail will determine the number and type of cells removed, and consequently the number and type of cells recovered for any further separation such as FACS. Extensive depletion of lineage-committed cells will give a greater enrichment of stem cells than a partial lineage depletion. One must determine what degree of enrichment (and consequently the number of recovered cells) is optimal in the lineage depletion step for the overall stem-cell isolation strategy. *See* **Note 4** for a discussion of sample size-estimation of cell yield. A basic lineage depletion with anti-glycophorin A, CD2, CD3, CD14, CD16, CD19, CD24, CD56, and CD66b will enrich LTC-IC approx 100-fold (depending on the sample) *(15)* and recover approx 1% of the nucleated cells. If anti-CD45R, CD36, and CD38 are added to the depletion cocktail the enrichment of LTC-IC is approx 1,000-fold, with 0.1% of the nucleated cells being recovered *(15)*. In both cases, the recovery of LTC-IC is excellent (100%) *(15)*. If the final step in the isolation strategy is a sort, one must consider what the optimal number/purity of cells to take to the sorter will be (*see* **Note 4**).

3.2.3. Immunomagnetic Labeling Procedure

1. Resuspend cells at approx 5×10^7 nucleated cells per mL (a range of 2–8×10^7 is acceptable) in medium with serum or protein (D-PBS or Hank's with 2–6% FBS or HSA). Add 100 µL of antibody cocktail for each mL of cells, and mix well.
2. Incubate on ice for 30 min or for 15 min at room temperature.
3. Add 60 µL of magnetic colloid for each mL of cells and mix well.
4. Incubate on ice for 30 min or 15 min at room temperature. During this incubation period, prepare columns as described in **Subheading 3.2.4.1., steps 1–15** (pump feed) or **Subheading 3.2.4.2., steps 1–16** (gravity feed). Cells are then ready for magnetic cell separation.

3.2.4. Magnetic Cell Separation

Caution: Do not let the column run dry at any time during the priming, washing, or loading of the column.

3.2.4.1. Procedure with Pump Feed System

1. Perform all procedures in a sterile environment.
2. Remove StemSep™ column from its sterile package without touching the luer fitting. (For column sizes, *see* **Table 1**).
3. Remove StemSep™ pump tubing from its sterile package.
4. Aseptically attach hub to luer fitting on column (**Fig. 3**).
5. Check all connections.

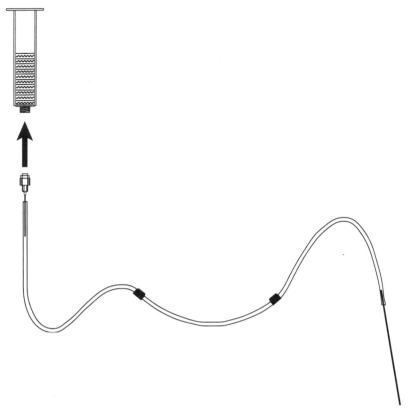

Fig. 3. StemSep™ Columns Assembly: Pump Feed. Reproduced with permission from StemCell Technologies Inc., Vancouver, BC, Canada.

6. Place magnet in stand.
7. Prepare column(s) for priming *(see* **Note 6**). Column(s) can be primed in place in the magnet, but it is difficult to check for air bubbles in the matrix. If the column(s) are placed in the magnet for priming, pull them out to check for air bubbles.
8. Insert pump tubing into peristaltic pump. *See* **Table 2** for pump settings.
9. Remove plug from top of column.
10. Remove paper cover from 10-cm metal end (probe) of pump tubing. Place into sterile PBS (without FBS or other protein).
11. Prime column: run pump to fill column from bottom to top *(upwards)*. *See* **Table 2** for flow rates. Do not disturb the column while priming.
12. When the level of PBS is above the stainless steel matrix of the column, stop the pump.
13. Remove column from rack on side of magnet. Place column in the magnet by holding magnet and slowly lowering column from above down into the gap. **Do not insert the column from the front. Caution**: the magnet will grab the column.

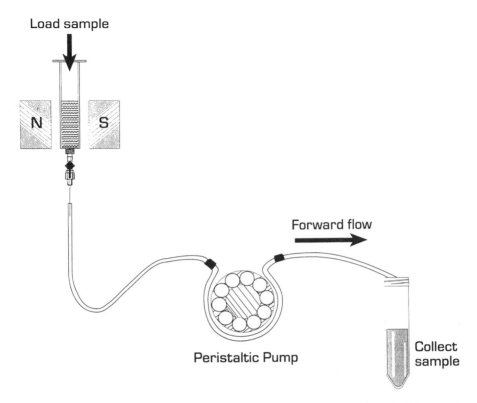

Fig. 4. StemSep™ Separation Procedure: Pump Feed. Reproduced with permission from StemCell Technologies Inc., Vancouver, BC, Canada.

14. To wash column, increase pump speed (**Table 2**) and reverse the pump direction to draw liquid down through the column (*downwards*). Add medium to top of column until you have collected three column volumes (1.0" column: collect 90 mL; 0.6" column: collect 25 mL; 0.5" column: collect 15 mL; 0.3" column: collect 8 mL).

15. Stop the pump when fluid level is just above column matrix and transfer the end probe to a collection tube. The column is now ready for the separation procedure (**Fig. 4**).

16. Load sample into top of column.

17. Start pump in downward direction and allow sample to run into matrix of column. Add medium to top of column until you have collected three column volumes of media (1.0" column: collect 90 mL; 0.6" column: collect 25 mL; 0.5" column: collect 15 mL; 0.3" column: collect 8 mL) plus the volume of your start sample. Do not allow top of fluid level to reach the matrix.

18. Stop the pump. The collected flowthrough fraction is the enriched cell fraction.

19. Pump all remaining fluid from the column into a waste container.

20. Remove used column from top of magnet.

0.1" column   0.6", 0.5", 0.3" columns

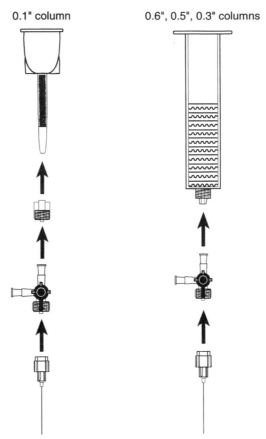

Fig. 5. StemSep™ Column Assembly: Gravity Feed. Reproduced with permission from StemCell Technologies Inc., Vancouver, BC, Canada.

21. Discard used column, pump tubing, and other materials into a biohazardous waste container.

3.2.4.2. Procedure with Gravity Feed System

1. Place magnet in stand.
2. Perform all procedures in a sterile environment.
3. Remove StemSep™ column from its sterile package without touching the luer fitting. *See* **Note 7** for information on 0.1" columns.
4. Place column in magnet. Be careful not to touch any surface with the tip of the luer lock. **Caution**: the magnet will grab the column.
5. Remove three-way stopcock from its sterile package and aseptically attach to the column or column extender (0.1" column only, *see* **Note 7**) (**Fig. 5**).
6. Remove blunt-end needle from its sterile package, keeping the cover on the end of the needle until **step 14** (washing the column), and aseptically attach hub to

WASH AND
CELL SEPARATION
Load sample

PRIME COLUMN

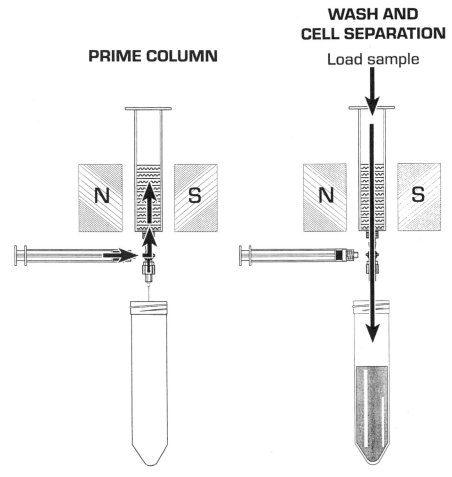

Fig. 6. StemSep™ Separation Procedure: Gravity Feed. Reproduced with permission from StemCell Technologies Inc., Vancouver, BC, Canada.

    luer fitting on the stopcock directly below the column (22 gauge blunt-end needle for 0.6" columns; 23-gauge blunt-end needle for 0.5", 0.3", and 0.1" columns) (*see* **Fig. 5**).

7. Check all connections.
8. Remove plug from top of column (0.6", 0.5", and 0.3" columns only).
9. Set three-way stopcock to allow flow from the side connection into column.
10. Fill a sterile syringe (included in kit) with PBS without FBS or other protein, remove air bubbles, and attach to the side connection of three-way stopcock (*see* **Fig. 6**).
11. For 0.6", 0.5", and 0.3" columns: **Slowly** depress plunger of syringe to deliver PBS up the column until the level of PBS is above the stainless steel matrix of column. Do not allow air bubbles to enter the mesh matrix.

12. For 0.1" column: Rapidly depress plunger of syringe with firm, even pressure to deliver PBS up the column. Deliver the entire 1 mL of PBS.
13. Remove any air bubbles trapped in the column matrix by gently moving the plunger of the side syringe in and out. Repeat 5 to 10 times, making sure that the level of PBS does not fall below the top of the column matrix (more PBS may be added to the top if needed). End the priming by pulling back 500 μL of PBS and any air bubbles into the side syringe.
14. To wash the column, place a waste container below the blunt-end needle, remove cover from needle, and add medium to top of column. Turn three-way stopcock so the flow is from the column down through the needle (as shown in **Fig. 6**; i.e., side exit closed). For information on correcting flow problems, *see* **Note 8**.
15. Continue adding media until you have collected three column volumes (0.6" column: collect 25 mL; 0.5" column: collect 15 mL; 0.3" column: collect 8 mL; 0.1" column: collect 1.0 mL). **Caution: Do not let the column run dry at any time.**
16. Turn stopcock to stop flow of media from the column when the fluid level is just above the column matrix. The column is now ready for the separation procedure (*see* **Fig. 6**).
17. Load sample into top of column.
18. Turn stopcock to start the flow of media down through the needle into collection tube. Allow sample to run into column matrix. Add medium to top of column until you have collected three column volumes (0.6" column: collect 25 mL; 0.5" column: collect 15 mL; 0.3" column: collect 8 mL; 0.1" column: collect 1.5 mL) plus the volume of your start sample. For information on correcting flow problems *see* **Note 8**. Turn stopcock to stop the flow of media. This collected flowthrough fraction is the enriched cell fraction.
19. Let remaining fluid drain from the column into a waste container.
20. Disconnect three-way stopcock.
21. Remove column from top of magnet.
22. Discard used column, syringes, stopcocks, and other materials into a biohazardous waste container.

3.3. Fluorescence-Activated Cell-Sorting

3.2.3. Staining Reagents

Refer to **Table 3** for clones, catalog numbers, and concentration of staining reagents. *See* **Note 9** for comments with respect to each reagent. Note that PI cannot be used together with phycoerythrin without replacement of filters in most standard single-laser flow cytometers.

3.3.2. Cell Staining Procedure

1. Resuspend cells in Hank's + FBS at 10^7/mL.
2. Remove samples of cells for controls (~10^5 cells/tube) as follows: Unstained cells; Irrelevant antibody controls for FITC, phycoerythrin, and Cy5; Single-color

positive controls for FITC, phycoerythrin, and Cy5. *See* **Table 3** for the appropriate reagents and quantities. *See* **Note 10** for a discussion of the purpose of each control.

3. To the remaining cells, add the appropriate antibodies for the chosen procedure, as outlined in **Table 3**. Incubate cells for 30 min at 4°C.
4. Wash cells twice and resuspend in Hank's + FBS containing 2 µg/mL propidium iodide (PI). Cells are now ready for sorting.

3.3.4. FACS Instrument Sterilization Procedure

For most applications, the sorted cells must be kept sterile. The following procedure can be used to provide a sterile fluid path:

1. Before the fluidic system is turned on, remove the fluid filter and use a syringe and blunt needle to inject a sufficient volume of filtered 10% bleach to flood the sample line (~10 mL for the Becton Dickinson FACStar⁺).
2. Remove the syringe, attach a new, clean filter, and reassemble the fluidic system.
3. Turn on the fluidic system and run a sample tube of filtered 10% bleach for approx 10 min.
4. Remove the bleach tube and back flush the sample line with sterile sheath fluid.
5. Rinse the outside of the sample line with alcohol, and then with sterile D-PBS.

Steps 3–5 should be repeated between each sample sorted, and to clear the system if it becomes clogged.

3.3.5. FACS Instrument Alignment Procedure and Instrument Settings

The instrument must be aligned using procedures recommended by the manufacturer. The use of calibration beads that mimic fluorescently labeled human cells facilitates selection of instrument settings in the range of the human cells to be sorted. For example, in the laboratory of the authors, 2-µ beads are used to set FL1 and FL 2, 10-µ beads are used for forward-scatter and side-scatter, and a human cell line (KG1A) stained with a Cy5-labeled antibody is used to align the Helium-Neon laser. Of course, the setting and results of cell-sorting experiments (purity, yield, speed, and data format) will vary to some extent with the cell sorter that is used. Several instruments are available from different manufacturers such as Becton Dickinson, Coulter and Cytomation. For the technique described in the chapter, access to a two-laser (Argon 488 nm, Helium-Neon 633 nm) instrument capable of sorting cells on the basis of seven independent variables is recommended. If a single-laser (488-nm) instrument is used, PE-Cy5 rather than Cy5 alone is required, and PI cannot be used simultaneously with this dye to discriminate viable and nonviable cells. In these circumstances, a CD34⁺CD38⁻ sort would be recommended.

A

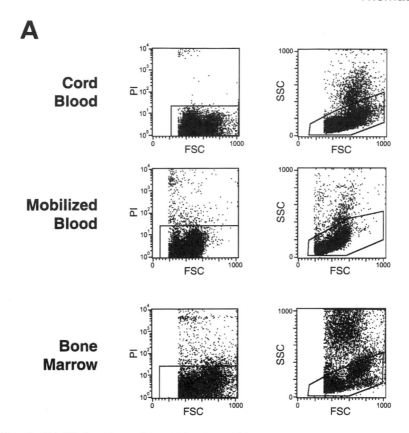

Fig. 7. FACS dot plots of cord blood, mobilized peripheral blood, and bone marrow after Ficoll density separation (**A**) and after StemSep™ lineage depletion (removal of cells which express glycophorin A, CD2, CD3, CD14, CD16, CD19, CD24, CD56, or CD66b). (**B**). Cells are gated for forward/side scatter (FSC, SSC) properties (*right column*) and viability (PI-) (*left column*).

3.3.6. Sort Windows: CD34+CD45RA^lo^CD71^lo Sort

Cells are gated on forward- and side-scatter and PI staining (PI-viable cells) as shown in **Fig. 7**. Cells are then gated for high expression of CD34 (**Fig. 8A**) and low expression of CD45RA and CD71 (**Fig. 8B**). If cells are re-sorted to select for Thy-1$^+$ cells the sort gates are given in **Fig. 8C**.

3.3.7. Sort Windows: CD34+CD38− Sort

Cells are gated on forward- and side-scatter and phycoerythrin and PI staining as shown in **Fig. 7**. CD34$^+$CD38$^−$ cells are gated as shown in **Fig. 9**.

B

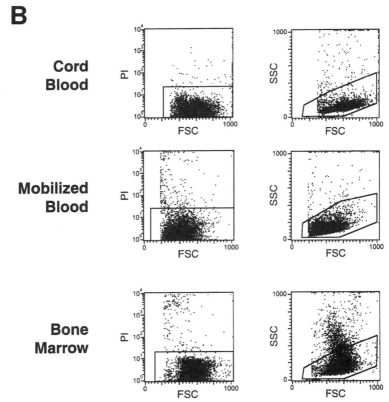

Fig. 7. (*Continued*) FACS dot plots of cord blood, mobilized peripheral blood, and bone marrow after Ficoll density separation (**A**) and after StemSep™ lineage depletion (removal of cells which express glycophorin A, CD2, CD3, CD14, CD16, CD19, CD24, CD56, or CD66b). (**B**). Cells are gated for forward/side scatter (FSC, SSC) properties (*right column*) and viability (PI-) (*left column*).

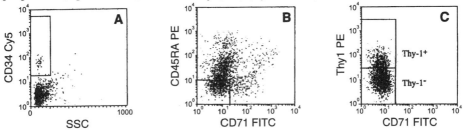

Fig. 8. Selection of CD34$^+$CD45RA^{lo}CD71^{lo} cell subpopulations from human umbilical cord blood by flow cytometry. (**A**) Low-density mononuclear cells with a low side scatter and expressing CD34 were selected. (**B**) Among the gated CD34$^+$ cells, those expressing low/undetectable levels of both CD45RA and CD71 (CD34$^+$CD45RA^{lo}CD71^{lo} cells) were selected. (**C**) CD34$^+$CD45RA^{lo}CD71^{lo} cells were further subdivided into those expressing intermediate/high (Thy-1$^+$) and low/undetectable (Thy-1$^-$) levels of Thy-1.

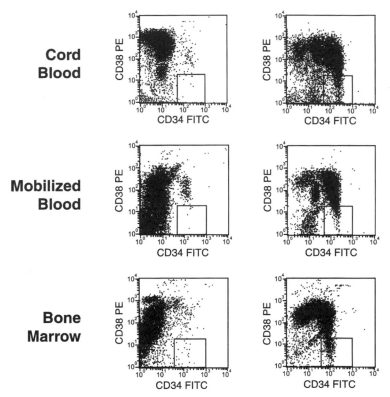

Fig. 9. FACS dot plots of cord blood, mobilized peripheral blood, and bone marrow after Ficoll density separation (*left column*) and after StemSep™ lineage depletion (removal of cells which express glycophorin A, CD2, CD3, CD14, CD16, CD19, CD24, CD56, or CD66b) (*right column*). Cells are gated for CD34⁺CD38⁻.

3.3.8. Collection Vessels and Media

The choice of collection tube and media will depend on the intended use of the sorted cells, and on the expected cell recovery. Single cells can be deposited directly into multi-well plates, or cells can be collected into appropriately sized tubes (e.g., 0.5 mL of media in a microfuge tube would be suitable for collecting 10^5 sorted cells, while for 10^6 cells a 12×75-mm tube is required). Suitable collection media includes FBS, long-term-culture (LTC) media, culture media containing FBS, or serum free media.

4. Notes

1. Samples and anticoagulants: The single most significant variable affecting the efficiency of an established cell separation (assuming protocols are strictly ad-

hered to) is the quality of the single-cell suspension available at the start of the procedure. Each tissue source offers unique challenges, but there are some general rules. All samples should be obtained with informed consent and/or approval of appropriate ethical review committees, and the processing of human tissue should strictly adhere to guidelines for processing of biohazardous human materials. Samples should be as fresh as possible. If a sample must be stored, it is usually better to delay all manipulation and store the sample "as is" at room temperature or at 4°C. (Bone-marrow samples containing a large amount of fat may be clumpy and difficult to work with if stored at 4°C). To optimize cell viability during processing, one should minimize exposure to conditions which will cause clumping and cell death (e.g., being in contact with medium without serum/protein, or prolonged contact with Ficoll). The use of heparin tends to cause clumping and to lower separation efficiency. If the cells are collected in heparin, wash twice with PBS (without Ca^{++} or Mg^{++}) and continue the procedure using medium without heparin. Ensure that a sufficient concentration of anticoagulant, such as Citrate or ACD, in all wash media exists. For example, use ACD-A at a 1/10 dilution.

2. Characteristics of different hematopoietic tissues.

Fresh whole blood: The abundance of mature erythrocytes in whole blood will interfere with FACS and most antibody-mediated bulk cell-separation techniques. Red cells are readily removed by a lysis step or by density separation (e.g., Ficoll). The advantage of using Ficoll rather than red-cell lysis is that it removes granulocytes as well as red cells. The nucleated cells in whole blood are up to 90% mature granulocytes. Removal of these cells gives a 10-fold enrichment of light-density cells, including stem cells.

Mobilized leukapheresis preparation of peripheral blood: Leukapheresis preparations are depleted of red cells and granulocytes. The number of red cells varies, depending on the collection method, and may be high enough to warrant a removal step. A general rule of thumb is that greater than 20 erythrocytes per nucleated cell will interfere with immunoabsorption techniques. Either lysis or Ficoll-density separation are suitable, but it is important to consider that most of the granulocytes have already been removed, so a Ficoll separation will not enrich the stem cells relative to the other nucleated cells.

Whole bone marrow: Whole aspirated bone marrow is essentially always contaminated with variable amounts of peripheral blood, and therefore has a high red-cell content. Whole bone marrow may be lysed or Ficoll-density-separated.

Bone-marrow buffy-coat suspensions: Buffy-coat suspensions vary greatly in erythrocyte content. If there are greater than 20 erythrocytes per nucleated cells, lyse or Ficoll.

Fetal liver: The following procedure can be used with fresh tissue to obtain a single-cell suspension of fetal liver cells:
a. Place the liver on a 60-mm sterile dish and remove any attached organs.

b. Add 2–3 mL of dispase II (Boehringer Mannheim 165 859, add one 5-mg vial to 1 L of D-PBS and filter-sterilize).

c. Dissect the liver into small pieces, using an 18-gauge needle attached to a 1-cc syringe.

d. Pour into a 50-cc tube containing 10–20 cc prewarmed dispase II and 0.5–1.0 mL DNase (*see* **Subheading 2.1.5.**).

e. Pipet up and down gently using a 16-gauge blunt needle and a 20-cc syringe.

f. Incubate 20 min at 37°C. If clumps are sill present, repeat pipetting procedure. If necessary, large clumps can be transferred to a sterile dish and further dissected.

g. Wash cells once with D-PBS.

h. Resuspend in 10–20 mL prewarmed Cell Dissociation Buffer (EGTA/ ethylenediaminetetraacetate, Gibco BRL B150–016) with 0.5–1.0 mL DNase. Repeat pipetting procedure.

i. Incubate 20 min at 37°C. If clumps are sill present, repeat pipetting procedure.

j. Filter through a coarse (70–100 μ) filter, adding D-PBS as necessary.

k. Spin, remove supernatant, and resuspend in D-PBS with FBS for ficolling.

Cord blood: Cord blood samples are especially difficult to process, as the density of the cells can vary over a wide range. Cord blood may also have very high platelet counts which lead to clumping, despite the presence of anticoagulants. Cells should be suspended in 10% anticoagulant citrate dextrose (ACD) or 5% ACD plus 1% Human Albumin in saline. One of the following is recommended for preparing samples of cord blood and samples with excessive platelets:

a. 1 Spin at 120*g* (about 800 rpm on Beckman GS6R benchtop centrifuge) for 10 min at room temperature with the brake off.

   2. Remove supernatant, resuspend, and repeat **step 1**.

   3. Resuspend in desired media.

b. 1. Spin at 360*g* (about 1,300 rpm in a Beckman GS6R benchtop centrifuge) for 3 min at room temperature with the brake off.

   2. Remove supernatant and repeat **step 1** twice.

   3. Wash twice with PBS (spin at 360*g* for 3 min).

   4. Resuspend in desired media.

There are several methods to remove red cells from cord blood. Initial attempts to remove red cells by sedimentation, centrifugation, or density-gradient procedures resulted in considerable loss of progenitor cells *(25)*. Since then, many groups have successfully removed red cells from cord blood using sedimentation *(26)* and Ficoll-density separation *(27,28)*. In all cases, it is important to first ensure that the sample is a good single-cell suspension and does not have excessive platelets. The lysing protocol outlined in **Subheading 3.1.3., steps 1–4** will typically reduce the red-cell content of fresh cord blood to the level (<10^9 red cells per mL) acceptable for StemSep™ magnetic cell separation.

3. Freezing and thawing of samples: When a sample cannot be separated within 48 h, it is usually preferable to freeze the cells. Red cells and granulocytes lyse upon

freezing/thawing, and it is therefore preferable to remove the red cells and granulocytes prior to freezing. Ficoll-density separation is recommended. The protocol for freezing cells is as follows:

Before beginning: have all media COLD.
1. Make up 15% dimethyl sulfoxide (DMSO) in FBS and filter-sterilize using a 0.2-μm filter. Keep on ice.
2. Leave cells in medium plus 10% FBS, on ice (2×10^8 cells per mL).
3. Mix cells gently with 15% DMSO in FBS at a ratio of 1:1 (the final cell suspension will be 47.5% FBS/7.5% DMSO in medium). Transfer into cryovials.
4. Place cryovials immediately into a precooled 70% isopropanol freezing container. Place container in a –80°C or –135°C freezer overnight. (Do not let cells sit in freezing media at room temperature. Keep on ice and transfer immediately into the freezing container).
5. Remove frozen vials from the freezing container and store in –135°C freezer or liquid nitrogen freezer.

For processing, thaw cells as follows:
1. Thaw cells quickly in a 37°C water bath or beaker of warm water. In a tissue-culture hood, wipe cryovial with 70% ethanol.
2. Do not vortex cells at any time.
3. Gently transfer cells into a larger tube (0.5–5.0 mL of cells into a 50-mL tube).
4. Slowly add 15 mL D-PBS dropwise while holding tube and gently swirling.
5. Fill tube to 50 mL with D-PBS. Gently invert tube to mix.
6. Spin down cells at 300g (1,200 rpm with a Beckman GS6R benchtop centrifuge) for 6 min.
7. Discard supernatant and flick tube gently to resuspend the pellet.
8. Resuspend cells at desired concentration in medium.
   Note: If cells are expected to be clumpy, add 0.25–0.5 mL of 1 mg/mL DNase per mL of cells, drop-wise, while gently swirling the tube. After the first wash, resuspend the pellet in 1 mL of 1 mg/mL DNase. DNase may be added finally to the cell suspension at 0.1 mg/mL.

4. Sample size—estimation of cell yield: There are cell losses with each step of a multi-step cell purification protocol. It is useful to estimate how many cells are likely to be available for the final FACS. If the starting sample is close to that which can be sorted in a reasonable amount of time (approx 10^7 cells can typically be sorted per hour), it may be possible to eliminate the pre-enrichment step. **Fig. 10** is a very rough guide to the number of nucleated cells that may be recovered with each step in the protocol described in this chapter. The number of cells available and the capacity of the FACS instrument will influence the choice of pre-enrichment strategy (i.e., basic lineage depletion vs a more extensive depletion, including markers such as CD38 and CD45RA). Tissue source, frequency

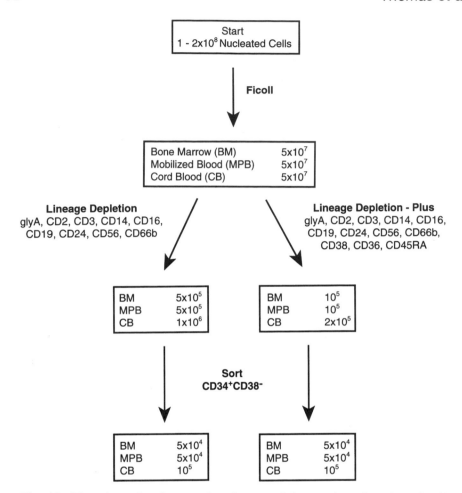

Fig. 10. Flowchart showing rough estimates of the number of nucleated cells re-covered at each processing step (Ficoll density separation, pre-enrichment-lineage depletion, and FACS). Estimates are given for starting samples of cord blood, mobilized peripheral blood, and bone marrow with $1-2 \times 10^8$ nucleated cells.

of primitive cells, and specific and nonspecific cell loss all affect the final cell yield. The overall message can be summarized as follows: If you need 10^6 puri-fied candidate stem cells, you should start with 2×10^9 bone marrow or mobi-lized peripheral blood cells or 10^9 cord blood cells. It should be emphasized again that this is only a rough guide, especially with respect to cord blood and mobi-lized peripheral blood suspensions which vary widely (up to 10-fold) in the con-tent of cells with a primitive phenotype. The frequency of these cells is typically lower in samples from patients who have been heavily pretreated as compared to normal samples.

5. Factors affecting purity and recovery in the lineage depletion procedure: Poor antibody binding to unwanted cells reduces the purity of the recovered cells. This could result, for example, from incubating the cells with the antibody and tetrameric antibody complexes at the wrong temperature and/or time, or using antibodies that are too dilute. Other factors affecting purity and recovery are as follows:
    1. Overloading the column may also decrease cell purity.
    2. An excess of red blood cells can reduce cell purity.
    3. Cell purity may be decreased if the column is not washed or primed correctly, if air bubbles are lodged in the column, or if the column is allowed to run dry at any time.
    4. Poor cell recovery may result from underloading the column.
    5. The protein in the wash solution blocks any protein-binding sites on the mesh in the column, thus preventing cells from binding nonspecifically to the column. Using wash solutions without a source of protein will decrease recovery.
    6. If cells are not in a single-cell suspension (i.e., if they are "clumpy"), cell recovery may be reduced. Poor cell suspensions may affect flow rates in the gravity feed system. If necessary, filter the cell suspension through a 70-m mesh.

6. Column priming: Columns can be primed in place in the magnet, but it is difficult to check for air bubbles in the matrix. Columns may be pulled out of the magnet to check for air bubbles. Air bubbles in the column matrix can be dislodged by sharply tapping the side of the column. If a large amount of air (0.5–1 mL bubble) remains in the column, do not use—prime a new column. Air bubbles lodged in the 3-way stopcock (gravity feed system) can be removed by adding PBS to the top of the column, and then bubbles can be pulled out into the side syringe. Continue if the bubble cannot be removed; it will likely remain in the stopcock and not interfere with separation.

7. Special considerations for 0.1" columns: The 0.1" column comes with an extender. This is required for use with the green magnet and red magnets purchased before January 1999. Aseptically attach extender if required (for column sizes, *see* **Table 2**). For 0.1" columns being used with a green magnet: the whole column will sit in the gap of the magnet with the column rim resting on the top of the magnet.

8. Correcting flow problems with gravity feed system: If the column stops running at any point, introduce a small volume of PBS from the side syringe into the column. This should remove any air bubbles trapped at the top of the column, which disrupt the flow. An air lock in the needle may be removed by redirecting the flow of buffer from the side syringe out through the needle. The 0.1" column will not run dry, but for best performance the separation procedure should not be prolonged unnecessarily.

9. Staining reagents for FACS: Optimal staining for FACS requires a strong fluorescent signal in the designated wavelength and good discrimination between

specific staining (to the specified cell-surface antigen) or nonspecific staining. The staining reagent concentrations given in **Subheading 3.** have been optimized for particular antibody clones. Other conjugates and clones may be used with the restrictions mentioned here, but each new reagent must be titrated for optimal staining.

CD34 antibodies: Use clones which recognize the class II and III epitopes. 8G12 (HPCA2), Qbend 10 and 581 are recommended. 8G12 (HPCA2) is the most reliable FITC conjugate. Most experience in the laboratory of the authors with respect to CD34-Cy5 is with a reagent prepared in-house. Commercially available PE-Cy5 reagents can be substituted; however, PI cannot be used with PE-Cy5 reagents on a single-laser FACS instrument.

CD38 antibodies: Specific staining with anti-CD38 typically reaches only moderate fluorescent intensity. Discrimination between specific and nonspecific staining is especially poor with FITC conjugates. Therefore, we recommend the combination of anti-CD34 FITC and anti-CD38 PE, especially if available cell sorters are equipped with an Argon (488 nm) laser only.

CD45RA, CD71: Most experience in the laboratory of the authors is with OKT9-FITC (anti-CD71) and 8D2-PE (anti-CD45RA) prepared in-house. Commercially available fluorochrome-labeled antibodies can be used instead of these particular reagents.

Propidium Iodide: The use of PI next to phycoerythrin-labeled antibodies requires appropriate filters and dichroic mirrors to separate dead cells from phycoerythrin-labeled cells. We use a 560 short-pass dichroic and a 575/26 band pass filter for FL1/2, and a 610 short pass dichroic for FL1/3 for this purpose. Note that PI cannot be used with PE-Cy5 on cell sorters equipped with an Argon (488 nm) laser only. Dead cells will be removed during the StemSep™ magnetic pre-enrichment.

10. FACS control samples: The purpose of the controls is to evaluate autofluorescence at each fluorescence wavelength (tube without antibody); evaluate nonspecific binding (tube with irrelevant isotype control for each labeled antibody); and set compensation between fluorescence channels on the cell sorter appropriately. Some of these controls may be excluded if sufficient experience with the cells, antibodies, and cell sorter has been obtained.

Acknowledgments

This work was supported in part by the Science Council of British Columbia. Work in the laboratory of PML is supported by grants from the National Institutes of Health (USA), and by a grant from the National Cancer Institute of Canada with funds from the Terry Fox Run. The authors would like to thank Maureen Fairhurst for preparing the FACS profiles.

References

1. Szilvassy, S. J., Humphries, R. K., Lansdorp, P. M., Eaves, A. C., and Eaves, C. J. (1990) Quantitative assay for totipotent reconstituting hematopoietic stem cells by a competitive repopulation strategy. *Proc. Natl. Acad. Sci. USA* **87**, 8736–8740.
2. Miller, C. L., and Eaves C. J. (1997) Expansion *in vitro* of adult murine hematopoietic stem cells with transplantable lympho-myeloid reconstituting ability. *Proc. Natl. Acad. Sci. USA* **94**, 13,648–13,653.
3. Ploemacher, R. E., van der Sluijs, J. P., Voerman, J. S. A., and Brons, N. H. C. (1989) An *in vitro* limiting-dilution assay of long-term repopulating hematopoietic stem cells in the mouse. *Blood* **74**, 2755–2763.
4. Sutherland, H. J., Eaves, C. J., Eaves, A. C., Dragowska, W., and Lansdorp P. M. (1989) Characterization and partial purification of human marrow cells capable of initiating long-term hematopoiesis in vitro. *Blood* **74**, 1563–1570.
5. Sutherland, H. J., Lansdorp, P. M., Henkelman, D. H., Eaves, A. C., and Eaves, C. J. (1990) Functional characterization of individual human hematopoietic stem cells cultured at limiting dilution on supportive marrow stromal layers. *Proc. Natl. Acad. Sci. USA* **87**, 3584–3588.
6. Terstappen, L. W. M. M., Huang, S., Safford, M., Lansdorp, P. M., and Loken, M. R. (1991) Sequential generations of hematopoietic colonies derived from single nonlineage-committed CD34$^+$CD38$^-$ progenitor cells. *Blood* **77**, 1218–1227.
7. Udomsakdi, C., Eaves, C. J., Sutherland, H. J., and Lansdorp, P. M. (1991) Separation of functionally distinct subpopulations of primitive human hematopoietic cells using rhodamine-123. *Exp. Hematol.* **19**, 338–342.
8. Lansdorp, P. M. and Dragowska W. (1992) Long-term erythropoiesis from constant numbers of CD34$^+$ cells in serum-free cultures initiated with highly purified progenitor cells from human bone marrow. *J. Exp. Med.* **175**, 1501–1509.
9. Craig, W., Poppema S., Little, M.-T., Dragowska, W., and Lansdorp, P. M. (1994) CD45 isoform expression on human haemopoietic cells at different stages of development. *Br. J. Haematol.* **88**, 24–30.
10. Civin, C. I., Strauss, L. C., Brovall, C., Fackler, M. J., Schwartz, J. F., and Shaper, J. H. (1984) Antigenic analysis of hematopoiesis. III. A hematopoietic progenitor cell surface antigen defined by a monoclonal antibody raised against KG-1a cells. *J. Immunol.* **133**, 157–165.
11. Bender, J. G., Williams, S. F., Myers, S., Nottleman, D., Lee, W. J., Unverzagt, K. L., et al. (1992) Characterization of chemotherapy mobilized peripheral blood progenitor cells for use in autologous stem cell transplantation. *Bone Marrow Transplant.* **10**, 281–285.
12. Udomsakdi, C., Lansdorp, P. M., Hogge, D. E., Reid, D. S., Eaves, A. C., and Eaves C. J. (1992) Characterization of primitive hematopoietic cells in normal human peripheral blood. *Blood* **80**, 2513–2521.
13. Siena, S., Bregni, M., Brando, B., Ravagnani, F., Bonadonna, G., and Gianni, A. M. (1989) Circulation of CD34$^+$ Hematopoietic Stem Cells in the peripheral blood of high-dose cyclophosphamide-treated patients: enhancement by intravenous

recombinant human granulocyte-macrophage colony-stimulating factor. *Blood* **74,** 1905–1914.

14. Yin, A. H., Miraglia, S., Zanjani, E., Almeida-Porada, G., Ogawa, M., Leary ,A. G., et al. (1997) AC133, a novel marker for human hematopoietic stem and progenitor cells. *Blood* **90,** 5002–5012.

15. Thomas, T. E., Fairhurst, M. A., and Lansdorp, P. M. (1997) Rapid single step immunomagnetic isolation of highly enriched primitive human hematopoietic progenitors. *Blood* **9,** 347b (Abstract).

16. Hogge, D. E., Lansdorp, P. M., Reid, D., Gerhard, B., and Eaves, C. J. (1996) Enhanced detection, maintenance, and differentiation of primitive human hematopoietic cells in cultures containing murine fibroblasts engineered to produce human steel factor, interleukin-3, and granulocyte colony-stimulating factor. *Blood* **88,** 3765–3773.

17. Bhatia, M., Bonnett, D., Murdoch, B., Gan, O. I., and Dick, J. E. (1998) A newly discovered class of human hematopoietic cells with SCID-repopulating activity. *Nat. Med.* **4,** 1038–1045.

18. Zanjani, E., Almeida-Porada, G., Livingston, A. G., Flake, A. W., and Ogawa, M. (1998) Human bone marrow CD34⁻ cells engraft in vivo and undergo multilineage expression that includes giving rise to CD34⁺ cells. *Exp. Hematol.* **26,** 353–360.

19. Craig, W., Kay, R., Cutler, R. L., and Lansdorp, P. M. (1993) Expression of Thy-1 on human hematopoietic progenitor cells. *J. Exp. Med.* **177,** 1331–1142.

20. Baum, C. M., Weissman, I. L., Tsukamoto, A. S., Buckle, A.-M., and Peault, B. (1992) Isolation of a candidate human hematopoietic stem-cell population. *Proc. Natl. Acad. Sci. USA* **89,** 2804–2808.

21. Mayani, H., Dragowska, W., and Lansdorp, P. M. (1993) Cytokine-induced selective expansion and maturation of erythroid versus myeloid progenitors from purified cord blood precursor cells. *Blood* **81,** 3252–3258.

22. Goodell, M. A., Rosenzweig, M., Kim, H., Marks, D. F., DeMaria, M., Paradis, G., et al. (1997) Dye efflux studies suggest that hematopoietic stem cells expressing low or undetectable levels of CD34 antigen exist in multiple species. *Nat. Med.* **3,** 1337–1345.

23. Lansdorp, P. M., Aalberse, R. C., Bos, R., Schutter,W. G., and Van Bruggen, E. F. J. (1986) Cyclic tetramolecular complexes of monoclonal antibodies: a new type of cross-linking reagent. *Eur. J. Immunol.* **16,** 679–683.

24. Lansdorp, P. M. and Thomas, T. E. (1990) Purification and analysis of bispecific tetrameric antibody complexes. *Mol. Immunol.* **27,** 659–666.

25. Broxmeyer, H. E., Douglas, G. W., Hangoc, G., Cooper, S., Bard, J., English, D., et al. (1989) Human umbilical cord blood as a potential source of transplantable hematopoietic stem/progenitor cells. *Proc. Natl. Acad. Sci. USA* **86,** 3828–3832.

26. Rubinstein, P., Dobrila, L., Rosenfield, R. E., Adamson, J. W., Migliaccio, G., Miggliaccio, A. R., et al. (1995) Processing and cryopreservation of placental/umbilical cord blood for unrelated bone marrow reconstitution. *Proc. Natl. Acad. Sci. USA* **92,** 10,119–10,122.

27. Harris, D. T., Schumacher, M. J., Rychlik, S., Booth, A., Acevedo, A., Rubinstein, P., et al. (1994) Collection, separation and cryopreservation of umbilical cord blood for use in transplantation. *Bone Marrow Transplant.* **13,** 135–143.
28. Regidor, C., Posada, M., Monteagudo, D., Garaulet, C., Somolinos, N., Forés, R., Briz, M., and Fernández, M.-N. (1999) Umbilical cord blood banking for unrelated transplantation: evaluation of cell separation and storage methods. *Exp. Hematol.* **27,** 380–385.

4

Method for Purification of Human Hematopoietic Stem Cells by Flow Cytometry

Michael J. Reitsma, Brenda R. Lee, and Nobuko Uchida

1. Introduction

Human hematopoietic stem cells (HSCs) and progenitors can be isolated by enriching for a rare cell population with a combination of monoclonal antibodies (MAbs). Such an isolation scheme involves multi-step procedures including ficoll-density fractionation and presort enrichment followed by cell sorting. Over the past decade, various cell-surface and metabolic markers have been identified and used to isolate human HSCs and progenitors as summarized in **Table 1**. Among them, CD34 has become the most critical cell-surface marker for positively selecting a rare cell population *(1,2)*. Within the $CD34^+$ cell population, the differential expression of Thy-1, CD38, and AC133 have been used to fractionate HSCs and progenitors. In order to subfractionate CD34+ cells by these markers, the cells can be further purified by flow cytometry. HSCs can be further enriched into a Thy-1$^+$ *(3–7)*, CD38^{-lo} *(8–10)*, Thy-1+ CD38^{-lo} *(11)*, or AC133+ *(12,13)* fraction of CD34+ cells.

Recent clinical studies of autologous transplantation of positively selected $CD34^+$ cells or purified $CD34^+$ Thy-1$^+$ HSC confirms that HSCs contribute to the early phase of engraftment. Dose-response studies of human $CD34^+$ cell-enriched transplants indicate that rapid engraftment can be regularly achieved if $>2 \times 10^6$ $CD34^+$ cells /kg are transplanted *(14–19)*. Mobilized peripheral blood (MPB) $CD34^+$ Thy-1$^+$ cells have been purified by flow cytometry and used in autologous transplantation. Rapid and consistent neutrophil and platelet recovery was achieved when patients were transplanted with $>0.8 \times 10^6$ $CD34^+$ Thy-1$^+$ HSC/kg *(20,21)*.

From: *Methods in Molecular Medicine, vol. 63: Hematopoietic Stem Cell Protocols*
Edited by: C. A. Klug and C. T. Jordan © Humana Press Inc., Totowa, NJ

Table 1
Commercially Available Cell-Surface and Metabolic Markers
for Isolation of Human HSC and Progenitor Cells

Marker	Expression/ remark	Fluorochrome conjugate recommended	Reference
Positive marker			
CD34	Positive	FITC, PE, APC, BIO	*1,2,33*
Thy-1	Positive	PE, BIO	*3,4*
AC133	Positive	PE	*12,34*
Negative/low marker			
CD38	Negative /low	FITC, PE, APC	*8,9*
HLA-DR[a]	Negative to low	FITC, PE	*35,36*
Mature lineage marker, Lin-			
CD2	T-cell lineage	FITC, PE, BIO	*3*
CD3	T-cell lineage	FITC, PE, APC, BIO	*3*
CD19	B-cell lineage	FITC, PE, APC, BIO	*3*
CD16	NK-cell lineage	FITC, PE, APC, BIO	*3*
CD14	Myeloid lineage	FITC, PE	*3*
CD15	Myeloid lineage	FITC, PE	*3*
Glycophorin A	Erythroid lineage	FITC, PE	*3*
2nd Step reagent			
Avidin/Streptavidin	For BIO MAb	FITC, PE, APC, TXRD, PharRed, Cy-chrome[d]	
Metabolic marker[b]			
Rhodamine 123[c]	Low	Mitochondria-binding dye	*37,38*
Hoechst 33342[c]	Low	DNA-binding dye	*39,40*
Pyronin Y	Low	RNA-binding dye	*39,40*
Propidium iodide	Negative to low	Dead-cell exclusion	

Abbreviations: FBM, fetal bone marrow; MPB, mobilized peripheral blood; ABM, adult bone marrow; HSC, hematopoietic stem cells; FITC, fluorescein; PE, phycoerythrin; APC, allophycocyanin; TXRD, Texas red; BIO, biotinylated.

[a] FBM, MPB HSCs express HLA-DR *(41,42)*.

[b] To isolate quiescent HSC.

[c] Substrates for p-glycoprotein, encoded by MDR-1. HSC possess high levels of p-glycoprotein efflux activity.

[d] Recommended for single laser flow cytometry only, lineage marker positive and PI positive cells can be excluded simultaneously.

Table 2
Positive and Negative Depletion Reagents Commercially Available

Product	Selection for	Vender
CD34 progenitor-cell isolation kit	Positively select CD34$^+$ cells	Miltenyi Biotech
Isolex-300	Positively select CD34$^+$ cells	Nexell Therapeutics
StemSep CD34$^+$ enrichment	Deplete lineage + cells	Stem Cell Technology

Flow cytometry allows for the purification of HSCs and primitive progenitors to near homogeneity. Separation by defined cell-surface markers can reveal different classes of rare populations, including those with extensive self-renewal capacity *(22–24)*, a multi-potent progenitor with limited self-renewal capacity *(25,26)*, or a common lymphoid progenitor population *(27,28)*. An understanding of the stem cell/progenitor hierarchy and evaluation of the role of these cells in stem-cell transplantation will be important for future clinical application, including autologous and allogeneic stem-cell transplantation, as well as ex vivo stem-cell expansion and gene therapy.

In this chapter, isolation of CD34$^+$ Thy-1$^+$ Lin$^-$ cells as a source of human HSCs is described, with emphasis on labeling and flow cytometric procedures. One option is to augment the four-color protocol described here, with the addition of CD38. **Note 7** offers suggestions for incorporating an additional immunofluorescent reagent in the staining panel. The authors also recommend some references regarding the enumeration of CD34$^+$ cells *(29,30)*, cell processing *(31)*, and presort enrichment *(30,32)*.

2. Materials

2.1. Cell Processing

1. Phosphate-buffered saline (PBS) (JRH Biosciences, Leneka, KS, #59321–79P) or Hank's Balanced Salt Solution (HBSS) (Life Technologies, Grand Island, NY, #14065–056) supplemented with 2% heat-inactivated fetal calf serum (FCS) or 0.5–1% human/bovine serum albumin (HSA/BSA).
2. Ficoll-Paque PLUS (Pharmacia Biotech, #17–1440–02).
3. Positive or negative selection reagents.

Table 2 summarizes options for positive or negative selection reagents used for presort enrichment.

2.2. Immunofluorescent Staining

1. Staining buffer: PBS or HBSS, supplemented with 2% FCS or 0.1–0.5% human/BSA.

2. Blocking buffer: 5% γ-immune (Miles-Bayer, # 640–12).
3. Sorting buffer: 0.5–1.0 g/mL propidium iodide (PI) in staining buffer. (0.5 mg/mL propidium iodide (PI) stock solution, Molecular Probes, # P-3566).
4. Falcon, polystyrene, round-bottom 12 × 75-mm tube with 35-μm strainer cap (Becton Dickinson, # 2235). (Although this product is packaged as "nonsterile," we have never experienced post sort contamination when using this product for presort filtration.)

2.3. Monoclonal Antibodies

Table 1 summarizes a panel of MAbs available for HSC isolation. In this chapter, only direct fluorochrome-conjugate or biotin-conjugate antibodies are listed. A combination of antibody panels can be chosen based on the objective of the experiment and the specific requirements for a given flow cytometer. In general, a combination of positive and negative (lineage) markers with dead-cell exclusion are recommended. Linscott's Directory of Immunological and Biological Reagents provides further information for antibody purchases. In this chapter, the following MAb reagents are used.

1. Fluroescein-5-isothiocyanate (FITC)-conjugated mouse immunoglobulins: IgG_1, IgG_{2a}, IgG_{2b}, and IgM isotype controls (Pharmingen cat. no. 33814X, 33034X, 33804X, 33064X).
2. Phycoerythrin-conjugated mouse IgG_1 (Pharmingen #33815X).
3. Sulforhodamine (TXRD)-conjugated anti-human CD34 (SyStemix) or APC-conjugated CD34 (Becton-Dickinson # 348053) (*see* **Note 2**).
4. Phycoerythrin-conjugated anti-human Thy-1 (Pharmingen #33085A).
5. Fluroescein-5-isothiocyanate (FITC)-conjugated anti-human CD2 (Becton-Dickinson #347593).
6. Fluroescein-5-isothiocyanate (FITC)-conjugated anti-human CD3 (Becton-Dickinson #349201).
7. Fluroescein-5-isothiocyanate (FITC)-conjugated anti-human CD14 (Becton-Dickinson #347493).
8. Fluroescein-5-isothiocyanate (FITC)-conjugated anti-human CD15 (Becton-Dickinson #347423).
9. Fluroescein-5-isothiocyanate (FITC)-conjugated anti-human CD16 (Becton-Dickinson #347523).
10. Fluroescein-5-isothiocyanate (FITC)-conjugated anti-human CD19 (Becton-Dickinson #340409).
11. Fluroescein-5-isothiocyanate (FITC)-conjugated anti-human GlycophorinA (Beckman-Coulter, #IM 2212).

2.4. Flow Cytometry

1. Dual-laser flow cytometer with sorting capability, such as the Becton Dickinson FACS Vantage (BDB, San Jose, CA) or the Cytomation MoFlo (Cytomation, Fort Collins, CO).

    a. Primary laser is a Coherent Innova 70, 90, or 300 series Argon Ion laser tuned to emit 200 mW of 488-nm laser light (Coherent Inc., Santa Clara, CA).

    b. Secondary laser is a CR599 Standing Wave Dye laser (Coherent Inc., Santa Clara, CA) tuned to emit 500 mW of 600-nm laser light. *(see* **Notes 1,2** regarding secondary laser configuration options*)*.

    c. We recommend utilizing a 70-μm nozzle tip for sorting HSCs.

2. Reference beads, Rainbow Fluorescent Particle, 3.2 m (Spherotech, Libertyville, IL, #RFP30-5A).

3. Epi-fluorescence microscope equipped with excitation and emission optics that permit visualization and quantitation of the reference particles. (i.e., UV excitation filter, 460/50-nm emission filter).

4. Glass microscope slides (Fisher Scientific, #12–544–15).

5. Biological control samples. (*See* **Subheading 3.4.** for instructions on preparing the appropriate biological control samples to be used in setting up the instrument.)

6. Sort sample-cell suspension at 5×10^6 cells/mL. (*See* **Subheading 3.5.** for instructions on preparing the sample from which the HSC will be isolated.)

7. FieldMaster™ laser power meter with LM-10 detector head (Coherent Instruments, Auburn, CA, #33–0506 and #33 0977, respectively).

8. Sheath fluid: 4 L PBS, Ca^{++}/Mg^{++} free, sterile-filtered, pH 7.0–7.4 (JRH Biosciences, Leneka, KS, #59321–79P).

9. Falcon, polystyrene, round-bottom 12×75-mm tube with cap (Becton Dickinson, #2058).

3. Methods

3.1. HSC Isolation Flowchart

Isolation of HSCs is achieved by a multi-step procedure beginning with tissue receipt, followed by cell processing, presort enrichment, sorting, and reanalysis. **Fig. 1** illustrates the flowchart for such a procedure. **Subheading 3.2.** describes detailed protocols for each step.

3.2. Tissue Sources for HSC, Cell Processing, and Presort Enrichment

Tissue sources used for HSC sorting can be heterogeneous, and may include unwanted cells, platelets, and debris which require some preliminary cell processing prior to presort enrichment for optimal recovery of HSCs. In general, the purpose of the initial step in cell processing is to remove residual erythrocytes, neutrophils, dead cells, and debris, which often cause instability of the fluid jet and/or occlusion of the nozzle orifice.

While apheresed mobilized peripheral blood samples require no processing prior to presort enrichment, adult bone marrow, fetal liver, and cord blood should be fractioned by density-gradient sedimentation in order to enhance

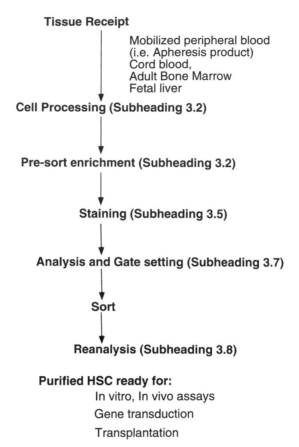

Fig. 1. Flowchart of human HSC purification.

recovery of HSCs. Cord-blood materials are often quite viscous compared to peripheral blood samples, and therefore require dilution with 2 vol of buffer (*see* **Subheading 2.1., item 1**) prior to fractionation by density-gradient sedimentation.

Presort enrichment involves either positive selection of target cells or depletion of unwanted cells, utilizing one of the selection devices summarized in **Table 2**. Refer to Chapter 3 or the individual manufacturer's recommendations for a specific procedure.

3.3. Antibody Titration

Prior to staining, specific titers for each monoclonal reagent should be established with the appropriate cell types. Determine the proper dilution of the MAbs by evaluating each immunofluorescent reagent for maximum resolution of the mean fluorescence intensities between negative and positive cells. Once the titers have been established, the concentration can be extrapolated for the actual cell number and volume of the sample to be stained. For more details, refer to **Note 1, ref. *31***.

3.4. Isotype and Compensation Control Staining (see Note 3)

The following is a list of control samples required to establish the gates for the HSC sort. Use a small aliquot of the postenrichment sample to make the following stained controls:

1. Cells stained with PI only.
2. Isotype-FITC/Isotype-phycoerythrin stained with PI.
3. CD34-FITC for FITC compensation control.
4. CD34-PE for phycoerythrin compensation control.
5. CD34-TXRD (or CD34-APC), lineage-FITC, isotype-phycoerythrin, stained with PI.

3.5. Sort Sample Staining

Throughout the staining procedure, it is important to maintain immunofluorescence-stained cell preparations on ice, protected from bright light. Keeping antibody-labeled cells cold helps to minimize the capping and internalization or shedding of surface antigen/antibody complex, and shielding immunofluorescent reagents from bright light will prevent the fluorochrome molecules from bleaching prior to laser excitation.

1. Determine the cell concentration of the sample with a hemocytometer or automated cell counter.
2. Perform Fc-receptor blocking by treating cells with human -globulin (γ-immune) reagent. Incubate cells in 0.1% γ-immune (1:50 dilution of 5 % γ-immune) in the staining buffer for 15 min on ice.
3. Centrifuge cells at 200–400g for 10 min at 4°C. Aspirate the supernatant, taking care not to disturb the cell pellet. Loosen the pellet by gentle vortexing.
4. Resuspend the cells in cold buffer and dispense 25,000-50,000 cells into 12 × 75-mm tubes for each isotype and compensation control.
5. In a 15-mL test tube, resuspend the remaining sample in a minimal volume of staining buffer at a concentration of $10^7 – 10^8$/mL. If the number of cells in the sample exceeds 10^8, use a 50-mL test tube to accommodate the appropriate volume of buffer required in the wash steps which follow.
6. Add each antibody (lineage-FITC, Thy-1-phycoerthrin, and CD34-TXRD) individually to the sample being stained. Alternatively, for convenience and consistency between experiments, a cocktail of these antibodies may be prepared in advance. Following the addition of each immunofluorescent staining reagent, mix the sample thoroughly by vortexing.
7. Incubate the samples on ice for 20–30 min.

8. Add 10–20 vol of cold staining buffer to each tube to wash (i.e., 1 mL staining vol requires 10–20 mL of buffer to adequately wash the cells). Vortex and centrifuge cells at 200–400g for 10 min at 4°C. Aspirate the supernatant, taking care not to disturb the cell pellet. Loosen the pellet by gentle vortexing.

9. Resuspend the cells in an appropriate volume of sorting buffer. An optimal cell concentration for sorting should be 4–8 × 10^6 cells/mL.

10. We highly recommend filtering the sample immediately prior to the sort to reduce the incidence of nozzle clogs during sort (*see* **Subheading 2.2., item 4**).

3.6. Instrument Setup

Although specific references to the flow cytometry instrumentation described in this chapter pertain to the Becton Dickinson FACS Vantage as used in our laboratory, analogous flow cytometry instrumentation from other manufacturers such as Cytomation can be used in order to achieve a similar endpoint. Investigators should also consider the scale of the stem-cell purification with respect to the design of the flow cytometry instrumentation to be utilized. Standard-speed commercial instrumentation typically allows for the processing of cells at a rate of several thousand events per second. From a sample that has been pre-enriched for CD34, one could reasonably expect to sort several million HSC in a normal workday, sorting at standard processing rates. Clinical scale HSC sorts may demand up to 10-fold more product than research-scale processes would typically yield. This requirement cannot be achieved in a reasonable period of time without the aid of specialized "high-speed" flow cytometry instrumentation. To address the specific performance demands of high-throughput sorting, instrumentation has been developed (*43,44*) which permits the processing of cells at a much greater speed than conventional flow cytometers.

In this protocol we employ a set of three (or four, *see* **Note 7** on CD38 staining option) immunofluorescent reagents, one DNA binding fluorescent dye for dead-cell exclusion and, two light-scatter parameters, for the discrimination of human HSCs. Both forward and orthogonal angle light-scatter signals are detected through 488-nm bandpass filters, amplified and measured on a linear scale. All fluorescent signals are amplified and measured over a four-decade log scale as specified in the **Table 3**.

3.7. Gate Setting

Purification of HSCs presumes a working definition of the stem-cell phenotype as characterized by prior flow cytometric analyses. In this chapter, we define the phenotype of the human hematopoietic stem cells as lineage-, Thy-1$^+$, and CD34$^+$. Dead cells are distinguished by excluding those cells that have taken up PI, while other cellular debris are excluded by light-scatter gating.

Table 3
Instrumentation Setup Requirements for Flow Cytometry

Fluorochrome label	Antibody conjugate	PMT parameter	Excitation wavelength	Emission maximum	Optical filter
FITC	Lin	FL1	488	514	530/30
PE	Thy-1	FL2	488	575	575/26
PI	PI	FL3	488	617	630/22
APC[a]	_	FL4	600/633	660	675/20
TXRD (SR)	CD34	FL5	600	615	630/25

[a] Option to use CD34 APC instead of CD34-TXRD (*see* **Note 2**).

Table 4
Region and Logical Gate Definition for HSC Sorting

Region	Associated Parameters
R1	Lineage FITC vs Propidium Iodide
R2	Thy-1 PE (–) vs CD34 TXRD
R3	Thy-1 PE (+) vs CD34 TXRD
R4	Forward Scatter vs Side Scatter

Gate	Logical gate Definition	Population Description
G1	G1 = R1	Viable Lin⁻ cells
G2	G2 = R1 and R2	Viable CD34⁺ Thy-1⁻ Lin⁻ cells
G3	G3 = R1 and R3	Viable CD34⁺ Thy-1⁺ Lin⁻ cells
G4	G4 = R4 and R1	Viable Lin⁻ cells in lymphoblastoid size
G5	G5 = R1 and R2 and R4	Viable CD34⁺ Thy-1⁻ Lin⁻ lymphoblastoid cells
G6	G6 = R1 and R3 and R4	Viable CD34⁺ Thy-1⁺ Lin⁻ lymphoblastoid cells

For convenience, we utilize a combination of rectangular regions derived from bivariate dot plots. The placement of a region boundary should be determined so that >99% of an isotype-stained control is contained within the region. In this way, the isotype control defines the staining intensity of cells that are negative for a given marker. We employ small aliquots of the CD34-enriched sample described in **Subheading 3.5, step 4.** for the gate-control samples. Refer to **Fig. 2** for an example of typical sort regions used in this protocol. **Table 4** contains details of the region and gate definitions we will refer to below.

1. Utilizing the flow cytometer's acquisition software, construct the following bivariate dot plots:
   a. Forward scatter vs side scatter.
   b. Lineage-FITC vs viability dye-PI.

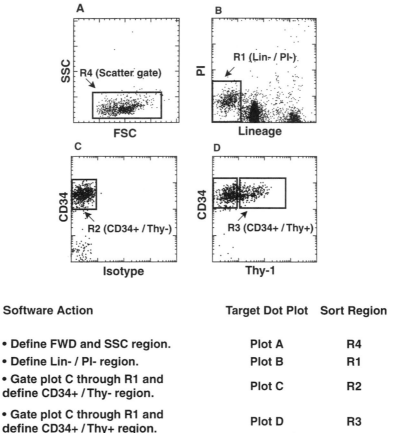

Software Action	Target Dot Plot	Sort Region
• **Define FWD and SSC region.**	Plot A	R4
• **Define Lin- / PI- region.**	Plot B	R1
• **Gate plot C through R1 and define CD34+ / Thy- region.**	Plot C	R2
• **Gate plot C through R1 and define CD34+ / Thy+ region.**	Plot D	R3
• **Gate plot A through both R1 and R2. Refine scatter region as needed.**	Plot A	R4

Fig. 2. Gate setting for CD34+ Thy-1+ Lin⁻ cell sorting (*see* **Subheading 3.7.** for details).

    c. Iso-phycoerythrin vs CD34-Texas Red (or CD34 APC).
    d. Thy-1-PE vs CD34-Texas Red (or CD34 APC).
2. Analyze the control sample described in **Subheading 3.4.** and identify the lymphocyte cluster in scatter plot A. Utilize the acquisition software controls to perform the following steps.
    a. Adjust the gain of the forward-scatter amplifier in order to position the lower end of the lymphocyte cluster near channel 300 on the forward-scatter axis. Positioning the lymphocyte cluster in this manner allows a space of approx 100 channels above the forward-scatter threshold so that smaller cells such as pre-B lymphocytes and erythrocytes are detected by the instrument's electronics. (**Fig. 2A**).

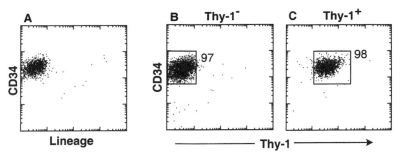

Fig. 3. Reanalysis of CD34+ Thy-1⁻ Lin⁻ and CD34+ Thy-1⁺ Lin⁻ cells after a successful cell sorting.

    b. In a similar manner, adjust the side-scatter amplifier in order to position the top end of the lymphocyte cluster near channel 300 on the side-scatter axis. Positioning the lymphocytes in the lower portion of the side-scatter axis allows space for cells such as monocytes and granulocytes, which exhibit a relatively higher side-scatter signal than lymphocytes (**Fig. 2A**).

3. Analyze the isotype control sample (*see* **Subheading 3.4., step 5**)(CD34-TXRD, Lineage-FITC, Isotype-PE, PI). Observe bivariate plot B (**Fig. 2**) and verify that the unstained cells reside in the lower left quadrant of this plot. On plot B construct rectangular **region R1** about the negative cells in the lower left quadrant.

4. Using the same isotope control sample (CD34-TXRD, Lineage-FITC, Isotype-PE, PI), construct rectangular **regions R2** and **R3** for the CD34+ Thy- and Thy+ subsets, respectively (*see* plots C and D in **Fig. 2**).

5. Define logical gate G2 as R1 and R2 (*see* **Table 4**). Using the same isotype control sample (CD34–TXRD, Lineage-FITC, Isotype-PE, PI), gate plot A (**Fig. 2**) with logical gate G2 and construct a rectangular region R4. The scatter region R4 should include the majority of cells residing in both the CD34+ and the Lineage-PI-compartments while excluding contaminating components such as residual RBCs and other cellular debris (*see* Plot A in **Fig. 2**).

6. Define the remaining logical gates G1–G6 as specified in **Table 4**. Analyze the sort sample (CD34-TXRD, Lineage-FITC, Thy-PE, PI) and verify that the CD34+ Thy+ cells reside in region R3. Download logical gate G6 (*see* **Table 4**) to the flow cytometer for sorting the viable CD34+ Thy+ Lineage-HSC. Observe the sort sample in plots A, B, and D (**Fig 2**) and make any necessary adjustments to the constructed regions. Depending on the experimental design, the researcher may choose to collect the nonstem cell progenitors as defined by logical gate G5 (*see* **Table 4**). If so, download gate (G5) to sort these sells in the opposing direction.

7. Install a covered collection container, turn on the deflection plates, and check the targeting of the side streams with respect to the opening of the container. Adjust the trajectory of the deflected side stream(s) as needed, using the left and right stream controls.

8. Remove the cover(s) from the collection container(s) and begin the sort.

3.8. Reanalysis Method

With experience, the researcher can expect to use flow cytometry to reliably sort an HSC product of high purity with an acceptable yield. Aside from product purity, other considerations in sorting cells by flow cytometry include recovery and viability of the product. In order to assess these variables, the end product must be subjected to further analyses. We recommend postsort analysis of the product by flow cytometry as well as an independent quantitative analysis of the product using a hemocytometer with Trypan blue *(31)*. For the purpose of determining the purity and viability by flow cytometry, a small aliquot of the sorted product should be reanalyzed, in the presence of propidium iodide, on the same instrument on which it was sorted. Purity can then be determined as the percentage of the target subset (implicitly defined by the sort regions) in the sorted product. Assessment of recovery requires determination of the cell concentration, pre- and postsort, in a known volume of buffer. Recovery may be described as the fraction of the desired cells that were sorted from the total sample. Actual recovery can be estimated using information provided by the instrument's electronic counters, while theoretical recovery can be calculated by utilizing Poisson statistics. Yield is defined as the quotient of the actual recovery divided by the theoretical recovery. *(See* **Note 4** regarding considerations and calculations employed in determining sort recovery.) Ideally, a viable HSC product can be recovered efficiently, and the reanalysis will exhibit high fidelity with respect to the defined sort regions. In our experience, the purity of the sorted product should typically be greater than 85%. *(See* **Note 5** for troubleshooting samples that fall below these expectations.)

1. Following the sort and prior to reanalysis, purge the fluidics path of any residual sort sample cells by running a tube containing only PBS (at high differential pressure) until the event rate approaches zero.
2. Using the reference beads, verify that the optical alignment is still optimized. Make adjustments as needed to bring the instrument alignment back to the specifications that were observed prior to initiating the sort.
3. Resuspend an aliquot of the sort product in a small volume of buffer containing PI and collect a data file. Evaluate the viability by exclusion of PI. Evaluate the purity of the product by observing the fraction of cells that fall within the regions used for sorting.
4. For issues related to contamination and biosafety, *(see* **Note 6**).

4. Notes

1. The 600-nm laser line is obtained using a pump-and-dye configuration in the secondary position. Typically, an Argon laser (Coherent I90, I70–4 or 305) capable of putting out up to 5W in multi-line visible mode is used to pump a

CR599 tuneable standing wave-dye laser (Coherent, San Jose, CA). The dye employed in the dye laser is rhodamine 6G, prepared according to the manufacturer's instructions.

2. Another option for a secondary laser is to use a HeNe laser (Model #127, Spectra-Physics, Mountain View, CA) instead of the pump-and-dye configuration described in **Note 1**. While the HeNe laser cannot be used for exciting the Texas red fluorochrome, it will emit 35 mW of 633-nm light, which is sufficient to excite other commercially available fluorochromes such as APC and APC-Cy7. It should be noted that fluorescence emissions in the red and far-red domain of the spectrum are measured more precisely with a photomultiplier optimized for the detection of red light, such as the Hamamatsu R3896 (personal communication from D. Sasaki).

3. Ideally, each fluorescent probe we measure on a multi-parameter flow cytometer could be detected in a separate detector so that optical (and spatial) filtering would allow that a given detector measured only the signal from a single probe. Unfortunately, the behavior of most fluorescent reporters commonly employed in flow cytometry does not adhere to this ideal. Instead, the emission spectra from some of the fluorochromes we utilize overlap to some degree. Spectral overlap occurs when a signal from a given fluorochrome "bleeds," or leaks into the detection range of another fluorochrome. In each fluorescence detector or channel, we attempt to measure as accurately as possible the signal contributed from only one type of fluorochrome or dye. In order to achieve this one-to-one correlation in signal measurement, each instrument manufacturer has implemented a methodology for fluorescence compensation. Please refer to the manufacturer's instructions for implementing the protocol appropriate for your instrument.

4. For the purpose of determining actual recovery by flow cytometry, the instrument's electronic counters should be set to display both sorted and aborted events. Actual recovery can be calculated as: Actual = sorted / (sorted + aborted). Theoretical recovery may be calculated by applying Poisson statistics according to the Pinkel and Stovel model *(45)*.

Recovery = (event rate × fraction of target particles)
    × exp (-event rate × deflection envelope × [1/drive frequency])

5. **Table 5** summarizes troubleshooting for HSC sorting.

6. Maintaining a clean flow cytometer significantly reduces the potential for bacterial contamination of the sorted product, and more importantly, will help minimize pathogen-associated risk to the instrument operator. It should be noted that the jet-in-air design of most commercial sorters leads to the production of aerosols. It has been demonstrated that some viruses can be transmitted through aerosols *(46)*. In addition to basic BSL2 safety precautions employed in handling human-derived tissues, certain precautions should be taken, because contamination of the air and surrounding surfaces with the material being sorted presents a potential biohazard to personnel working in the sorter laboratory. Utilize an industrial disinfectant (Lysol Professional Disinfectant, National Laboratories, Montvale, NJ) to decontaminate surrounding surfaces daily. While the instrument

Table 5
Troubleshooting

Symptom	Possible causes	Suggestions
High abort rate	Cell aggregates in sample	Filter sample, use DNase in sample
	High level of contaminating RBCs in sample	Reduce contaminating erythrocytes by lysis or density gradient centrifugation
	Coincidence error aborts	Try a lower cell concentration in the sample
		Try using a higher drop drive frequency
		Lower sample differential pressure -> lower event rate
Poor recovery	High abort rate	See high abort rate
	Inaccurate drop delay setting	Correct for drift in drop breakoff point
		Recalculate drop delay setting
	Unstable drop breakoff point	Reduce large aggregates in sample
		Purge air bubbles and/or debris from fluidics path
		Increase the size of the drop deflection envelope
	Inappropriate sort mode	Refer to the manufacturer's recommendations for choosin an optimal sort mode
Poor purity on re-analysis	Contamination in fluidics path	Clean fluidics path more rigorously
		Replace sample tubing
	Fluorochrome bleaching	Minimize exposure of fluorochrome-labeled antibodies to bright light
	antibody capping/shedding	Keep antibody-labeled cells on ice
		Employ a temperature regulation device at sample deliver and collection vessels
Poor product viability	Induction of apoptosis	Try a more nourishing media in sample and collection vessels
		Check sheath fluid for optimal pH and osmolarity
		Keep sort sample and product cold

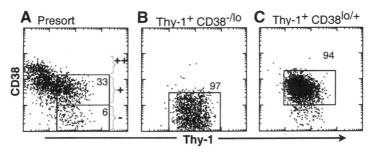

Fig. 4. MPB CD34⁺ Lin⁻ Thy-1⁺ CD38⁻/ˡᵒ and CD38ˡᵒ/⁺, and CD34⁺ Lin⁻ Thy-1⁻ cells were sorted as described. The Thy-1 vs CD38 profile of CD34⁺ Lin⁻gated cells revealed that the CD38 negative cells were highly enriched in Thy-1⁺ cells, and CD38⁺⁺ cells were virtually Thy-1⁻ (**A**). Reanalysis of CD34⁺ Lin⁻ Thy-1⁺ CD38⁻/ˡᵒ (**B**) and CD34⁺ Lin⁻ Thy-1⁺ CD38ˡᵒ/⁺ (**C**) populations shows that we could not eliminate the redistribution of CD38 signal intensity, although sorting gates were defined to separate CD38⁻ and CD38⁺ cells. With single-step sorts, the purity of CD38⁻/ˡᵒ and CD38ˡᵒ/⁺ subsets were 97–1 (SE) % and 91–2 %, respectively, by the gates shown. These sorted cells were highly enriched for Thy-1⁺ expression (99–0.08 %, without CD38 gate). The mean fluorescent intensity of the Thy-1 profile on the CD38⁻/ˡᵒ subset is consistently brighter (80–8 fluorescence units) than the CD38ˡᵒ/⁺ subset (53–3) ($p<0.05$). (Reprinted with permission from Uchida et al., *Proc. Natl. Acad. Sci. USA* 95, 11,939–11,944 [1998] in **ref. 11.**)

is in operation, a barrier should be in place between the operator and the fluid jet. If no such barrier has been implemented in the instrument's design—or as is more often the case, the built-in protective barriers have been removed or modified in some way—the operator should seriously consider wearing a face shield. Whether or not the experimental design necessitates a sterile HSC product, a routine cleaning protocol for the cell-sorter fluidics path is indicated. Relying on antibiotics to ensure sterility of the sheath fluid will eventually result in colonization of the system by resistant organisms, and is not recommended. Instead, we suggest sterilization of the entire fluidics path by introducing an antiseptic solution from the sheath reservoir. The instrument operator may find it more convenient to utilize a dedicated tank for the sole purpose of delivering disinfectant to the instrument. Some of the more commonly employed disinfectant solutions include dilute chlorine bleach, alcohol, and hydrogen peroxide solutions. For both research and clinical HSC sorting, we routinely utilize a solution of 6% hydrogen peroxide. Following human-cell sorting, we run 6% peroxide solution (STERI-PEROX™, Paxxis Inc., Belmont, CA) through the entire fluidics system for a minimum of 30 minutes. Following disinfection, thoroughly purge the antiseptic solution from the fluidics system with sterile sheath fluid before re-introducing live cells. Refer to the published biosafety guidelines for sorting formulated by the International Society of Analytical Cytology *(47)*.

7. Four-color immunofluorescent staining + PI can be performed to further subset CD34+ Thy-1+ Lin⁻ cells based on CD38 expression. An example of the staining and reanalysis is shown in **Fig. 4** *(11)*. To achieve this with commercially available reagents, one can use CD38-APC with either biotinylated Thy-1 or CD34 MAb. The biotinylated MAB will be revealed by either streptavidin TXRD or PharRed (*see* **Table 1**).

References

1. Strauss, L. C., Rowley, S. D., La Russa, V. F., Sharkis, S. J., Stuart, R. K., and Civin, C. I.. (1986) Antigenic analysis of hematopoiesis. V. Characterization of My-10 antigen expression by normal lymphohematopoietic progenitor cells. *Exp. Hematol.* **14,** 878–886.

2. Civin, C. I., Strauss, L. C., Brovall, C., Fackler, M. J., Schwartz, J. F., and J. H. Shaper. (1984) Antigenic analysis of hematopoiesis. III. A hematopoietic progenitor cell surface antigen defined by a monoclonal antibody raised against KG-1a cells. *J. Immunol.* **133,** 157–165.

3. Baum, C. M., Weissman, I. L., Tsukamoto, A. S., Buckle, A. M., and Peault, B. (1992) Isolation of a candidate human hematopoietic stem-cell population. *Proc. Natl. Acad. Sci. USA.* **89,** 2804–2808.

4. Craig, W., Kay, R., Cutler, R. L., and Lansdorp, P. M. (1993) Expression of Thy-1 on human hematopoietic progenitor cells. *J. Exp. Med.* **177,** 1331–1342.

5. Murray, L., Chen, B., Galy, A., Chen, S., Tushinski, R., Uchida, N., et al. (1995) Enrichment of human hematopoietic stem cell activity in the CD34+Thy-1+Lin-subpopulation from mobilized peripheral blood. *Blood* **85,** 368–378.

6. Humeau, L., Bardin, F., Maroc, C., Alario, T., Galindo, R., Mannoni, P., et al. (1996) Phenotypic, molecular, and functional characterization of human peripheral blood CD34+/THY1+ cells. *Blood* **87,** 949–955.

7. Cashman, J. D., Lapidot, T., Wang, J. C., Doedens, M., Shultz, L. D., Lansdorp, P., et al. (1997) Kinetic evidence of the regeneration of multilineage hematopoiesis from primitive cells in normal human bone marrow transplanted into immunodeficient mice. *Blood* **89,** 4307–4316.

8. Terstappen, L. W., Huang, S., Safford, M., Lansdorp, P. M,. and Loken, M. R. (1991) Sequential generations of hematopoietic colonies derived from single nonlineage-committed CD34+CD38– progenitor cells. *Blood* **77,** 1218–1227.

9. Petzer, A. L., Zandstra, P. W., Piret, J. M., and Eaves, C. J. (1996) Differential cytokine effects on primitive (CD34+CD38–) human hematopoietic cells: novel responses to Flt3–ligand and thrombopoietin. *J. Exp. Med.* **183,** 2551–2558.

10. Prosper, F., Stroncek, D., and Verfaillie, C.M. (1996) Phenotypic and functional characterization of long-term culture-initiating cells present in peripheral blood progenitor collections of normal donors treated with granulocyte colony-stimulating factor. *Blood* **88,** 2033–2042.

11. Uchida, N., Sutton, R. E., Friera, A. M., He, D., Reitsma, M. J., Chang, W. C., et al. (1998) HIV, but not murine leukemia virus vectors mediate high efficiency

gene transfer into freshly isolated G0/G1 human hematopoietic stem cells. *Proc. Natl. Acad. Sci. USA* **95,** 11,939–11,944.

12. Yin, A. H., Miraglia, S., Zanjani, E. D., Almeida-Porada, G., Ogawa, M., Leary, A. G., et al. (1997) AC133, a novel marker for human hematopoietic stem and progenitor cells. *Blood* **90,** 5002–5012.

13. de Wynter, E. A., Buck, D., Hart, C., Heywood, R., Coutinho, L. H., Clayton, A., et al. (1998) CD34+AC133+ cells isolated from cord blood are highly enriched in long-term culture-initiating cells, NOD/SCID-repopulating cells and dendritic cell progenitors. *Stem Cells* **16,** 387–396.

14. Brugger, W., Henschler, R., Heimfeld, S., Berenson, R. J., Mertelsmann, R., and Kanz, L. (1994) Positively selected autologous blood CD34+ cells and unseparated peripheral blood progenitor cells mediate identical hematopoietic engraftment after high-dose VP16, ifosfamide, carboplatin, and epirubicin. *Blood* **84,** 1421–1426.

15. Gorin, N. C., Lopez, M., Laporte, J. P., Quittet, P., Lesage, S., Lemoine, F., et al. (1995) Preparation and successful engraftment of purified CD34+ bone marrow progenitor cells in patients with non-Hodgkin's lymphoma. *Blood* **85,** 1647–1654.

16. Cottler-Fox, M., Cipolone, K., Yu, M., Berenson, R., O'Shaughnessy, J., and Dunbar, C. (1995) Positive selection of CD34+ hematopoietic cells using an immunoaffinity column results in T cell-depletion equivalent to elutriation. *Exp. Hematol.* **23,** 320–322.

17. Bensinger, W. I., Buckner, C. D., Shannon-Dorcy, K., Rowley, S.,Appelbaum, F. R., Benyunes, M., et al. (1996) Transplantation of allogeneic CD34+ peripheral blood stem cells in patients with advanced hematologic malignancy. *Blood* **88,** 4132–4138.

18. Civin, C. I., T. Trischmann, N. S. Kadan, J. Davis, S. Noga, Cohen, K., et al. (1996) Highly purified CD34–positive cells reconstitute hematopoiesis. *J. Clin. Oncol.* **14,** 2224–2233.

19. Handgretinger, R., Lang, P., Schumm, M., Taylor, G., Neu, S., Koscielnak, E., et al. 1998. Isolation and transplantation of autologous peripheral CD34+ progenitor cells highly purified by magnetic-activated cell sorting. *Bone Marrow Transplant.* **21,** 987–993.

20. Archimbaud, E., Philip, I., Coiffier, B., Michallet, M., Salles, G., Sebban, C., et al. 1997. Selected autologous peripheral blood CD34+Thy-1+Lin- hematopoietic stem cell (HSC) transplantation in multiple myeloma: a European study. *Blood.* **90(Suppl. 1),** 394(Abstract).

21. Negrin, R., Tierney, K., Stockerl-Goldstein, E., Hu, W., Shizuru, J., Johnston, L., et al. (1997) Rapid hematopoietic engraftment following transplantation of purified CD34+Thy1+ stem cells in patients with metastatic breast cancer. *Blood* **90(Suppl. 1),** 593a(Abstract).

22. Morrison, S. J. and Weissman, I. L. (1994) The long-term repopulating subset of hematopoietic stem cells is deterministic and isolatable by phenotype. *Immunity* **1,** 661–673.

23. Larochelle, A., Vormoor, J., Hanenberg, H., Wang, J. C., Bhatia, M., Lapidot, T.,

et al. (1996) Identification of primitive human hematopoietic cells capable of re-populating NOD/SCID mouse bone marrow: implications for gene therapy. *Nat. Med.* **2,** 1329–1337.

24. Conneally, E., Cashman, J., Petzer, A., and Eaves, C. (1997) Expansion in vitro of transplantable human cord blood stem cells demonstrated using a quantitative assay of their lympho-myeloid repopulating activity in nonobese diabetic-scid/scid mice. *Proc. Natl. Acad. Sci. USA* **94,** 9836–9841.

25. Punzel, M., Wissink, S. D., Miller, J. S., Moore, K. A., Lemischka, I. R., and Verfaillie, C. M. (1999) The myeloid-lymphoid initiating cell (ML-IC) assay assesses the fate of multipotent human progenitors in vitro. *Blood* **93,** 3750–3756.

26. Morrison, S. J., Wandycz, A. M., Hemmati, H. D., Wright, D. E., and Weissman, I. L. (1997) Identification of a lineage of multipotent hematopoietic progenitors. *Development* **124,** 1929–1939.

27. Galy, A., Travis, M., Cen, D., and Chen, B. (1995) Human T, B, natural killer, and dendritic cells arise from a common bone marrow progenitor cell subset. *Immunity* **3,** 459–473.

28. Kondo, M., Weissman, I., and Akashi, K. 1997. Identification of clonogenic common lymphoid prognitor in mouse bone marrow. *Cell* **91,** 661–672.

29. Keeney, M., Chin-Yee, I., Weir, K., Popma, J., Nayar, R., and Sutherland, D. R. (1998) Single platform flow cytometric absolute CD34+ cell counts based on the ISHAGE guidelines. International Society of Hematotherapy and Graft Engineering. *Cytometry* **34,** 61–70.

30. Wunder, E., Sovalat, H., Henon, P., and Serke, S. (1994) Hematopoietic Stem Cells: The Mulhouse Manual (Serke, S., ed.), AlphaMed Press, Dayton, OH, p. 125.

31. Robinson, J. P., Darzynkiewicz, Z., Dean, P. N., Orfao, A., Rabinovitch, P. S., Stewart, C. C., et al. (1997) Current Protocol in Cytometry, in *Current Protocol in Cytometry*, John Wiley & Sons, New York, NY.

32. Nieto, Y. and Shpall, E. J. (1998) CD34+ blood stem cell transplantation, in *Blood stem cell transplantation* (Reiffers, J., Goldman, J. M., and Armitage, J. O., eds.) Mosby, St. Louis, MO, pp 187–200.

33. Andrews, R. G., Singer, J. W., and Bernstein, I. D. (1986) Monoclonal antibody 12–8 recognizes a 115–kd molecule present on both unipotent and multipotent hematopoietic colony-forming cells and their precursors. *Blood* **67,** 842–845.

34. Miraglia, S., Godfrey, W., Yin, A. H., Atkins, K., Warnke, R., Holden, J. T., et al. (1997) A novel five-transmembrane hematopoietic stem cell antigen: isolation, characterization, and molecular cloning. *Blood* **90,** 5013–5021.

35. Srour, E. F., Brandt, J. E., Leemhuis, T., Ballas, C. B., and Hoffman R. (1992) Relationship between cytokine-dependent cell cycle progression and MHC class II antigen expression by human CD34+ HLA-DR- bone marrow cells. *J. Immunol.* **148,** 815–820.

36. Brandt, J., Briddell, R. A., Srour, E. F., Leemhuis, T. B., and Hoffman, R. (1992). Role of c-kit ligand in the expansion of human hematopoietic progenitor cells. *Blood* **79,** 634–641.

37. Udomsakdi, C., Eaves, C., Sutherland, H., and Lansdorp, P. (1991) Separation of

functionally distinct subpopulations of primitive human hematopoietic cells using rhodamine-123. *Exp. Hematol.* **19**, 338–342.

38. Uchida, N., Combs, J., Chen, S., Zanjani, E., Hoffman, R., and Tsukamoto, A. (1996) Primitive human hematopoietic cells displaying differential efflux of the rhodamine 123 dye have distinct biological activities. *Blood* **88**, 1297–1305.

39. Ladd, A. C., Pyatt, R., Gothot, A., Rice, S., McMahel, J., Traycoff, C. M., et al. (1997) Orderly process of sequential cytokine stimulation is required for activation and maximal proliferation of primitive human bone marrow CD34+ hematopoietic progenitor cells residing in G0. *Blood* **9,** :658–668.

40. Gothot, A., Pyatt, R., McMahel, J., Rice, S., and Srour, E. F. (1997) Functional heterogeneity of human CD34(+) cells isolated in subcompartments of the G0 /G1 phase of the cell cycle. *Blood* **90**, 4384–4393.

41. Tsukamoto, A., Weissman, I., Chen, B., DiGiusto, D., Baum, C., Hoffman, R., et al. (1995) Phenotypic and functional analysis of hematopoietic stem cells in mouse and human, in *Hematopoietic Stem Cells: Biology and Therapeutic Applications* (Levitt, D. and Mertelsmann, R. eds.), pp 85–124.

42. Waller, E. K., Huang, S., and Terstappen, L. (1995) Changes in the growth properties of CD34+, CD38– bone marrow progenitors during human fetal development. *Blood* **86,** 710–718.

43. Sasaki, D. T., Tichenor, E. H., Lopez, F., Combs, J., Uchida, N., Smith, C. R., et al. (1995) Development of a clinically applicable high-speed flow cytometer for the isolation of transplantable human hematopoietic stem cells. *J. Hematother.* **4,** 503–514.

44. Rehse, M. A., Corpuz, S., Heimfeld, S., Minie, M., and Yachimiak, D. (1995) Use of fluorescence threshold triggering and high-speed flow cytometry for rare event detection. *Cytometry* **22**, 317–322.

45. Van Dilla, M. A., Dean, P. N., Laerum, O. D., and Melamed, M.R. (1985) Flow cytometry: Instrumentation and data analysis, Academic Press, New York, NY.

46. Merrill, J. T. (1981) Evaluation of selected aerosol-control measures on flow sorters. *Cytometry* **1**, 342–345.

47. Schmid, I., Nicholson, J. K., Giorgi, J. V., Janossy, G., Kunkl, A., Lopez, P.A., et al. (1997) Biosafety guidelines for sorting of unfixed cells. *Cytometry* **28,** 99–117.

48. Linscott's Directory of Immunological and Biological Reagents.

5

Noninvasive Measurement of Hematopoietic Stem Cell Cycling and Turnover by In Vivo Bromodeoxyuridine Incorporation

Gillian B. Bradford and Ivan Bertoncello

1. Introduction

The hematopoietic system comprises a concatenated series of stem- and transit-progenitor-cell compartments of progressively restricted potentiality and proliferative capacity *(1–5)*. Analysis of hematopoietic regulation in transplantation models and in marrow regeneration following cytotoxic challenge suggests that normal steady state blood-cell production is ultimately maintained by the progeny of only a few stem-cell clones. The majority of primitive hematopoietic stem cells (PHSC) in the steady state are either highly quiescent or dormant, and are transiently recruited only in times of unusual demand resulting from hematopoietic stress caused by infection, hemorrhage, myelotoxicity, or following transplantation where transiting progenitor-cell compartments need to be replenished. The relative quiescence or dormancy of the stem-cell compartment greatly increases the probability of survival of continuously renewing cell populations by providing a protected stem-cell reserve, thus reducing differentiative pressure and maintaining lifelong genetic stability and integrity of stem cells by facilitating repair *(2,6)*.

Whether stem cells *in situ* are truly dormant and in a G_0 state, or whether the relative quiescence of the stem cell compartment is caused by variations in cell-cycle transit times primarily regulated by the length of G_1 phase *(2)* is not a semantic question. This remains a key issue in experimental hematology, with significant implications for modeling and predicting stem cell behavior, and manipulating stem cell fate. For example, in hematopoietic models invok-

From: *Methods in Molecular Medicine, vol. 63: Hematopoietic Stem Cell Protocols*
Edited by: C. A. Klug and C. T. Jordan © Humana Press Inc., Totowa, NJ

ing absolute self-renewal as a fundamental stem cell property, dormancy is not an obligatory requirement of "stemness." While quiescence confers a survival advantage, the stem-cell reserve is primarily maintained by physiological mechanisms that regulate the probability of symmetric renewal or asymmetric differentiative divisions in the stem cell pool. On the other hand, clonal succession models—and the generation-age model in particular *(1,3,4)*—propose that the stem cell reserve comprises a finite pool of dormant cells, where cell division is synonymous with the loss of proliferative and differentiative potential.

Our knowledge of the kinetics of the stem cell compartment has primarily relied on analysis of the selective toxicity of cell-cycle active cytotoxic drugs, irradiation, and thymidine suicide utilizing surrogate stem and progenitor cell assays in mice. These invasive techniques have the potential to activate and modulate stem-cell activity during the process of measurement. Analysis with these techniques is compromised by their inability to reliably quantify the turnover rate of rare, unperturbed, putatively quiescent stem cell populations *in situ*, long-term. Recent advances and refinements in stem-cell separative techniques, combined with the adaptation of methods for the delivery and measurement of incorporation of the nontoxic thymidine analog bromodeoxyuridine (BrdU) into specific stem- and progenitor-cell subsets, has led to the development of a powerful experimental approach that permits noninvasive long-term monitoring of the kinetics of defined, closely related stem- and progenitor-cell populations *in situ*.

Incorporation of BrdU into DNA provides a specific measure of cell cycling. BrdU is a thymidine analog in which the methyl group of thymine is replaced by bromine *(7,8)*. Since rodent cells demonstrate a preference for thymidine to BrdU incorporation, with an average ratio of 2.35:1 *(9)*, BrdU substitution of DNA is not complete. The resultant low levels of BrdU substitution generally do not interfere with cellular proliferation, and are noninvasive even following long-term continuous infusion in vivo *(10–12)* (*see* **Note 1**).

The development of monoclonal antibody (MAb) reagents which detect BrdU incorporated in single-stranded DNA *(13,14)* has enabled high throughput flow cytometric analysis of cell cycling. When administered as a pulse label, BrdU incorporation provides an instantaneous measurement of the proportion of cells which are in S phase at any point in time *(15,16)*. When combined with propidium iodide (PI) staining, the cell-cycling status of cell populations can be determined from pulse-labeling experiments with great precision (**Fig. 1**).

Since BrdU is retained during cellular proliferation, and is passed on to the daughter cells with each cell division *(9)*, it can also be administered continuously over extended periods to investigate population turnover rates

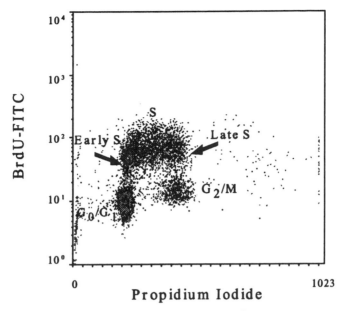

Fig. 1. BrdU/PI staining of pulse-labeled FDCP-1 cells: FDCP-1 cells were pulse-labeled with BrdU (100 μM, 37°C, 30 min), and fixed and stained with FITC-conjugated anti-BrdU antibody and PI. The bivariate dot-plot shows the ability of the technique to discriminate cells in each phase of cell cycle.

(7,11,12,17). This method enables rare populations of cells which cycle infrequently to be identified (**Fig. 2**), and their proliferation history to be assessed. Because the fixation method used in these analyses does not excessively disrupt the physical characteristics of the cells, it is possible to simultaneously determine the immunophenotypic characteristics, light-scattering properties, and kinetic status of discrete cell subsets within a population, providing great power of analysis in complex populations such as the bone marrow or peripheral blood.

Continuous BrdU administration has often been achieved using subcutaneous osmotic pumps *(11,17)*. However, insertion of osmotic pumps requires minor, yet invasive surgery, and long-term BrdU administration requires removal and replacement of pumps at weekly or biweekly intervals. Fluctuations in steady state hematopoiesis and stem cell cycling as a result of these invasive procedures must be considered.

In 1990, Forster and Rajewsky *(12)* demonstrated that long-term continuous infusion of BrdU could be achieved by administration of BrdU in the drinking water of mice. This alternative route of administration allowed the noninvasive assessment of proliferation and turnover of long-lived murine lymphocyte

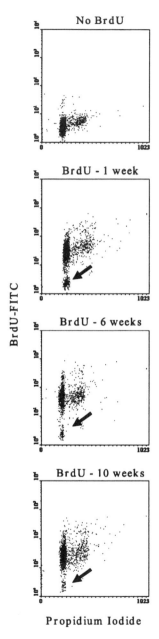

Fig. 2. BrdU/PI staining of unseparated bone-marrow cells isolated from mice administered BrdU (0.5 mg/mL) for periods of 0–10 wk, demonstrating the capacity of this technique to detect highly quiescent cell populations indicated by the arrow.

populations in vivo. We have adapted and refined this technique for the analysis of stem-cell cycling and turnover *in situ (18)*. Analysis of BrdU incorporation in lineage negative (Lin⁻) PHSC sorted on the basis of rhodamine 123 (Rh) and Hoechst 33342 (Ho) dye uptake showed that PHSC cycle continuously throughout life, with an average turnover time of 30 d, and duration to 50% cycled of 19 d *(18)*. Recently, Cheshier et al. *(19)* have also utilized long-term BrdU administration in drinking water to confirm these observations in PHSC, defined on the basis of expression of a repertoire of stem cell associated cell-surface antigens (Kit⁺, Sca-1⁺, Thyˡᵒ, Lin⁻).

The BrdU feeding regime and the protocol for flow cytometric analysis of BrdU incorporation outlined in this chapter have been optimized for the long-term measurement of cycling and turnover of murine hematopoietic stem and progenitor cells in this laboratory. It is important to note that genetic background, the exquisite sensitivity of the hematopoietic system to perturbation, and environmental and experimental conditions are significant sources of variability in the measurement of hematopoietic parameters both within and between groups of mice.

Inbred strains of mice were initially developed to establish the existence and influence of genetic factors on the incidence of cancer *(20)*. Coincidentally, these genetic factors also influence hematopoiesis, immune-surveillance, and inflammatory responses. Different strains of mice vary markedly in total and differential leukocyte counts *(21)*, in their susceptibility to irradiation *(22)*, and in their propensity to mobilize stem and progenitor cells in response to cytokine administration *(23)*. Recent studies have also demonstrated that stem cell pool size and stem cell cycling characteristics are genetically controlled *(24,25)*.

Husbandry and environmental factors are also important yet often neglected variables in the measurement of physiological parameters in mice *(26,27)* *(see* **Note 2**). The kinetic status of hematopoietic cells will also be conditioned by the spectrum of environmental pathogens present in individual mouse colonies, and will differ in mice housed in a conventional animal house environment or under pathogen-free conditions.

Although the methods we describe are robust and reliable, it should be noted that the optimal dose of BrdU recommended for continuous long-term oral BrdU administration in mice should only be used as a guide, and must be validated empirically. This dose should be varied if necessary to account for strain differences and variability in environmental conditions which may influence the behavior of the hematopoietic system of mice in individual laboratories. BrdU does have some toxic side effects, which have been shown to be both species- and strain-specific *(12,28)*. Therefore, a dose-response experiment should be done prior to use, to determine the dose of BrdU which gives optimal levels of BrdU labeling, without toxicity (*see* **Note 3**).

2. Materials

1. BrdU Reagents: BrdU stock solution is made up from powder (Sigma, St. Louis, MO) at a concentration of 10mg/mL in sterile water, and stored protected from light at 4°C for up to 4 wk, or frozen at –20°C.
   BrdU supplemented drinking water (0.5 mg/mL in water); BrdU for in vivo pulse-labeling (100 mg/kg, made in PBS, administered intraperitoneally); and, BrdU for in vitro pulse-labeling of cell lines (100 μ*M* final concentration in media; 30.7 μg/mL) is made up fresh as required, by serial dilution of the BrdU stock solution (*see* **Note 4**).
2. Fluorescein-5-isothiocyonate (FITC)-conjugated anti-BrdU antibody (Clone B44, Cat #347583; Becton Dickinson, San Jose, CA) diluted in PBS-1% Tween-20 (made fresh each time). Antibody is stored at 4°C (*see* **Note 5**).
3. Phosphate-Buffered Saline (PBS: pH 7.4, 310 mosM). The following ingredients are required for 5 L of PBS:

40 g	NaCl
1.0 g	KCl
5.75 g	Na_2HPO_4
1.0 g	KH_2PO_4
1.0 g	glucose

   Dissolve NaCl in approx 4 L of distilled H_2O. Add the remaining salts and glucose separately, ensuring that each has fully dissolved before adding the next ingredient. The buffer is then adjusted to pH = 7.4 using HCl (1 N) or NaOH (1 N), and the volume is then adjusted to 5 L. The osmolarity is checked by osmometer and adjusted to 310 mosM with distilled H_2O. The buffer is then sterile-filtered (0.2 μm) and stored refrigerated at 4°C.
4. Heat-inactivated serum: PBS supplemented with 0.55% heat-inactivated fetal calf serum (FCS), or newborn bovine serum (PBS-0.55% HiSe) is used as a wash buffer for the preparation and manipulation of cell suspensions and antibody dilution. Serum is heat-inactivated at 56°C for a minimum of 1 h, then cooled and filtered through coarse filter paper to remove denatured protein. HiSe is then filtered through filters of progressively smaller pore size, and finally sterile-filtered (0.2 μm), aliquoted and stored frozen for use as required (*see* **Note 6**).
5. Fixing solution: Paraformaldehyde (0.5%; v/v) is made up in PBS, filtered through a Whatman #1 filter, and stored frozen at –20°C.
6. Denaturing solution: 2 *M* HCl-0.5% Tween-20 is made up fresh by addition of 0.5% Tween-20 (v/v) to 2 *M* HCl (diluted in water) and mix well. This solution is stored at room temperature.
7. Sodium borate: $Na_2B_4O_7 \cdot 10H_2O$ (0.1 *M*) is made up from powder in water, and stored at room temperature.
8. Propidium iodide: PI (5 μg/mL) is made up in PBS and stored at 4°C, protected from light.

9. FDCP-1 cells: The interleukin 3 (IL-3) dependent FDCP-1 cell line **(29)** in exponential growth phase is used as a positive control for BrdU labeling in each experiment (*see* **Note 7**). FDCP-1 cells are passaged weekly in 25-cm^2 flasks using α-MEM-10% FCS and 10% WEHI-3 CM as a source of IL-3.

3. Methods
3.1. Incorporation of BrdU in Defined Target Cells In Vivo

The cell-cycling status of defined hematopoietic stem- and progenitor-cell subpopulations in vivo is determined by BrdU pulse-labeling. In this protocol, BrdU (100 mg/kg, ip) is administered to mice 1 h prior to euthanasia. Bone-marrow cells are harvested by excising the femurs and tibiae, and flushing the bone marrow into PBS-% HiSe using a 23-gauge needle attached to a 1-mL syringe. For measurement of the turnover of hematopoietic stem- and progenitor-cell compartments long-term, BrdU is administered continuously to mice *ad libitum* via their drinking water, at a concentration of 0.5 mg/mL (*see* **Note 8**).

Defined hematopoietic stem- and progenitor-cell populations are purified using multiparameter cell-separative strategies, incorporating density gradient centrifugation, immunomagnetic selection, and flow cytometric analysis, and sorting utilizing stem cell reagents of choice (*see* **Note 9**).

An aliquot of sorted cells is set aside for functional stem- and progenitor-cell assays, and the remainder of cells are retained for detection and analysis of BrdU incorporation.

3.2. BrdU Pulse-Labeling In Vitro

Actively growing cultures of FDCP-1 cells in exponential growth phase are pulse-labeled with BrdU (100 µ*M*, 30 min, 37°C). Approx 1×10^6 cells are harvested from flasks and washed once in PBS-5% HiSe in preparation for fixation, labeling, and analysis.

3.3. Fixation, Staining, and Detection of BrdU Incorporation and DNA Content

1. Up to 1×10^6 cells are pelleted by centrifugation (1,350 rpm—250–300*g*, 4°C, 5 min), and the supernatant is discarded.
2. The cell pellet is loosened by gentle vortexing, and then fixed by adding 0.5 mL paraformaldehyde fixing solution. The cell suspension is then chilled on ice for 5 min (*see* **Note 10**).
3. Cells are equilibrated to room temperature. They are then centrifuged (1,350 rpm—250–300*g*, 5 min), the supernatant is discarded, and the cell pellet is loosened by gentle vortexing.
4. Denaturing solution (0.5 mL 2 *M* HCl containing 0.5% Tween-20) is added, and cells are incubated for 30 min at 37°C (*see* **Note 11**).

5. The cell suspension is centrifuged, the supernatant is discarded, and the cells are resuspended in 0.1 *M* sodium borate (0.5 mL) to neutralize residual acid.
6. Cells are centrifuged and washed in PBS.
7. Cells are incubated at room temperature (30 min in the dark) in 20 µL FITC-conjugated anti-BrdU antibody diluted in 50 µL PBS-1% Tween-20.
8. Cells are washed in PBS-5%HiSe and resuspended in PBS-5%HiSe containing PI (5 µg/mL) and incubated at room temperature (10 min in the dark) prior to flow cytometric analysis.

3.4. Flow Cytometry

Fluorochromes are excited at 488 nm and FITC-conjugated BrdU fluorescence is detected through a 530-nm bandpass filter with a bandwidth of ±15 nm. DNA-linked PI red fluorescence is detected through a red 600-nm wavelength filter. List files of up to 10,000 target cells are collected, and BrdU incorporation and DNA content are displayed as fluorescence histograms and bivariate dot plots of cells which have been gated on the basis of forward- and 90° light-scatter.

3.5. Analysis of Data

For pulse-labeling experiments, the cell-cycling status of target-cell populations can simply be determined by the analysis of bivariate BrdU-FITC/PI plots as shown in **Fig. 1**. BrdU incorporation by hematopoietic cells continuously labeled with BrdU (**Figs. 2** and **3**) is determined by comparison of the BrdU-FITC and PI fluorescence profiles of labeled cells with those of bone-marrow cells which have not been exposed to BrdU. A sample of FDCP-1 cells which have been exposed to BrdU (100 µM, 30 min, 37°C) during exponential growth phase is also included in each run as a positive control.

List files of labeled and negative control cells are displayed as BrdU-FITC/PI bivariate plots using flow cytometric analysis software (*see* **Note 12**). The BrdU-FITC/PI bivariate plot (**Fig. 3A**) is initially gated to exclude debris or aggregates which may distort the percentages of 2N DNA- and BrdU-positive cells. The percentage of 2N DNA (G_0/G_1 phase) cells is obtained from the PI fluorescence histogram by gating cells with >2N DNA within this region and subtracting that percentage (the percentage of $S/G_2/M$ cells) from 100 (**Fig. 3B**).

BrdU incorporation by labeled cells is analyzed by overlaying and comparing the BrdU-FITC histograms of stained and negative control samples (**Fig. 3C**). An electronic gate is set using the fluorescence histogram of unlabeled cells, so that background fluorescence is no greater than 5%. The percentage of BrdU-positive cells is then determined by subtracting background fluorescence from the value obtained by applying this gating strategy to the labeled target-

A

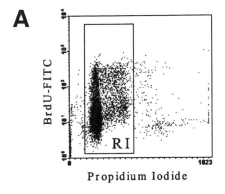

B

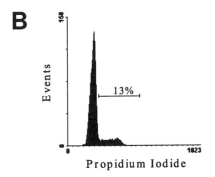

C

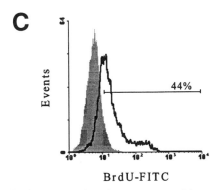

Fig. 3. Analysis of BrdU incorporation in unseparated bone marrow cells of mice administered BrdU (0.5 mg/mL) for 4 wk. BrdU/PI-stained bone-marrow cells were initially gated (RI) to exclude debris and aggregates (**A**). DNA content, and the percentage of cycling cells (S/G_2/M phase of cell cycle) was determined from the PI histogram of gated cells (**B**). BrdU incorporation (**C**) by labeled cells (*solid line*) was determined by comparison with the fluorescence profile of unstained cells (*shaded histogram*) where the gate was set so that background fluorescence was no higher than 5%.

cell population. In situations where the majority of cells have incorporated BrdU, the fluorescence histogram list file of the negative control cells is electronically scaled and reduced to fit prior to overlaying the histograms and applying the gating strategy.

We have found that the level of BrdU incorporation measured following continuous long-term BrdU administration at low doses is clearly underestimated. The extent to which BrdU incorporation is underestimated following long-term BrdU administration can be determined through analysis of BrdU incorporation in the mature granulocyte pool. Mature granulocytes have a very short half-life *(37)*, and are generated rapidly and continuously. Within days, the entire granulocyte pool will have turned over, and all granulocytes should be 100% BrdU-positive. Values for BrdU incorporation in specific hematopoietic cell subsets following long-term BrdU administration are adjusted by the conversion factor used to adjust the measured percentage of granulocytes determined to have fully incorporated BrdU to 100%.

4. Notes

1. BrdU substitution levels are highly dependent on cell type and the dose of BrdU, and are possibly also species- and strain-dependent *(12,29)*. Although BrdU is nontoxic at low doses, it has been shown to have adverse physiological effects at higher levels of substitution *(10,29–32)*. Studies in a canine model have also shown that adverse physiological interactions may occur when BrdU is combined with cytotoxic drugs commonly used in the analysis of hematopoietic stem cell function *(33)*. Consequently, it is necessary to determine empirically an appropriate noninvasive dose for continuous long-term BrdU administration under each new set of experimental conditions.

2. Excellent references *(26,27)* describing the impact of phenotypic, environmental, and experimental variability in animal research may be obtained from The Australian and New Zealand Council for the Care of Animals in Research and Teaching (ANZCCART). Details and addresses are available on the Web sites: http://www.adelaide.edu.au/ANZCCART/ or http://anzccart.rsnz.govt.nz

3. It is possible that accumulated damage to cells as a result of BrdU incorporation could result in recruitment of otherwise noncycling stem cells, giving a false impression of the cycling status and turnover rate of the PHSC compartment. Rajewski *(34)* controlled for this effect by using pulse chase to compare the rate of dilution of BrdU from the lymphocyte compartment with the rate of BrdU incorporation in these cells. It is also important to assess toxicity by analyzing the functional status of the hematopoietic system in mice fed BrdU for the length of time equivalent to that in the experimental groups. In our experience, certain doses of BrdU do not affect steady state hematopoietic parameters, but do compromise the ability of the hematopoietic system to recover when treated with myeloablative doses of 5-fluorouracil. Doses of BrdU should be tailored to exclude this effect.

4. BrdU concentrations quoted in the literature for pulse-labeling of cell cultures range from 10 μM-100 μM. We have routinely used 100 μM BrdU, but lower concentrations should be adequate.

5. Similar BrdU antibody reagents can be purchased from other suppliers. It is also possible to use a two-step labeling procedure using primary unconjugated anti-BrdU followed by labeling with fluorescent second-antibody conjugates.

6. We routinely use heat-inactivated serum as a buffer supplement for processing hematopoietic cells in our laboratory to prevent complement-mediated cell lysis. Because this protocol entails the labeling and analysis of fixed cells, the use of heat-inactivated serum is not strictly necessary.

7. We have used the FDCP-1 cell line as a positive control for flow cytometric analysis of BrdU labeling. However, any rapidly growing cell line pulse-labeled in the exponential phase of growth is suitable for this purpose.

8. Since it is commonly reported that BrdU solutions should be protected from light, and replaced every 3–5 days, the stability of 0.5 mg/mL BrdU solutions was tested under various storage conditions. No significant difference was found between the labeling obtained from solutions stored under different conditions (4°C and room temperature; exposed to and protected from light) and that obtained from a freshly made BrdU solution, suggesting that no detectable degradation occurred under any of these storage conditions. Consequently, BrdU was fed to the mice in clear water bottles, and changed weekly.

9. A description of cell separative procedures is beyond the scope of this chapter.

10. It is critical to ensure that cells are well-dispersed before addition of fixative to avoid aggregation. The presence of aggregates will compromise flow cytometric analysis of BrdU incorporation. Cell aggregation during fixation can be minimized by dropwise addition of fixative while gently vortexing the cell pellet. Once fixed, cells can be processed immediately, or can be stored at 4°C for a few days prior to analysis.

11. Since all currently available MAbs recognize BrdU only in single-stranded DNA, the DNA of the target cells must be denatured prior to labeling. Although a variety of protocols for denaturation have been described *(35)*, some methods which provide the best denaturation (e.g., heat) are too severe for use with hematopoietic cells. Treatment of these cells with HCl and mild heat is a successful compromise, providing adequate DNA denaturation for detection of BrdU incorporation and retaining cellular integrity *(15,35,36)*. Denaturation of the cells in 2 M HCl containing 0.5% Tween-20 at 37°C for 30 min yields optimal BrdU staining of murine hematopoietic cells. Lower HCl concentrations and denaturation temperatures and shorter denaturation times result in lower levels of BrdU staining, and higher HCl concentrations damage cells (especially at higher temperatures), as evidenced by the increased coefficient of variation of peaks in the PI fluorescence profiles.

12. We routinely use the WinMDI Software package (Joseph Trotter, Scripps Institute) for this purpose. Commercially available computer modeling programs such as Modfit (Verity Software House Inc., Topsham, Maine) may also be used.

Acknowledgments

We thank Brenda Williams and Ralph Rossi for their expert technical assistance with cell preparation and flow cytometry.

References

1. Kay, H. E. (1965) How many cell generations? *Lancet* **II,** 418–419.
2. Lajtha, L. G. (1979) Stem cell concepts. *Differentiation* **14,** 23–34.
3. Rosendaal, M., Hodgson, G. S., and Bradley, T. R. (1979) Organisation of haemopoietic stem cells: the generation-age hypothesis. *Cell Tissue Kinet.* **12,** 17–29.
4. Botnick, L. E., Hannon, E. C., and Hellman, S. (1979) Nature of the hemopoietic stem cell compartment and its proliferative potential. *Blood Cells* **5,** 195–210.
5. Potten, C. S. and Loeffler, M. (1990) Stem cells: attributes, cycles, spirals, pitfalls and uncertainties. Lessons for and from the crypt. *Development* **110,** 1001–1020.
6. Clarkson, B. D. (1974) The survival value of the dormant state in neoplastic and normal cell populations, in *Control of Proliferation in Animal Cells* (Clarkson, B. and Baserga, R., eds.), Cold Spring Harbor Laboratory, Cold Spring Harbor, NY, pp. 945–972.
7. Pietrzyk, M. E., Priestley, G. V., and Wolf, N. S. (1985) Normal cycling patterns of hematopoietic stem cell subpopulations: an assay using long term in vivo BrdU infusion. *Blood* **66,** 1460–1462.
8. Willis, M. C., Hicke, B. J., Uhlenbeck, O. C., Cech, T. R., and Koch, T. H. (1993) Photocrosslinking of 5–Iodouracil-substituted RNA and DNA to proteins. *Science* **262,** 1255–1257.
9. Kriss, J. P. and Revesz, L. (1962) The distribution and fate of bromodeoxyuridine and bromodeoxycytidine in the mouse and rat. *Cancer Res.* **22,** 254–265.
10. Tice, R. R., Schneider, E. L., and Rary, J. M. (1976) The utilization of bromodeoxyuridine incorporation into DNA for the analysis of cellular kinetics. *Exp. Cell Res.* **102,** 232–236.
11. Hagan, M. P. and MacVittie, T. J. (1981) CFUs kinetics observed in vivo by bromodeoxyuridine and near-UV light treatment. *Exp. Hematol.* **9,** 123–128.
12. Forster, I. and Rajewsky, K. (1990) The bulk of the peripheral B-cell pool in mice is stable and not rapidly renewed from the bone marrow. *Proc. Natl. Acad. Sci. USA* **87,** 4781–4784.
13. Gratzner, H. G. (1982) Monoclonal antibody to 5–bromo- and 5–iododeoxyuridine: a new reagent for detection of DNA replication. *Science* **218,** 474–475.
14. Gratzner, H. G. and Leif, R.C. (1981) An immunofluorescence method for monitoring DNA synthesis by flow cytometry. *Cytometry* **1,** 385–389.
15. Dolbeare, F., Gratzner, H. G., Pallavicini, M. G., and Gray, J. W. (1983) Flow cytometric measurement of total DNA content and incorporated bromodeoxyuridine. *Proc. Natl. Acad. Sci. USA* **80,** 5573–5577.
16. Lin, P. and Allison, D. C. (1993) Measurement of DNA content and of tritiated

thymidine and bromodeoxyuridine incorporation by the same cells. *J. Histochem. Cytochem.* **41**, 1435–1439.

17. Patt, H. M., Maloney, M. A., and Lamela, R. A. (1980) Hematopoietic stem cell proliferative behaviour as revealed by bromodeoxyuridine labeling. *Exp. Hematol.* **8**, 1075–1079.

18. Bradford, G. B., Williams, B., Rossi, R., and Bertoncello, I. (1996) Quiescence, cycling and turnover in the primitive hematopoietic stem cell compartment. *Exp. Hematol.* **25**, 445–453.

19. Cheshier, S. H., Morrison, S.J., Liao, X., and Weissman, I. L. (1999) In vivo proliferation and cell cycle kinetics of long-term self-renewing hematopoietic stem cells. *Proc. Natl. Acad. Sci. USA* **96**, 3120–3125.

20. Staats, J. (1966) The Laboratory Mouse, in *Biology of the Laboratory Mouse,* 2nd ed., (Green, E. L., ed.), McGraw-Hill, Inc., New York, NY, pp. 1–9.

21. Russell, E. S. and Bernstein, S. E. (1966) Blood and blood formation, in *Biology of the Laboratory Mouse,* 2nd ed., (Green, E. L., ed.), McGraw-Hill, Inc., New York, NY, pp. 351–372.

22. Yuhas, J. M. and Storer, J. B. (1969) On mouse strain differences in radiation resistance: hematopoietic death and the endogenous colony-forming unit. *Radiat. Res.* **39**, 608–622.

23. Roberts, A. W., Foote, S., Alexander, W. S., Scott, C., Robb, L., and Metcalf, D. (1997) Genetic influences determining progenitor cell mobilization and leukocytosis induced by granulocyte colony-stimulating factor. *Blood* **89**, 2736–2744.

24. Müller-Sieburg, C. E. and Riblet, R. (1996) Genetic control of the frequency of hematopoietic stem cells in mice: mapping of a candidate locus to chromosome 1. *J. Exp. Med.* **183**, 1141–1150.

25. de Haan, G. and Van Zant, G. (1997) Intrinsic and extrinsic control of hemopoietic stem cell numbers: mapping of a stem cell gene. *J. Exp. Med.* **186**, 529–536.

26. Harris, I. (1997) Variables in animal based research: Part 1. Phenotypic variability in experimental animals. (Facts Sheet). *ANZCCART News* **10(3)**, Insert 1–7.

27. Reilly, J. (1998) Variables in animal based research: Part 2. Variability associated with experimental conditions and techniques. (Facts Sheet). *ANZCCART News* **11(1)**, Insert 1–12.

28. Schneider, E. L., Sternberg, H., and Tice, R. R. (1977) In vivo analysis of cellular replication. *Proc. Natl. Acad. Sci. USA* **74**, 2041–2044.

29. Dexter, T. M., Garland, J., Scott, D., Scolnick, E., and Metcalf, D. (1980) Growth of factor-dependent hemopoietic precursor cell lines. *J. Exp. Med.* **152**, 1036–1047.

30. Latt, S. A., George, Y. S., and Gray, J. W. (1977) Flow cytometric analysis of bromodeoxyuridine-substituted cells stained with 33258 Hoechst. *J. Histochem. Cytochem.* **25**, 927–934.

31. Matsuoka, K., Nomura, K., and Hoshino, T. (1990) Mutagenic effects of brief exposure to bromodeoxyuridine on mouse FN3A cells. *Cell Tissue Kinet.* **23**, 495–503.

32. Ensminger, W. D., Walker, S. C., Stetson, P. L., Wagner, J. G., Knol, J. A.,

Lawrence, T. S., et al. (1994) Clinical pharmacology of hepatic arterial infusions of 5–bromo-2'-deoxyuridine. *Cancer Res.* **54,** 2121–2124.

33. Smith, D. E., Brenner, D. E., Knutsen, C. A., Deremer, S. J., Terrio, P. A., Johnson, N. J., et al. (1993) Mutual kinetic interaction between 5–fluorouracil and bromodeoxyuridine or iododeoxyuridine in dogs. *Drug Metab. Dispos.* **21,** 277–283.

34. Rajewsky, K. (1993) B-cell lifespans in the mouse—why to debate what? *Immunol. Today* **14,** p. 41.

35. Gray, J. W., Dolbeare, F., and Pallavicini, M. G. (1990) Quantitative cell-cycle analysis, in *Flow Cytometry and Sorting*, 2nd ed., (Melamed, M. R., Lindmo, T., and Mendelsohn, M. L., eds.), Wiley-Liss, Inc., New York, NY, pp. 445–467.

36. Dolbeare, F., Beisker, W., Pallavicini, M. G., Vanderlaan, M., and Gray, J. W. (1985) Cytochemistry for bromodeoxyuridine/DNA analysis: stoichiometry and sensitivity. *Cytometry* **6,** 521–530.

37. Micklem, H. S., Lennon, J. E., Ansell, J. D., and Gray, R. A. (1987) Numbers and dispersion of repopulating hematopoietic cell clones in radiation chimeras as functions of injected cell dose. *Exp. Hematol.* **15,** 251–257.

6

Isolation and Characterization of Primitive Hematopoietic Cells Based on Their Position in the Cell Cycle

Edward F. Srour and Craig T. Jordan

1. Introduction

Hematopoietic progenitor and stem cells are believed to lie dormant within the adult bone marrow microenvironment in a state characterized by both mitotic and metabolic quiescence. This state of cell-cycle quiescence has been the focus or target of many studies aimed at identifying cells with such mitotic properties for their eventual isolation and characterization. On the other hand, knowledge of the type, frequency, and primitive status of dividing cells in patients with malignant hematopoietic diseases is very important for the hematologist designing therapies aimed at targeting cycling cancer cells with cell-cycle-specific chemotherapuetic drugs that can spare noncycling normal hematopoietic stem cells (HSC).

The use of cell-cycle analysis in the field of experimental hematology has been an important tool in the study of HSC biology. However, the invasive nature of cell-cycle analysis has made it difficult to isolate viable candidate HSC based on their position in the cell cycle. It has not been possible to simultaneously investigate the functional properties and cell-cycle status of the same group of putative stem cells. Instead, cell-cycle analysis and assessment of hematopoietic potential of primitive progenitor cells have usually been conducted separately rather than concurrently. In addition, little attention has been given to differences between the G0 and G1 phases of the cell cycle (*see* **Subheading 1.1.**). Thus, cells determined by simple DNA staining (e.g., with propidium iodide [PI]) to belong to the G0/G1 phases of the cell cycle have

From: *Methods in Molecular Medicine, vol. 63: Hematopoietic Stem Cell Protocols*
Edited by: C. A. Klug and C. T. Jordan © Humana Press Inc., Totowa, NJ

been considered quiescent. Yet over the last few years, it has become increasingly evident that cells in either of these two phases of the cell cycle are functionally different. Perhaps the major difference between these two phases of the cell cycle is that only when cells are in G1 can they respond to extracellular signals and commit to progressing through G1 and ultimately cell division, or retreating away from the cycle and into a mitotically quiescent state such as G0 *(1)*. It is also within G1—specifically late G1—that the first restriction point controlling the transition of cells from G1 into S is located *(2)*. It is therefore critical that we are able to distinguish between these two stages of the cell cycle in order to separate cells committed to progression through the cell cycle from those withdrawn from cycling.

1.1. Cellular Changes During Cell Cycle Progression

As cells cycle, they undergo important changes essential for successful completion of cell division and production of two intact and complete daughter cells. Thus, a proliferating cell must duplicate its complement of DNA through a process involving DNA synthesis (S) to provide a full copy of its genetic material to each progeny cell during mitosis (M). These "phases" of the cell cycle, based on the observations of Howard and Pelc *(3)*, were interspersed by "gaps" characterized by a lack of DNA activity *(4)*. One such gap was observed to take place between S and M called G2, and another much longer gap was noted between the end of mitosis and the onset of a new cycle in the resulting daughter cells (G1). In 1963, Lajtha *(5)* coined the term G0 to describe another "gap" phase of the cell cycle to describe dormant hepatic cells responding to liver insult. Consequently, the G0 phase of the cell cycle was identified in most cells as a phase during which cells exit from cycle in response to an environmental stimulus, or caused by a genetic program, and cease to divide. The length of stay in G0, its relationship to G1, and how quickly cells exit G0 to begin active cell-cycle progression vary depending on the cell type, the environment, and growth stimuli received by cells. Any disturbance of cell-cycle progression or DNA replication is clearly detrimental—if not fatal—to cells. This is why nature devised an elaborate cell-cycle regulatory network, which controls both progression of cells through the cell cycle and DNA replication *(6–8)*.

The introduction of flow cytometry *(9,10)* sparked an interest in the automated detection of cancer cells that contained an elevated amount of DNA, and led to the rapid development of procedures capable of detecting and measuring the amount of cellular DNA. Various dyes which specifically stain cellular DNA were used over the years, as single agents, to generate a static "snapshot" of DNA content of individual cells. More sophisticated procedures were later introduced by several researchers who correlated the level of cellular DNA with other cell components such as mitochondria *(11–14)*, nuclear proteins *(15)* and RNA *(16,17)*. However, many of these procedures were unsuitable for the recovery of viable cells, because permeabilization was required or toxicity of one dye or another was encountered. With one such approach, Darzynkiewicz et al. *(18,19)*, using the metachromatic dye acridine orange, examined the amount of cellular RNA relative to that of DNA during the cell cycle and were able to identify subclasses of the G1 phase which they identified as G1A and G1B *(20)*. Cells containing RNA levels similar to those in early S were categorized as G1B cells, and those with lower RNA levels belonged to the G1A subcompartment of G1 *(18,19)*. These authors went on to show that when 3T3 cells are deprived of nutrients and are growth-arrested by contact inhibition, they enter a cell-cycle phase characterized by an RNA content lower than that seen in G1A cells *(21)*. Cells in this deep state of "quiescence" were labeled G1Q cells. G1Q cells differed from G1A cells in that they had very low metabolic activity and slow cell-cycle kinetics as assessed by their RNA content and the rate at which they progressed toward S phase, respectively. Although flow-cytometric analysis of the cell cycle using this approach or other staining regimens involving simultaneous DNA and RNA staining can be very informative, these procedures require cell fixation prior to staining or are extremely toxic, therefore prohibiting the isolation of viable cells in different phases of the cell cycle.

In 1981 Shapiro et al. *(16)* described a double DNA/RNA staining protocol with the aim of identifying cells in different phases of the cell cycle and the eventual isolation of viable and functional cells. To that end, Hoechst 33342 (Hst) was used to stain DNA and pyronin Y (PY) was used to stain RNA. Hst is a relatively nontoxic, water soluble, cell-permeable bisbenzimide dye that specifically binds to the minor groove of double-stranded DNA. Hst can be excited with ultraviolet (UV) light (350 nm), and has a large Stokes shift fluorescing at 460 nm. Pyronin Y is a nucleic acid dye that has affinity to both DNA and RNA, and can also stain mitochondrial membranes *(17,22)*. However, when cells are first stained with Hst, pyronin Y is prohibited from staining DNA, and at moderate concentrations will predominantly stain RNA rather than mitochondrial membranes. The combination of Hst and PY, as used by Shapiro et al. *(16)* proved to be toxic to the cells they stained with these dyes at the concentration used in their studies so that although quantitation of DNA and RNA was successful, viable cells could not be recovered. This led several researchers to search for a different dye in order to identify quiescent or metabolically inactive cells. Rhodamine 123 was successfully used *(12,13)* to isolate hematopoietic stem and progenitor cells with diminished mitochondrial activity.

1.2. Sorting of Cells in Different Phases of the Cell Cycle

Several years ago, we revisited the Hst and PY staining described by Shapiro and colleagues (16) and investigated whether this DNA/RNA staining could be applied to human hematopoietic progenitor cells (23). A readjusted PY concentration (see below) was capable of staining cellular RNA without any toxicity to human CD34+ cells (23). Furthermore, when cells were treated with RNase prior to staining with PY, the level of PY staining was diminished, indicating that PY was specifically staining RNA and not mitochondrial membranes (23). Whether successful staining of viable human CD34+ cells with PY is related to the "resistance" of these cells to the toxic effects of this dye relative to other cell types has not been investigated. This might be a plausible explanation, since our experience with this dye combination with murine cells is less favorable (E.F. Srour, unpublished observations). Hst and PY have been used in our laboratory to examine the functional capacity of human CD34+ cells in G0 both in vitro (24,25) and in vivo (26,26a).

The progression of cells through the cell cycle is a complex process requiring the interaction of a large number of regulatory molecules at different checkpoints throughout the cycle. The elaborate network of regulatory molecules ensures the orderly transition of cells from one phase of the cell cycle into another and the faithful replication of cellular DNA. To maintain proper regulation of cell-cycle progression, synthesis, activation, and degradation of most regulatory molecules is turned on or off in a cell-cycle phase-associated manner (2,27,28). The key molecules regulating cell-cycle progression and transition of dividing cells through the different checkpoints along the cell cycle are cyclins, cyclin-dependent kinases (Cdk), and Cdk inhibitors. The interaction of these molecules at different stages of the cell cycle and how they regulate cell division are not the focus of this chapter. This article presents a concise summary of the timing of appearance of these molecules within dividing cells in order to prepare for their cell-cycle-related detection by flow cytometric analysis.

Although nine types of cyclins have been described thus far, cyclins A, B, D, and E are the most prominent cell-cycle regulators. Expression of these cyclins is cyclic, and can therefore be associated with specific phases of the cell cycle. Members of the cyclin D family (D1, D2, and D3) are cell-type or tissue-specific, but are all expressed (each in its respective cell-type) as cells exit from G0 and in early G1. Cyclin E is expressed periodically in late G1 and into early S, while cyclin A begins to accumulate in mid S and into G2+M. Cyclin B accumulates in late S and reaches maximal levels in M (See Darzynkiewicz et al. (28) for further details). Through cell-cycle progression, these cyclins associate with specific Cdks which require the activity of Cdk-activating kinases (CAK) to acquire the catalytic activity essential for the formation of holoenzymes that phosphorylate key cell-cycle regulatory proteins. This phase-associated expression of cyclins prompted the proposal that expression of cyclin D, followed by the emergence of cyclin E, be considered as a molecular marker to delineate between cells in G0 and G1 *(28)*. Such a proposal may apply to normal cells only when expression of cyclins is scheduled, whereas expression of these molecules in cancerous cells is usually unscheduled and may not be cell-cycle phase-specific. Different cyclins bind to and activate different Cdks during the cell cycle. D type cyclins bind to Cdk4 and Cdk6, and are responsible for the phosphorylation of the retinoblastoma (RB) protein. Phosphorylated RB releases transcription factors that activate the DNA replication machinery, and therefore propels cells through the G1 checkpoint and into S. Cyclin E associates with Cdk2, while cyclin A associates with both Cdk2 and Cdk1 (previously identified as CDC2). Cyclin B1 associates with Cdk1. Cdk enzymatic activity can be inhibited by specific inhibitors which result in cell-cycle arrest. The most potent Cdk inhibitors are p21 and p27. p21-inhibitory activity is most potent when it is present as a single molecule associated with a cyclin-Cdk complex. The inhibitory activity of p21 decreases as the ratio of p21 to cyclin-Cdk complexes increases *(29)*. p27, also known as Kip1, inhibits the catalytic activity of Cdks in different cyclin-Cdk complexes including D-type cyclins-Cdk4 and cyclin E-Cdk2 complexes. In general, p27 levels are high in growth-arrested cells (in G0), and begin to diminish as cells begin to respond to mitogenic or growth-factor stimulation. All of these regulatory molecules can be detected flow-cytometrically, as described in **Subheading 2.2.**

2. Materials

2.1. Hoechst/Pyronin Sorting

Staining of cells with Hst and PY is simple. The procedure requires approx 2 h from the beginning of the staining procedure until cells are ready for analysis or cell sorting. Since cells become photosensitive when stained with Hst and PY, it is advisable to shield the cells during staining and sorting, and immediately after sorting from direct light.

1. Hst (Molecular Probes).
2. PY (Polysciences).
3. Verapamil (Sigma) (*see* **Note 4** for further details on reagents and vendors).
4. Hoechst buffer (Wolf et al.) *(30)*: Hank's Balanced Salt Solution (HBSS), 20 mM HEPES, 1 g/L glucose, 10% fetal calf serum (FCS), pH 7.2. Hst buffer can be prepared and stored for up to 6 wk at 4°C. Before staining, a fraction of this

buffer can be prepared with verapamil at 50–100 μM to be used within 24 h. Verapamil should be present in the Hst buffer for all subsequent staining and sorting steps.

5. Hst intermediate and working solutions: In order to prepare a working solution of Hst, the stock solution (*see* **step 6**) must be diluted extensively in Hst buffer. When diluted in PBS, Hst precipitates at concentrations of >30 μM. However, this process is not instantaneous, and therefore allows for the quick preparation of an intermediate solution (of a concentration >30 μM) followed by the final dilution into a working solution. Both the intermediate and working solutions should be prepared fresh for every application, kept in the dark, and used within a few hours of preparation. The two solutions are prepared as such:
   a. Intermediate solution: 20 μL of stock solution in 1.98 mL of Hst buffer.
   b. Working solution: 50 μL of intermediate solution in 4.95 mL of Hst buffer.
   These dilutions will result in a final concentration of 1 μg Hst per mL, which is equivalent to 1.6 μM.

6. PY working solution: PY is used for the second step of staining while the cells are still suspended in the Hst working solution (*see* **Subheading 3.**). Therefore, addition of a certain volume of the PY working solution to the cell suspension constitutes a dilution step which can be included in the dilution scheme of this dye.
   a. Working solution: Add 10 μL of the 10 mg/mL stock solution to 490 mL Hst buffer.
   Including the final dilution step (*see* below) this will result in a final concentration of 1 mg/mL PY, which is equivalent to 3.3 μM.

2.2. Analysis of Cell-Cycle Regulatory Molecules

A commercial source providing high-quality reagents for the staining of cell-cycle regulatory molecules is essential for successful flow-cytometric detection of these markers. Cross-reactivity of antibodies between different classes of cyclins is possible, and care should be taken in selecting minimally cross-reacting reagents. In our experience, reagents obtained through Pharmingen (10975 Torreyana Road, San Diego, CA 92121; Tel: 619-812-8800) are of high quality and specificity. Some common anti-human reagents and the names of the clones from which they are derived and the isotype of monoclonal antibodies (MAbs) obtained from Pharmingen are listed in **Table 1**.

2.3. Cell-Cycle Analysis Using Combined Surface, Intracellular, and DNA Labeling

1. Antibodies:
   CD38-Phycoerythrin (PE) (Becton Dickinson).
   CD34-Allophycocyanin (APC) (Becton Dickinson).
   Ki-67-Fluorescein isothiocyanate (FITC) (Coulter, MIB-1 clone).
   IgG-FITC isotype control (Becton Dickinson).

Table 1
Clones and Isotypes of Monoclonal Antibodies Recognizing
Key Molecules in Cell Cycle Regulation

	Protein	Clone	Isotype
Monoclonal antibody (MAb)			
	Cyclin D	G124–259[a]	Mouse IgG$_1$
	Cyclin E	HE12	Mouse IgG$_1$
	Cyclin A	BF683	Mouse IgE
	Cyclin B1	GNS-1	Mouse IgG$_1$
	P21	SX118	Mouse IgG$_1$
	P27	G173–524	Mouse IgG$_1$
	Cdk1	A-17	Mouse IgG$_{2a}$
	Cdk2	G120–72	Mouse IgM
	RB (underphosphorylated)	G99–549	Mouse IgG$_1$
	RB (phosphorylated)	G99–73	Mouse IgG$_1$
Polyclonal Ab			
	Cdk4		
	Cdk6		

[a] Clone G124–259 reacts with an epitope common among cyclins D1, D2, and D3, thus providing detection of any of the three D-type cyclins without the need to investigate the tissue-specific reagent for the cell type in question.

2. 16% Formaldehyde (ultrapure, EM grade from Polysciences, catalog #18814).
3. Triton-X-100 (Sigma).
4. 7-Aminoactinomycin D (7-AAD, Molecular Probes).
5. Phosphate-buffered saline (PBS): calcium- and magnesium-free tissue-culture grade (Gibco/BRL).
6. Staining buffer (SB): PBS with 1% albumin or serum (any source of human or bovine reagent is acceptable).
7. 2X permeabilization solution: PBS with 0.2% Triton-X-100.
8. 2X DNA staining solution: staining buffer with 1.0 µg/mL 7-AAD (made fresh on the day of analysis).

3. Methods

3.1. Sorting of Purified Populations Using the Hoechst/Pyronin Method

Cells to be stained with Hst and PY must first be selected for the final desired surface phenotype to ensure that all cells sorted on the basis of their cell-cycle status are homogeneous in their phenotypic makeup. When this staining procedure is applied to CD34+ cells, several options are available. Cells purified with any selection procedure to excess of 95% purity do not need to be selected further. A cell preparation consisting of CD34+ cells at less than 95% purity (or less than any other acceptable level of purity) must first be sorted on the basis of CD34 expression (or other cell-surface determinants, *see* **Subheading 3.2.**). Sorted cells can then be stained with Hst and PY for further selection.

The excitation and emission properties of Hst and PY allow for the use of Fluorescein-5-isothiocyanate (FITC) as a surface marker along with these two dyes and possibly for other fluorochromes if excitation and detection of additional fluorochromes is possible with a given instrument configuration. Our experience is that the use of FITC along with Hst and PY allows for the selection of cells in different phases of the cell cycle after gating on FITC-positive events, which are then analyzed for their Hst and PY fluorescence distribution. This approach circumvents the need for prior sorting of CD34+ cells that are not of high or acceptable purity levels. The staining protocol for Hst and PY is described for pure populations of cells, and a modification for staining with Hst, PY, and a surface marker is presented.

1. Place cells to be stained in a 15-mL snap-cap tube.
2. Prepare two control tubes, each with 10 to 20×10^3 cells for single color controls (more cells can be used if available).
3. Wash cells in all three tubes with Hst buffer containing verapamil.
4. Decant supernatant and blot the mouth of the tubes dry on a sterile gauze.
5. Add 0.5 mL of Hst buffer to the PY control tube.
6. Add 0.5 mL of the Hst working solution to the Hst control tube.
7. Add 1.5 mL of the Hst working solution to the sort tube. In general, 1.5 mL of the Hst working solution can be used to stain up to 5×10^6 cells. For larger numbers of cells, the volume can be doubled to 3 mL. For cell numbers in excess of 25×10^6, the volume can be increased to 4.5 mL.
8. Vortex all three tubes gently, and incubate in a 37°C water bath in the dark for 45 min. Vortex gently every 15 min.
9. At the end of the 45-min incubation period, add 2.5 μL of the PY working solution to the PY control tube and 7.5 μL (or equivalent volume) to the sort tube. Add 2.5 μL Hst buffer to the Hst control tube. Vortex all three tubes and incubate in a 37°C water bath in the dark for 45 min. Vortex gently every 15 min.
10. After the second incubation period, add 2–3 mL of Hst buffer to each tube and centrifuge. Decant the supernatant and resuspend the cell pellet in an appropriate volume of Hst buffer. These tubes are now ready for analysis and cell sorting.

3.2. Staining of Partially Purified Populations of Cells with Hst, Pyronin Y, and a Cell-Surface Marker

Partially purified cell populations (e.g., CD34+ cells) will yield non-CD34+ cells in specific phases of the cell cycle if stained and sorted based on their uptake of Hst and PY. Expression of CD34 can be incorporated into the sorting decisions if cells are first stained with Hst and PY, followed by staining with CD34. The following staining protocol can be used when a FITC-conjugated cell surface marker is needed (**Fig. 1**).

1. Stain the cells to be sorted with Hst and PY as described in **steps 1–9**. At the end of the second incubation period, fill all the staining tubes with ice-cold Hst buffer (with verapamil).
2. Pellet cells by centrifugation and decant the supernatant, leaving behind 50–100 μL of medium. Add up to 0.5 mL of Hst buffer to Hst and PY control tubes and leave on ice.
3. Add the required volume of FITC-conjugated test antibody to cells stained with Hst and PY, vortex, and incubate on ice for 15–20 min. Vortex once or twice during incubation. In the event that the test antibody used for this step is unconjugated, a second-step reagent can be used to develop the primary antibody with FITC.
4. At the end of the 15-min incubation period, wash the cells with cold Hst buffer, decant, and resuspend the cells in the appropriate volume of Hst buffer.

Several control tubes which are essential for adequate identification of background fluorescence and identification of positive events should be prepared for this procedure. These include:

1. Cells stained with Hst, PY, and FITC-conjugated isotype control to be used for establishing background FITC fluorescence.
2. Cells stained with the FITC-conjugated test antibody to be used only in adjusting the required level of compensation between green and red fluorescence. The PY control tube can be used for the reverse compensation.

A flow cytometer providing 50 mW of UV light at a wavelength of approx 350 nm is required for the excitation of Hst. Both PY and FITC can be excited by 100 mW of 488-nm light emitted from an argon laser. FITC is the easiest fluorochrome to be simultaneously used with Hst and PY to provide a third fluorescence signal. Optical filters required for the detection of forward and orthogonal (side) light scatter, and FITC signals are identical to those used for other applications. PY, which has a λ max 552 nm, can be detected through a 575 ± 13 nm dichroic filter, and Hst can be detected through a 424 ± 22 nm dichroic filter.

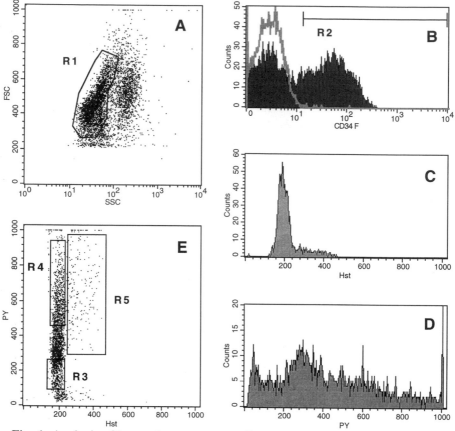

Fig. 1. Analysis of human bone marrow cells stained with FITC-conjugated CD34, Hst, and PY. Low-density bone-marrow cells were selected for CD34+ cells using the MACS system, and only one wash of the positive fraction attracted to the magnet was applied to recover a partially purified fraction of CD34+ cells. These cells were first stained with Hst and PY as described in **Subheading 3.1.**, then chilled, washed, and stained with FITC-conjugated CD34. (**A**) represents light-scatter distribution of selected low-density bone marrow cells. Gate R1 in (**A**) was established to contain "small" cells, where the majority of CD34+ cells are found. Histogram (**B**) shows the FITC-CD34 fluorescence of R1–gated events. The light-colored overlaid histogram represents background fluorescence of R1–gated events established with an isotype-matched FITC-conjugated control antibody. Events contained within R2 were considered CD34+ and were processed for further analysis. Events satisfying the selection criteria of gates R1 and R2 combined were then analyzed for their Hst (histogram **C**) and PY (histogram **D**) fluorescence distributions separately, or simultaneously (dot plot **E**). Dot plot E depicts a typical two-dimensional distribution of DNA (X axis) and RNA (Y axis) content of freshly isolated BM CD34+ cells with few cells in S and G2+M phases of the cell cycle (gate R5). The majority of BM CD34+ cells have 2 n DNA, and are therefore located within the traditional G0/G1 peak of a DNA histogram appearing in dot plot **E** as the vertical population to the left. PY distribution (along the Y axis) differentiates between cells with low RNA content (G0 cells contained within gate R3) and cells expressing higher levels of RNA as they progress through G1 (gate R4). Sort windows similar to those shown in dot plot **E** (R3, R4, and R5) are normally constructed for the isolation of G0, G1, or S/G2+M cells, respectively.

3.3. Flow-Cytometric Detection of Cell-Cycle Regulatory Molecules

Staining protocols for the visualization of cyclins, Cdks, and Cdk inhibitors are not universal. Since these molecules are predominantly in the nucleus (some are in both the nucleus and the cytoplasm), permeabilization of cells prior to staining is required. It is the permeabilization step which must be customized to enhance the detection of certain intracellular antigens. The most peculiar of the cyclins in terms of the fixative required for optimal detection are the D-type cyclins *(31)*. Whereas most cyclins, Cdks, and Cdk inhibitors can be adequately detected if cells are fixed and permeabilized with 80% ethanol at –20°C for 2 h or overnight, D-type cyclins are best detected if cells are fixed in 1% methanol-free formaldehyde in PBS for 15 min on ice *(31)*. Following this initial step, all molecules can be appropriately stained following a unified protocol (*see* below). Quantitation of cell-cycle regulatory molecules is most meaningful in the context of cell-cycle analysis, so that precise localization of different molecules in different phases of the cell cycle becomes possible. Thus, cells are usually stained with a DNA dye following staining with cell-cycle regulatory molecules.

1. Fix cells to be stained with D-type cyclins in a 1% methanol-free formaldehyde solution in PBS for 15 min at 4°C, then wash in cold PBS supplemented with 0.1% bovine serum albumin (BSA) (Wash Buffer).
2. Fix cells to be stained with other cyclins, Cdks, Cdk inhibitors, or RB overnight or up to 30 d in cold 75% ethanol at –20°C.
3. When ready to complete the staining procedure, wash cells with wash buffer once.
4. Resuspend cells in 1 mL of cold 0.25% solution of Triton-X-100 for 5 min at 4°C and rinse in wash buffer.
5. Incubate cells with appropriate Ab (anticyclins, Cdks, or Cdk inhibitors) for 30 min at room temperature and wash with wash buffer.
6. Incubate cells requiring a second-step Ab with appropriate fluorochrome-conjugated Ab for 30 min at room temperature and wash with wash buffer.
7. Resuspend all cells in 0.5 mL solution of 7-AAD at 5 µg/mL for at least 15 min before running on the flow cytometer for cell-cycle analysis. In most cases, propidium iodide (PI) can be substituted for 7-AAD.

3.4. Cell-Cycle Analysis Using Combined Surface, Intracellular, and DNA Labeling

For analytical studies in which viable cells are not required, there is an alternative protocol for the characterization of primitive hematopoietic cells that permits specific examination of the G0 to G1 transition event. This strategy has previously been termed Surface, Intracellular, and DNA (SID) labeling, and allows simultaneous analysis of cell-cycle activity in multiple subpopulations *(15)*. The method can be applied in the context of multiple fluorescence parameters (i.e., four- or five-color analysis), and because specific cellular subsets can be readily defined, it is not necessary to start with a highly purified population of stem cells. Rather, phenotypically defined primitive cells can be examined along with other more mature cells. This strategy has been useful for characterization of cells derived from human bone marrow, peripheral blood, and cord blood. Central to the method is labeling of the nuclear antigen Ki-67. The expression of this molecule has previously been shown to be closely associated with entry into cell cycle *(33,34)*. Thus, in conjunction with developmentally regulated markers such as CD34 and CD38, and a DNA dye, it is possible to analyze varying cycle stages for primitive subpopulations. The strategy may also be applicable to analysis of nonhuman stem cells; however, the Ki-67 antigen has not been well defined for other species, and preliminary tests should be performed to establish its utility as a cycle marker.

The protocol described in **steps 1–4** is for four-color labeling of hematopoietic cells, but the specific method employed will depend largely on the configuration of available flow cytometry equipment. The four-color strategy requires a two-laser instrument with lines at 488 and 633 nm. The technique can also be readily adapted to a five-color method, but requires the additional use of a UV laser. Although the method allows examination of minor subsets, it is usually not practical to perform detailed analysis of primitive cells in unfractionated tissues. Therefore, it is generally necessary to employ a pre-enrichment step for CD34+ cells before labeling samples for cycle analysis. Although any type of CD34+ cell immunoaffinity selection system is appropriate to enrich primitive cells (e.g., Miltenyi, Dynal, and StemSep), some types of magnetic beads can interfere with subsequent flow-cytometry procedures. This point should be clarified prior to using the procedure described below. For our studies, good results have been obtained using the Miltenyi MiniMACS or VarioMACS systems (detailed discussion of CD34 selection is presented in Chapter 3).

1. Suspend viable CD34-enriched cells in SB at a concentration of $1–5 \times 10^6$/mL and prepare 6 tubes (12×75 mm) with 0.5 mL of the cell suspension per tube. Add appropriate amounts of the surface antigen or control antibodies (as indicated in **Table 2**) and incubate on ice for 30 min. Wash cells once with SB.
2. Pellet the surface-labeled cells and resuspend in 0.5 mL of cold PBS. Add 33 µL of 16% formaldehyde for a final concentration of 1%. Incubate on ice for 30 min, then add an equal volume of 2X permeabilization solution and incubate for a further 15 minutes on ice.
3. Pellet the cells and resuspend in 0.5 mL of SB (it is not necessary to wash the

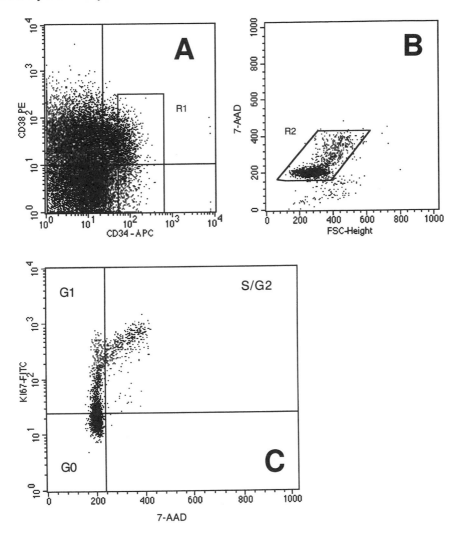

Fig. 2. Representative SID staining of Leukemic human BM cells.

cells before proceeding). Add appropriate amounts of the Ki-67 or control antibodies and incubate for 45 min at 4°C.

4. Wash cells once in SB and resuspend samples #1–3 in 0.5 mL SB. Resuspend samples #4–6 in 0.25 mL of staining buffer and add an equal volume of 2X DNA staining solution. Incubate cells at 4°C for 2 h to overnight. Proceed to flow cytometry.

The samples in tubes #1–4 provide standard single-color controls for background staining and compensation that are required for any type of flow

Table 2
Staining Protocol for Cell Surface Antigens and Cell Cycle Status

Tube	Step 1	Step 2	Step 3	Step 4
1	NA	Fix/Permeabilize	NA	NA
2	NA	Fix/Permeabilize	Ki-67–FITC	NA
3	CD38–PE	Fix/Permeabilize	FITC control	NA
4	NA	Fix/Permeabilize	NA	7–AAD
5	CD34–APC/CD38–PE	Fix/Permeabilize	FITC control	7–AAD
6	CD34–APC/CD38–PE	Fix/Permeabilize	Ki-67–FITC	7–AAD

NA = nothing added.

cytometry. Most aspects of the flow cytometry setup are standard; however, it is important to note that the DNA signal must be collected with the PMT in linear mode. To collect sample data, it is recommended that a gate first be set using a dot-plot of the surface-antigen staining. An example is shown in **Fig. 2A**, where the gate designated R1 encompasses the CD34+ subset of a primary leukemia sample. Next, use the R1 gate to visualize forward light scatter (FCS) vs DNA (7-AAD) staining on a second dot plot (**Fig. 2B**). On the FCS vs 7-AAD dot plot draw a second gate around the main population (*see* R2 gate). This allows the primary population to be defined and excludes the aggregates and debris that are commonly found in fixed samples. Finally, using both the surface antigen (R1) and FCS vs DNA (R2) gates together, display the Ki-67 (FITC) vs DNA (7-AAD) dot-plot (**Fig. 2C**). Cells that fall in the lower left quadrant are in G0; upper left quadrant is G1; and upper right quadrant is S and G2. At this stage, the sample from tube #5 becomes an important control. Tube #5 contains all the antibodies required for complete labeling, except for Ki-67 (substituted with the IgG-FITC isotype control). This allows one to set the gates described above and determine the background staining of CD34+ cells in the FITC channel. Once this level is established, the fully stained sample (tube #6) can be run, and the relative proportions of cells in G0, G1, or G2, S, and M phases can be established.

4. Notes

4.1. Hoechst/Pyronin Staining Method

1. The most important criterion in selecting a source for Hst and PY is the purity of the reagent. Both Hst and PY are inexpensive, and therefore the amount of reagent supplied by the vendor is not of practical concern. A very reliable source for Hst is Molecular Probes (Eugene, OR 97402–9165) which supplies Hst in

different quantities and forms including a 10 mg/mL solution (dissolved in water). This solution is the stock solution of Hst referred to in **Subheading 2.1.** and should be stored at 4°C in the dark. As for PY, the most reliable source of PY is probably Polysciences, which is located in Warrington, (400 Valley Road) PA 18976. Polysciences provides PY in 5-g quantities (Cat # 18614), which can be dissolved in water to prepare a 10 mg/mL stock solution. PY stock solution should also be stored in the dark at 4°C. Verapamil can be obtained from Sigma Chemical Company, P.O. Box 14508, St. Louis, MO. Verapamil is supplied in 1.0-g amounts of verapamil HCl (catalogue number V4629), and should be dissolved in DMSO prior to diluting it out in Hst buffer.

4.2. Surface, Intracellular, and DNA Method

2. The overall cell viability of the sample must be reasonably good (i.e., 85–90% or better). Samples with poor viability will yield false staining patterns.

3. Although the procedure can be used for any cell population, results tend to be somewhat better on samples that have been cultured. Therefore, the technique is particularly well-suited for in vitro time-course studies in which the induction of cycle activity is monitored.

4. In addition to its primary excitation by the 488-nm laser, 7-AAD can also be excited to some degree by the 633-nm laser. Therefore, it must be used at a low concentration when APC is to be used simultaneously. When used at a final concentration of 0.5 µg/mL, reasonably good DNA staining can be obtained with only a low background fluorescence in the APC channel. If the CV for DNA is poor, the 7-AAD concentration can be increased to at least 1.0 µg/mL. Less than 0.5 µg/mL gives poor DNA staining. Also, at higher concentrations, 7-AAD appears to partially quench phycoerythrin fluorescence.

5. The concentration of formaldehyde is important, with 0.4–0.5% yielding good CVs for DNA, and reasonably good antibody staining. Higher concentrations (i.e., 0.5–1.0%) will give somewhat better antibody staining, but progressively worse CVs.

6. Samples should be run at a low differential pressure to get the best DNA CV (i.e., standard procedure for DNA analysis).

7. 7-AAD is made as a 1.0 mg/mL stock in 50% ethanol (store at –20°C). The stock solution is not exceptionally stable, and should only be used for approx 2–3 mo. When the 7-AAD gets too old, the CV for the DNA staining deteriorates. Also, increased staining time tends to improve DNA staining. Thus, samples can be run after a few hours, but will generally look better after overnight 7-AAD staining.

8. Cell concentrations listed for fixation and staining are approximate values. It is unlikely that there is a lower limit for cell concentration, but going higher than described is probably not a good idea.

9. In some cases the post-fixation cells do not pellet well. It is not uncommon for the pellets to be diffuse or difficult to see.

10. To perform five-color SID staining, the following modifications can be employed: For surface-antigen staining, use CD38-APC (Becton Dickinson) and CD34-biotin (Coulter, Qbend-10 clone) with streptavidin-Red 613 (Gibco/BRL). For Ki-67 labeling, use the PE conjugated reagent from Dako. For DNA labeling, use 4,6-Diamidino-2-phenylindole (DAPI, Molecular Probes) in place of 7-AAD (final concentration of 2.0–10 µmol). This configuration leaves the FITC channel available for a reagent of the investigator's choice. Of course, a FITC-conjugated antibody is appropriate, and we have also had good results using this channel to detect expression of the green fluorescent protein (GFP).

11. The relatedness of the expression of Ki-67 to the mitotic status of any cell allows for the use of the MIB-1 antibody to verify the cell-cycle position of cells isolated by the dual DNA/RNA sorting technique described in **Subheading 3.1.** *(26)*. In this regard, sorted cells determined by their staining pattern with Hst and PY to be in G0, G1, or S/G2+M can be stained as described in **Subheading 3.4.** with Ki-67. Analysis of stained cells should reveal a distinct pattern of expression of Ki-67 by these cell fractions. Cells in G0 should be predominantly negative for the expression of Ki-67 because their quiescent nature. As cells enter into active phases of cell cycle and progress into G1, expression of Ki-67 is elevated so that cells isolated in G1 or S/G2+M should be mainly positive for the expression of Ki-67. The use of this technique to verify the cell-cycle status of sorted cells can also be used to examine the effectiveness and accuracy of the chosen sort windows in defining cells in G0. Expression of Ki-67 on a large fraction of cells sorted as G0 cells is in most cases indicative of a liberal sorting window, which most likely allows for the separation of cells in early G1. Although the construction of a sort window for cells in G0 is empirical, monitoring of isolated cells with Ki-67 provides a vehicle for future adjustments of selection criteria.

For this particular analysis, the settings used on a FACStar plus were:

Table 3
Potential Instrument Settings Suitable for the Detection of FITC, Hst, and PY on a FACStar Plus Flow Cytometer

Parameter	Signal	Detector	Voltage	AmpGain
P1	Light scatter	FSC	—	1
P2	Light scatter	SSC	400	Log
P3	CD34 FITC	FL1	600	Log
P4	PY	FL2	800	1
P6	Hst	FL4	410	1

Compensation applied between FL1 and FL2 was: FL1 − 0.8% FL2 and FL2 − 17.2% FL1.

References

1. Sherr, C. J. (1996) Cancer cell cycles. *Science* **274,** 1672–1677.
2. Elledge, S. J. (1996) Cell cycle checkpoints: preventing an identity crisis. *Science* **274,** 1664–1672.
3. Howard, A. and Pelc, S. R. (1953) Synthesis of deoxyribonucleic acid in normal and irradiated cells and its relation to chromosomal breakage. *Heredity* **6,** 261–273.
4. Puck, T. T. and Steffen, J. (1963) Life cycle analysis of mamalian cells. Part I. *Biophys. J.* **3,** 379–397.
5. Lajtha, L. G. (1963) On the concept of the cell cycle. *J. Cell. Comp. Physiol.* **62,** 143–149.
6. Stillman, B. (1996) Cell cycle control of DNA replication. *Science* **274,** 1659–1664.
7. Grafi. G. (1998) Cell cycle regulation of DNA replication: the endoreduplication perspective. *Exp. Cell Res.* **244,** 372–378.
8. Schafer, K.A. (1998) The cell cycle: a review. *Vet. Pathol.* **35,** 461–478.
9. Hulett, H. R., Bonner, W. A., Barret, J., and Herzenberg, L. A. (1969) Cell sorting: automated separation of mamalian cells as a function of intracellular fluorescence. *Science* **166,** 747–749.
10. VanDilla, M. A., Trujillo, T. T., Mullaney, P. F., and Coulter, J. R. (1969) Cell microfluorometry: a method for rapid fluorescence measurements. *Science* **169,** 1213–1214.
11. Johnson, L. V., Walsh, M. L., and Chen, L. B. (1980) Localization of mitochondria in living cells with rhodamine 123. *Proc. Natl. Acad. Sci. USA* **77,** 990–994.
12. Bertoncello, I., Hodgson, G. S., and Bradley, T. R. (1985) Multiparameter analysis of transplantable hematopoietic stem cells. I. The separation and enrichment of stem cells homing to marrow and spleen on the basis of rhodamine 123 fluorescence. *Exp. Hematol.* **13,** 999–1006.
13. Visser, J. W. M. and deVries, P. (1988) Isolation of spleen-colony forming cells (CFU-S) using wheat germ agglutinin and rhodamine 123 labeling. *Blood Cells* **14,** 369–384.
14. Darzynkiewicz, Z., Traganos, F., Staiano-Coico, L., Kapuscinski, J., and Melamed, M. R. (1982) Interactions of rhodamine 123 with living cells studied by flow cytometry. *Cancer Research* **42.**
15. Jordan, C. T., Yamasaki, G., and Minamoto, D. (1996) High-resolution cell cycle analysis of defined phenotypic subsets within primitive human hematopoietic cell populations. *Exp. Hematol.* **2,** 1347–1352.
16. Shapiro, H. M. (1981) Flow cytometric estimation of DNA and RNA content in intact cells stained with Hoechst 33342 and Pyronin Y. *Cytometry* **2,** 143–151.
17. Darzynkiewicz, Z., Kapuscinski, J., Traganos, F., and Crissman, H. A. (1987) Application of pyronin Y (G) in cytochemistry of nucleic acids. *Cytometry* **8,** 138–145.
18. Darzynkiewicz, Z., Evenson, L., Staiano-Coico, L., Sharpless, T., and Melamed, M. (1979) Relationship between RNA content and progression of lymphocytes through S-phase of cell cycle. *Proc. Natl. Acad. Sci. USA* **76,** 358–365.

19. Darzynkiewicz, Z., Traganos, F., and Melamed, R. M. (1980) New cycle compartments identified by multiparameter flow cytometry. *Cytometry* **1**, 98–105.
20. Darzynkiewicz, Z., Evenson, D. P., Staiano-Coico, L., Sharpless, T., and Melamed, M. R. (1979) Correlation between cell cycle duration and RNA content. *J. Cell. Physiol.* **100**, 425–438.
21. Darzynkiewicz, Z., Sharpless, T., Staiano-Coico, L., and Melamed, M. R. (1980) Subcompartments of the G1 phase of cell cycle detected by flow cytometry. *Proc. Natl. Acad. Sci. USA* **77**, 6696–6700.
22. Cowden, R. R. and Curtis S. K. Supravital experiments with pyronin Y, a fluorochrome of mitochondria and nucleic acids. *Histochemistry* **77**.
23. Ladd, A. C., Pyatt, R., Gothot, A., Rice, S., McMahel, J., Traycoff, C. M., and Srour, E. F. (1997) Orderly process of sequential cytokine stimulation is required for activation and maximal proliferation of primitive human bone marrow CD34+ hematopoietic progenitor cells residing in G0. *Blood* **90**, 658–668.
24. Gothot, A., Pyatt, R., McMahel, J., Rice, S., and Srour, E. F. (1997) Functional heterogeneity of human CD34+ cells isolated in subcompartments of the G0/G1 phase of the cell cycle. *Blood* **90**, 4384–4393.
25. Gothot, A., Pyat,t R., McMahel, J., Rice, S., and Srour, E. F. (1998) Assessment of proliferative and colony-forming capacity after successive in vitro divisions of single human CD34+ cells initially isolated in G0. *Exp. Hematol.* **26**, 562–570.
26. Gothot, A., van der Loo, J. C. M., Clapp, D. W., and Srour, E. F. Cell cycle-related changes in repopulating capacity of human mobilized peripheral blood CD34+ cells in non-obese diabetic/severe combined immune-deficient mice. *Blood* **92**, 2641–2649.
26a.Wilpshaar, J., Falkenburg, J. H. F., Tong, X., Noort, W. A., Breese, R., et al. (2000) Similar repopulating capacity of mitotically active and resting umbilical cord blood CD34+ cells in NOD/SCID mice. *Blood* **96**, 2100–2107.
27. Hartwell, L. H. and Kastan, M. B. (1994) Cell cycle control and cancer. *Science* **266**, 1821–1823.
28. Darzynkiewicz, Z., Gong, J., Juan, G., Ardelt, B., and Traganos, F. (1996) Cytometry of cyclin proteins. *Cytometry* **25**, 1–13.
29. Sherr, C. J. and Roberts, J. M. (1995) Inhibitors of mammalian G1 cyclin-dependent kinases. *Genes Dev.* **9**, 1149–1163.
30. Wolf, N. S., Kone, A., Priestley, G. V., and Bartelmez, S. H. (1993) In vivo and in vitro characterization of long-term repopulating primitive hematopoietic cells isolated by sequential Hoechst 33342–rhodamine 123 FACS selection. *Exp. Hematol.* **21**, 614–622.
31. Gong. J., Traganos, F., and Darzynkiewicz, Z. (1995) Threshold expression of cyclin E but not D type cyclins characterizes normal and tumour cells entering S phase. *Cell Prolif.* **28**, 337–346.
32. Neering, S. J., Hardy, S. F., Minamoto, D., Kaye Spratt, S., and Jordan, C. T. (1996) Transduction of primitive human hematopoietic cells with recombinant adenovirus vectors. *Blood* **88**, 1147–1155.
33. Gerdes. J., Lemke, H., Baisch, H., Wacker, H. H., Schwab, U., and Stein, H.

(1984) Cell cycle analysis of a cell proliferation-associated human nuclear antigen defined by the monoclonal antibody Ki-67. *J. Immunol.* **133,** 1710–1715.

34. Schluter, C., Duchrow, M., Wohlenberg, C., Becker, M. H., Key, G., Flad, H. D., and Gerdes, J. (1993) The cell proliferation-associated antigen of antibody Ki-67: a large, ubiquitous nuclear protein with numerous repeated elements, representing a new kind of cell cycle-maintaining proteins. *Journal of Cellular Biology* **123,** 513–522.

7

Hematopoietic Colony-Forming Cells

Makio Ogawa and Anne G. Livingston

1. Introduction

The hematopoietic progenitors that can be assayed in clonal culture systems represent a continuum of differentiation, which includes multipotential progenitors and very late-committed progenitors with only limited cell-division capabilities *(1)*. The late-committed progenitors, such as day-2 erythroid colony-forming cells (CFU-E) produce, after brief incubation, small colonies consisting of a few mature cells. Earlier progenitors, such as day-7 erythroid burst-forming cells (BFU-E) produce bigger colonies consisting of mature cells at later times of incubation. There are no universally accepted dates of incubation that define differentiation stages of progenitors. Since the rate of colony growth can be affected by multiple cell-culture conditions, direct comparison between two different laboratories is sometimes difficult. Therefore, investigators must have their own internal controls in all experiments. There is a general correlation between length of incubation and colony size. An exception to this rule is blast-cell colonies that will be described in **Subheading 3.3.** Since the progenitors of the blast-cell colonies are in the cell-cycle dormancy state, a long incubation period is needed to observe formation of small blast-cell colonies.

The primary purpose of the use of a clonal-culture assay is to obtain information on the developmental stages and differentiation potentials of progenitors producing the colony growth. The standard method for determination of colony types depends on identification *in situ* of mature cells possessing unique morphology, such as normoblasts containing hemoglobin, large-sized megakaryocytes, and highly refractile mast cells. One problem with this method is that it does not recognize the presence of cells which have not matured enough

From: *Methods in Molecular Medicine, vol. 63: Hematopoietic Stem Cell Protocols*
Edited by: C. A. Klug and C. T. Jordan © Humana Press Inc., Totowa, NJ

to exhibit the characteristics of mature cells. The major feature of hematopoiesis is asymmetric cell divisions regarding both differentiation and proliferative potentials *(1)*. Survival of the mature cells also varies depending on their lineages. For example, mature neutrophils do not survive long in culture, whereas macrophages and mast cells persist throughout a long incubation period. Together, these constitute the reasons for nonsynchronized lineage expression in the colonies. One example is multilineage colonies consisting of neutrophilic granulocytes, macrophages, and megakaryocytes (GMM) *(2)*. While progenitors for some GMM colonies have proven to be committed to the expression of only these three lineages, others are derived from earlier multipotential progenitors, because the replating of such colonies produces erythroid growth in the secondary culture. In order to obtain complete information on the differentiation programs of the colonies, it is often necessary to score colonies in the same dishes at different times of incubation and to replate colonies to identify hidden lineages.

Sequential scoring and replating of all colonies may not guarantee identification of all lineages if lineage identification was performed only by *in situ* identification on an inverted microscope. We have documented extremely skewed ratios of lineage expression in both mouse and human colonies. For example, only a few macrophages may be present in what appears to be a pure erythroid burst *(3)*. To identify such bipotential erythroid macrophage progenitors, it is necessary to carry out total cell differentials of all colonies in some experiments. For cytochemical and functional characterization of the cells grown in clonal culture, methylcellulose is far better than other types of semisolid materials such as plasma clot or agar. Cells in an entire dish may be centrifuged by diluting methylcellulose with culture media. Individual colonies may be easily harvested from methylcellulose media with a micropipet. Micromanipulation of single cells is also possible *(4)*, and methylcellulose does not interfere with polychrome staining of the cultured cells. For these reasons, we have used methylcellulose culture exclusively for studies of human and murine hematopoietic progenitors. Unless studies are directed to cells of specific lineages, the culture conditions should be permissive to all lineages, and the identification methods—such as cytochemistry—must be inclusive of all lineages. Cultures supported by lineage-specific cytokines or special staining for a certain lineage exclude information on multipotential progenitors, and may erroneously overestimate the incidence of progenitors.

Blast-cell colonies provide a unique material for studies of commitment and differentiation of hematopoietic progenitors. Murine blast-cell colonies were first identified as small colonies consisting only of blast cells on day 16 of culture *(5)*. Studies have revealed that the progenitors for blast-cell colonies are dormant in the cell cycle. Analysis of the secondary replating potential of the cells within the colony indicates that the majority are colony-forming cells (CFC), including multipotential colonies. The incidence of blast-cell colonies in normal bone marrow was very low, and enrichment of the population was necessary for detection. One effective method for the murine system is IV injection of high-dose 5-fluorouracil (5-FU), which preferentially kills the cycling progenitors. It is important to note that the blast-cell colonies represent transient populations of cells, which may have varying differentiation and proliferation potentials. Small colonies usually contain a large population of multipotential progenitors, and larger colonies identified later in culture usually have less replating ability and fewer multipotential progenitors. Just as in culture of committed progenitors, the cytokine combinations used for blast-cell colony development and analysis of replating potentials should be permissive for all lineages.

Identification of blast-cell colonies in human bone marrow presents unique challenges, such as the question of how to decrease the incidence of cycling progenitors. We employed the technique of low-serum culture and delayed addition of cytokines to populations of enriched progenitors to achieve selective growth of blast-cell colonies *(6)*. In both human and murine blast-cell colonies, the progenitors are dormant in the cell cycle. However, the replating ability and incidence of multipotential progenitors is much higher in murine blast-cell colonies. This may be a technical problem caused by the selective culture conditions for human blast cell colonies. An alternative approach is to separate the dormant progenitors and add cytokines at the initiation of culture. Other investigators have achieved limited success with the use of elutriation *(7)*.

This chapter focuses on serum-containing culture for murine and human progenitors. However, serum-free culture is preferable for certain purposes. **Subheading 3.2.** describes methods for the modification of the culture ingredients and special care necessary for serum-free culture of small numbers of purified cells. The blast-cell colony assay is described in **Subheading 3.3.**

2. Materials

2.1. Serum-Containing Clonal Culture

Media: Both α-modification of Minimum Essential Media (α-MEM) (ICN Biomedicals, Costa Mesa, CA) and Iscove's modification of Dulbecco's medium (IMDM) (Gibco, Grand Island, NY) have been used for the growth of murine and human colonies in culture. While colony formation is comparable in serum-containing culture, our observations indicate that a-MEM is superior to IMDM for the serum-free culture of a small number of purified cells.

The α-MEM is prepared according to the manufacturer's instructions with the addition of 100,000 u penicillin, 100 mg streptomycin, and 2.2 g of $NaHCO_3$. The pH of α-MEM depends upon the concentration of $NaHCO_3$ in the medium and the CO_2 content in the air. When this medium is exposed to 5% CO_2 in the air, the pH of the medium is 7.4. To establish the optimal concentrations of $NaHCO_3$ in the medium and CO_2 in the air, the pH of the medium must be measured after equilibrating it in an incubator. A CO_2 incubator with an injection system must be monitored periodically using Fyrite (Bacharach Instrument Co., Pittsburgh, PA). The quality of CO_2 also has a major influence on colony growth in culture, particularly when purified target cells are grown under low-serum conditions. We have compared CO_2 of commercial grades with 99.5% purity and 99.9% purity, with the latter having less than 1 ppm carbon monoxide (CO). A reduction CO concentration has a very positive effect on colony formation.

Sera: Selection of the appropriate fetal bovine serum (FBS) is a critical step, which may require the screening of many lots of sera. Once an appropriate batch is identified, the purchase of a large quantity is recommended, since the serum may be stored for years at −70°C. Mouse serum (or plasma) provides comparable colony growth to the best FBS. Pooled human serum and autologous plasma are used by some investigators for growth of human colonies. The complement in the serum should be denatured by incubating at 56°C for 30 min, and the sera should be divided into 100–mL aliquots and frozen. To achieve maximum colony growth, we use 30% (v/v) final concentration of FBS.

Bovine Serum Albumin: The selection of bovine serum albumin (BSA) also requires considerable effort in screening various lots. Cohn's fraction V requires deionization, while highly purified BSA may not. The following is the deionization protocol used in our laboratory:

1. Add 10 g of BSA powder (Sigma) to 44.2 mL of distilled water in a 100-mL beaker and allow to stand at 4°C until the BSA completely dissolves. Do not shake or stir the beaker.
2. To deionize the BSA solution, add 1.0 g of fresh analytical-grade mixed bed resin. (Bio Rad AG501- X8)
3. Remove the resin by passing the solution through gauze, and repeat the procedure. Measure the volume and add an equal volume of 2X α-MEM.
4. Sterilize by filtering the solution through a 0.45-μm filter, divide into 10-mL aliquots, and store at -20°C.
5. After thawing an aliquot, add 0.4 mL of 7% $NaHCO_3$ to each 10 mL of 10% BSA solution to adjust to a neutral pH. The addition of $NaHCO_3$ is necessary, because deionized BSA has a low pH. Store the remaining BSA solution at 4°C until it is depleted.

Methylcellulose: By providing viscosity, methylcellulose supports the three-dimensional growth of hematopoietic colonies. Methylcellulose is miscible in water at near-boiling temperatures, and dissolves at low temperatures. If air bubbles are not eliminated from the fibers, the methylcellulose cannot dissolve completely, thus leaving undigested fibers in the media. Methylcellulose in two fiber lengths have been used for hematopoietic cell culture: 4000 and 1500 centipoise (cp). Empirically, 0.8–0.9 % (w/v) of methylcellulose 4000 cp and 1.0–1.2% of methylcellulose 1500 cp provide comparable viscosities. It is important to test the lots of methylcellulose for selection of batches that support the maximal colony growth.

1. Slowly boil 500 mL of distilled water for about 30 min.
2. Pour 300 mL of boiling water into a sterilized 2-L flask containing a sterilized magnetic stirrer.
3. Add 30 g of 1500-cp methylcellulose (Shinetsu Chemical Co., Chiyoda-ku, Tokyo, Japan) into the flask slowly while stirring continuously. Mix for approx 30 min to ensure that all the particles are wet.
4. Add 200 mL of cold sterile distilled water (4°C) followed by 500 mL of cold 2X α-MEM.
5. Shake the flask vigorously to separate large clumps of gel.
6. Stir for 24–48 h at 4°C until the solution is visibly clear.
7. Divide the mixture into 100-mL quantities and store at -20°C until use.
8. Store thawed methylcellulose at 4°C (*see* **Note 1**).

Culture dishes: It is important to use tissue-culture-grade Petri dishes, because they do not promote the cellular attachment which is detrimental to colony formation. We use Falcon #1008 in the 35-mm × 10-mm size.

Reagents for Polychrome Staining: We have found that the May Grunwald Giemsa stain yields the best color balance for cultured cells. A commercial preparation of May Grunwald stain is available from Gaillard Schlessinger #35025. Several preparations of Giemsa stain are available, but each new batch must be titrated to achieve the proper color balance.

2.2. Serum-Free Clonal Culture

Serum and fraction V BSA both contain growth factors, and allow endogenous production of growth factors. Whenever it is necessary to critically evaluate the effect of growth factor, serum-free culture should be used. However, it is important to note that serum-free culture is not "chemically defined" culture, and variable amounts of growth factors may still be present in the culture. Described next are the materials used in our serum-free culture method which is a modification of the method of Gilbert and Iscove *(8)*. All water used in preparation of reagents should be greater than 10 mega ohms/cm resistance.

BSA: 99% pure, fatty acid-free, globulin-free BSA from Sigma (#A7638) is used. It is not necessary to deionize this purified fraction, but it should be prepared using bicarbonate-free α-MEM. Aliquot and freeze the sample. Adjust to a neutral pH with 1 M NaOH just prior to use.

Iron-Saturated Human Transferrin:
1. Prepare 7.9×10^{-3} M FeCl$_3$ (Sigma) by dissolving 21.35 mg FeCl$_3 \cdot$ 6 H$_2$O in 10 mL of 1×10^{-3} M HCl.
2. Adjust the pH of bicarbonate-free α-MEM to 7.4 with 1 M NaOH.
3. Dissolve 360 mg of 98% pure human transferrin (Sigma) in 4 mL of pH 7.4 α-MEM. Add 1.5 mL of 7.9×10^{-3} MFeCl$_3$. Do not freeze.

Lecithin and Cholesterol:
1. Add 20 mg of lecithin (Sigma) and 12 mg of cholesterol (Sigma) to a 40-mL glass beaker.
2. Add 1 mL of chloroform and mix until the lipid is completely dissolved.
3. Use a stream of nitrogen gas to evaporate the chloroform.
4. Add 1 mL of purified BSA and 9 mL of bicarbonate-free α-MEM. Sonicate to remove the lipid from the surface of the beaker.
5. This reagent should not be used for longer than 2 wk.

Sodium Selenite: Prepare 10^{-1} M by dissolving 173 mg of sodium selenite (Fluka) in 10mL of bicarbonate-free α-MEM. Freeze the stock in small aliquots. Dilute 1×10^{-1} to 1×10^{-5} just prior to use with bicarbonate-free α-MEM.

2.3. Human Blast-Cell Colony Culture

All reagents for the culture of human blast-cell colonies are the same as those of serum-free culture, except for BSA. Although it is not recommended to use such a purified fraction of BSA as in the serum-free culture system, the fraction V BSA allows the growth of cycling progenitors. We have found that globulin-free crystallized BSA from Sigma (#A7638) produces the most consistent results. The choice of growth factors to use for the analysis of blast-cell colonies depends on the specific experimental design. Optimal growth is achieved with a combination of factors, such as IL-3 + IL-6 *(9)* or IL-3 + SF at 50–100 mg/mL. Most human and mouse growth factors may be purchased from R&D Systems.

3. Methods

3.1. Serum-Containing Culture

1. Add the following ingredients to a 17 × 100 mm polystyrene tissue culture tube (Falcon #2057):

   a. 1.5 mL FBS.
   b. 0.5 mL 10% BSA.
   c. 0.05 mL of $1 \times 10^{-2} M$ 2-mercaptoethanol (ME).
   d. Cells (for 5 mL).
   e. Growth factors (for 5 mL).
   f. 2 mL of 3% methylcellulose. Use a 15-gauge needle and 5mL syringe to dispense the methylcellulose.
2. Adjust the volume to 5 mL with α-MEM. Mix well and place 1 mL into each of four 35-mm Falcon dishes using a syringe fitted with an 18-gauge needle.
3. Incubate the dishes at 37°C in a humidified atmosphere of 5% CO_2 in air.

3.2. Serum-Free Culture

The instructions for reagent preparation are presented in **Subheading 2.2.**

1. Add the following ingredients to a 17×100 polystyrene tube.
   a. 0.5 mL of 10% BSA.
   b. 0.25 mL of a 1:11 dilution of fully iron-saturated human transferrin. (0.021 mL transferrin + 0.229 mL bicarbonate-free α-MEM).
   c. 0.025 mL of lecithin-cholesterol.
   d. 0.05 mL of $1 \times 10^{-2} M$ 2-ME.
   e. Cells (for 5 mL).
   f. Growth factors (for 5 mL).
   g. 2.0 mL 3% methylcellulose.
2. Adjust the volume to 5 mL with α-MEM and place 1 mL into each of four 35-mm culture dishes.
3. We have found that low oxygen culture is superior to culture in ambient oxygen tension. Dishes are incubated at 37°C in a humidified atmosphere of 5% CO_2, 5% O_2, and 90% N_2.

3.3. Blast-Cell Colony Culture

3.3.1. Murine Blast-Cell Colonies

In order to enrich for progenitors for blast- cell colonies, mice are injected with 150 mg/kg 5-FU. We use Adrucil from Pharmacia at a concentration of 50 mg/mL. 5-FU is injected into the tail vein and the cells are harvested two days later. Prepare a single-cell suspension of bone-marrow cells by flushing the cells from the femurs and tibiae. Pool the cells and make a single-cell suspension by repeated flushing through a 25-gauge needle. Plate 2×10^4 to 5×10^4 cells per dish as described in **Subheading 3.1.** The time course of blast-cell colony formation and their functional heterogeneity is described in detail in **ref. 10**. We now recommend use of a combination of steel factor (SF)(c-kit ligand) and interleukin-11 (IL-11) at 10~100 ng/mL instead of the conditioned media.

3.3.2. Human Blast-Cell Colonies

The incidence of the progenitors for blast-cell colonies is very low in normal bone marrow. Cell suspensions should be enriched for target progenitors by cell sorting, immune adherence, selection with magnetic beads, and/or elutriation. A typical experiment would contain 1×10^4 CD34$^+$ cells per dish. Human blast-cell-colony culture is almost identical to serum-free culture (**Subheading 3.1**) with the following exceptions:

1. Add 0.1 mL of FBS.
2. Do not add growth factors at the initiation of culture. On d 14 of culture, carefully layer growth factors in 0.1 mL volume over the cultures. The optimal growth of blast-cell colonies is achieved with a combination of growth factors. See **Subheading 2.3.**

3.4. Identification of Colonies

3.4.1. In Situ Identification

In situ identification of colonies is not an exact science. Colony morphology is affected by types and concentrations of growth factors as well as batches of serum and methylcellulose (*see* **Note 2**). It may be particularly difficult for a novice to discriminate single- and multiple-lineage colonies. The major advantage of the use of methylcellulose clonal culture is that individual colonies may be easily harvested. The use of a Shandon Cytospin and polychrome staining allows easy confirmation of *in situ* identity. The method of May Grunwald - Giemsa staining is outlined as follows:

1. Prepare fresh PBS by diluting 66 mM PBS, pH 6.47, 1:10 with deionized water. Stock buffer is prepared by dissolving 6.36 g KH_2PO_4 in 700 mL of distilled H_2O. This is combined with 300 mL of solution containing 2.84 g of Na_2HPO_4.
2. Dilute the Giemsa stain 1:10 to 1:20, depending upon the batch, with fresh PBS.
3. Place 1.5 mL of May-Grunwald stain on the slide for 3–4 min.
4. Carefully add 1 mL of fresh buffer to the Giemsa stain for an additional 3 min.
5. Wash the slide with water and add 2–3 mL of fresh Giemsa stain for 20 min.
6. Rinse with water.

3.4.2 Blast-Cell Colonies

Blast-cell colonies are homogenous populations of small, round, refractile cells that reveal no signs of differentiation. When the cells are stained with May Grunwald Giemsa, blast cells with immature nuclei and prominent nucleoli are seen. Blast cells are negative for specific stains such as benzidine, acetylcholine esterase, or myeloperoxidase. When growth factors are added on d 14 of culture in the human blast-cell colony assay, there is usually very sparse background growth, and the emergence of new colonies is easy to detect. However, it is necessary to transfer human blast-cell colonies to permissive culture conditions as soon as they are identified.

3.4.3. Blast-Cell Colony Replating

1. Examine the dishes on an inverted microscope after growth factors are added on d 14 of culture.
2. When candidate blast-cell colonies containing 25 or more cells are identified, they are individually lifted from the dish using a 3-µL Eppendorf pipet.
3. Each colony is added to 100 µL of α-MEM in the bottom of a 35-mm culture dish.
4. Distribute the 100 µL volume evenly around the culture dish. Twenty small droplets is usually sufficient to dispense the 100 µL.
5. Add 0.9 mL of medium containing 30% FBS, 1% BSA, 1.2% methylcellulose, and a cocktail of growth factors that supports permissive growth of all lineages. A combination of GM-CSF, IL3 and SF, each at 50 ng/mL, should provide good colony growth.
6. Incubate dishes at 37°C in a humidified atmosphere of 5% CO_2 for an additional 10–14 days.

4. Notes

1. A commercial preparation of methylcellulose is available from StemCell Technologies. We have successfully used it for analysis of committed progenitors, but we have never used it for growth of blast-cell colonies.
2. Many variables can change colony morphology and thereby affect the ability to identify colonies *in situ*. One of the best ways to become competent is to "teach yourself." Observe the morphology of the colony on an inverted microscope. Then pick the colony from the culture with a 3 µL Eppendorf pipet and suspend it in 200 µL of 50% FCS in PBS. Centrifuge (Shandon Southern, Sewickly, PA) at 500 rpm for 5 min and stain. We have found that May-Grunwald Giemsa (*11*) stain is superior to Wright's stain for critical evaluation of cultured cells. **Refs. *12* and *13*** describe cytochemical methods that can be used to descriminate monocytes, neutrophils, basophils, and eosinophils. Also, a very comprehensive description of the *in situ* morphology of granulocyte and macrophage colonies is provided in **ref. *14*.**

References

1. Ogawa, M. (1993) Differentiation and proliferation of hematopoietic stem cells. *Blood* **81,** 2844–2853.
2. Nakahata, T. and Ogawa, M. (1982) Clonal origin of murine hemopoietic colonies with apparent restriction to granulocyte-macrophage-megakaryocyte (GMM) differentiation. *J. Cell Physiol.* **111,** 239–246.

3. Leary, A. G., Ogawa, M., Strauss, L. C., and Civin, C. I. (1984) Single cell origin of multilineage colonies in culture: Evidence that differentiation of multipotent progenitors and restriction of proliferative potential of monopotent progenitors are stochastic processes. *J. Clin. Investig.* **74,** 2193–2197.

4. Suda, T., Suda, J., and Ogawa, M. (1983) Single cell origin of mouse hemopoietic colonies expressing multiple lineages in variable combinations. *Proc. Natl. Acad. Sci. USA* **80,** 6689–6693.

5. Nakahata, T. and Ogawa, M. (1982) Identification in culture of a new class of hemopoietic colony-forming units with extensive capability to self renew and generate multipotential hemopoietic colonies. *Proc. Natl. Acad. Sci. USA* **79,** 3843–3847.

6. Leary, A. G. and Ogawa, M. (1987) Blast cell colony assay for umbilical cord blood and adult bone marrow progenitors. *Blood* **69,** 953–956.

7. Brandt, J. E., Baird, N., Lu, L., Srour, E., and Hoffman, R. (1988) Characterization of a human hematopoietic progenitor cell capable of forming blast cell containing colonies in vitro. *J. Clin. Investig.* **82,** 1017–1027.

8. Gilbert, L. J. and Iscove, N. N. (1976) Partial replacement of serum by selenite, transferrin, albumin and lecithin in haemopoietic cell cultures. *Nature* **26,** 594–595.

9. Leary, A. G., Ikebuchi, K., Hirai, Y., Wong, G. G., Yang ,Y-C., Clark, S. C., and Ogawa, M. (1988) Synergism between interleukin-6 and interleukin-3 in supporting proliferation of human hemopoietic stem cells: comparison with interleukin-1a. *Blood* **71,** 1759–1763.

10. Suda, T., Suda, J., and Ogawa, M. (1983) Proliferative kinetics and differentiation of murine blast cell colonies in culture: Evidence for variable G_0 periods and constant doubling rates of early pluripotent hemopoietic progenitors. *J. Cell. Physiol.* **117,** 308–318.

11. Osgood, E. and Ashworth, C. M. in *Diagnostic Laboratory Hematology* (2nd ed.), (Cartwright, G. E., ed.), New York, NY, Grune & Stratton, pp. 378–386.

12. Yam, L. T., Li, C. Y., and Crosby, W. H. (1971) Cytochemical identification of monocytes and granulocytes. *Am. J. Clin. Pathol.* **53,** 283–290.

13. Shoham, D., David, E. B., and Rozenszajn, L. A. (1974) Cytochemical and morphologic identification of macrophages and eosinophils in tissue cultures of normal human bone marrow. *Blood* **44,** 221–233.

14. Dao, C., Metcalf, D., Zittoun, R., and Bilski-Pasquier, G. (1977) Normal human bone marrow cultures in vitro: Cellular composition and maturation of the granulocytic colonies. *Br. J. Haematol.* **37,** 127–136.

8

Long-Term Culture-Initiating Cell Assays for Human and Murine Cells

Cindy L. Miller and Connie J. Eaves

1. Introduction

In normal adults, the majority of primitive hematopoietic cells are concentrated in the bone marrow, where they are in contact with a variety of molecules that influence their cell-cycle status, viability, motility, and differentiation. These include components of the extracellular matrix, soluble and bound growth-promoting factors and inhibitors, and adhesion molecules that mediate direct interactions between cells. The long-term culture (LTC) system initially developed to support the continued production of myeloid cells, *(1–3)* and subsequently for the production of lymphoid cells *(4–7)* has provided a unique approach for the investigation of the regulation and maintenance of early hematopoietic progenitors under conditions that reproduce many aspects of the marrow microenvironment. The LTC system has also provided a basis for the development of powerful assay procedures for quantitating and distinguishing cells at discrete stages of early hematopoietic cell differentiation.

Over 30 years ago, Dexter and colleagues first showed that serum-containing cultures initiated with high concentrations of murine bone marrow cells ($>10^7$/mL) rapidly form an adherent layer, which supports the generation of mature granulocytes and macrophages for many weeks in the absence of exogenously added cytokines beyond those present in the serum used *(1,2)*. It is now recognized that many parameters can influence both the types of cells produced in these cultures and the duration of their production. These include variables that can independently affect the establishment and maintenance of a supportive stromal cell-containing feeder layer, as well as the types and numbers of hematopoietic cells generated. For example, serum substitutes that

From: *Methods in Molecular Medicine, vol. 63: Hematopoietic Stem Cell Protocols*
Edited by: C. A. Klug and C. T. Jordan © Humana Press Inc., Totowa, NJ

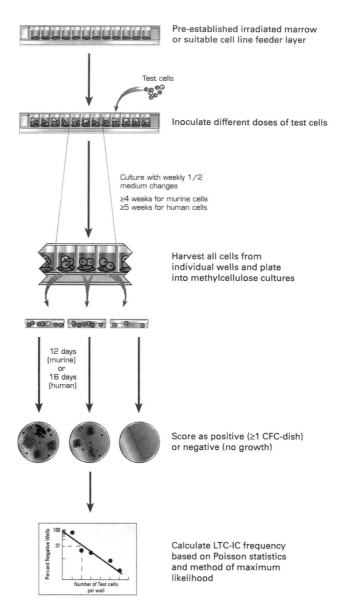

Pre-established irradiated marrow
or suitable cell line feeder layer

Test cells

Inoculate different doses of test cells

Culture with weekly 1/2
medium changes

≥4 weeks for murine cells
≥5 weeks for human cells

Harvest all cells from
individual wells and plate
into methylcellulose cultures

12 days
(murine)
or
16 days
(human)

Score as positive (≥1 CFC-dish)
or negative (no growth)

Calculate LTC-IC frequency
based on Poisson statistics
and method of maximum
likelihood

Percent Negative Wells
100
37

Number of Test cells
per well

Fig. 1. LTC-IC limiting dilution analysis. Adherent feeder layers are established in mini-cultures (flat-bottom 96–well culture plate). Doses of test cells are seeded into replicate wells. Cultures are maintained at 33°C for murine test cells on irradiated primary murine marrow feeders, and at 37°C for human cells on irradiated M2-10B4 or engineered M2-10B4: Sl/Sl feeders. Cultures are incubated for ≥4 wk for murine cells and ≥5 wk for human cells with weekly one-half medium exchanges. After harvest, adherent and nonadherent cells from each individual well are placed in methylcellulose cultures and scored as "positive" (≥1 CFC) or "negative" (no CFC), 12 d (murine LTC-IC) or 16–18 d (human LTC-IC) later. The LTC-IC frequency is derived using Poisson statistics and the method of maximum likelihood.

meet the needs of hematopoietic cells are not adequate to support the outgrowth of supportive marrow stromal cells, which require unknown factors in certain batches of horse serum. The addition of hydrocortisone to the medium also appears to be important *(3,8)*. Because both committed myeloid progenitor cells and their progeny have finite proliferative potentials, the continuing presence of such cells in LTC for extended periods has been used to infer their generation from a very primitive cell type present in the starting inoculum. These studies have prompted the use of pre-established irradiated LTC adherent layers as feeders to allow this system to be adapted for the quantitation of such primitive cells from both human *(9,10)* and murine *(11,12)* sources. The cells thus identified have been called LTC-initiating cells (LTC-IC).

A schematic illustration of the procedure used to measure LTC-IC frequencies is given in **Fig. 1**. Test cells, which may be unseparated cell preparations, mononuclear cells, or additionally purified subpopulations of hematopoietic cells subsets, are first seeded onto irradiated semi-confluent marrow feeders, or a cell line with equivalent supportive activity (*see* **refs. *13,14***). Committed progenitors present in the input test cell inoculum then rapidly mature and disappear during the initial 3–5 wk of culture. Successively, more primitive cells (LTC-IC) begin to proliferate and generate a new cohort of colony-forming cells (CFC), a process which may continue for several months. To determine the frequency of LTC-IC in a given hematopoietic cell population using limiting dilution analysis (LDA), varying doses of test cells are seeded into mini-cultures containing pre-established feeder layers. The cultures are supplemented with 50% LTC medium with fresh hydrocortisone at weekly intervals, and after a defined period (≥ 4 wk for murine cells and ≥ 5 wk for human cells), the cultures are assessed for the presence of later-stage hematopoietic cells. We recommend harvesting both adherent and nonadherent cells from each mini-culture and then placing them together in a single methylcellulose culture to determine whether CFC are present, and if so, the type and quantity found. Each LTC-IC assay well is scored as positive (≥ 1 CFC detected) or negative (no CFC detected), and the proportion of negative wells is calculated for each cell dose used. The frequency of LTC-IC is the reciprocal of the concentration of test cells that yields 37% negative cultures by the application of Poisson statistics and the method of maximum likelihood *(15)*. Once the LTC-IC frequency for a given population is determined, it can be used to derive the average CFC output per LTC-IC in that population. This value can then be used to derive LTC-IC frequencies from the total number of CFC generated from a given starting cell population in "bulk LTC" (**Fig. 2**) as long as the requirement for a linear relationship between CFC output and number of cells seeded is met (*see* **ref. *10***). However, it is important to emphasize that the proliferative potential exhibited by individual LTC-IC within a given popula-

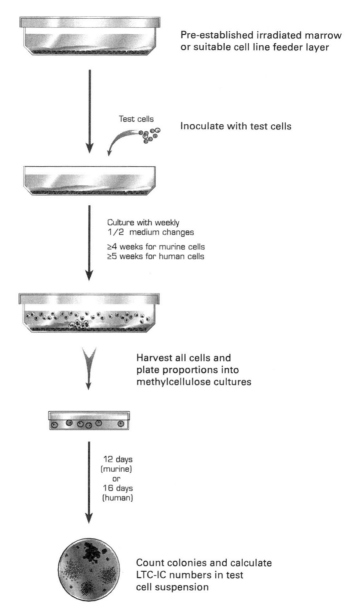

Pre-established irradiated marrow
or suitable cell line feeder layer

Test cells   Inoculate with test cells

Culture with weekly
1/2 medium changes

≥4 weeks for murine cells
≥5 weeks for human cells

Harvest all cells and
plate proportions into
methylcellulose cultures

12 days
(murine)
or
16 days
(human)

Count colonies and calculate
LTC-IC numbers in test
cell suspension

Fig. 2. Quantitation of LTC-IC in Bulk Cultures. Adherent feeder layers are established in culture plates (i.e., 35 mm dishes) and seeded with cell populations for analysis of LTC-IC content. Cultures are maintained as described in Fig. 1. After the culture period, the LTC (adherent and nonadherent cells) is harvested and proportions are placed in methylcellulose cultures for quantitation of total CFC numbers. The number of secondary CFC generated is linearly related to the number of LTC-IC present in the test-cell population (*see* text).

Table 1
Frequencies of LTC-IC in Human Hematopoietic Cell Populations

Cell population	LTC-IC (%)[a]	References
Light-density BM	0.005–0.05	*10, 14, 21, 22*
Lin⁻ CD34⁺ BM	0.2–1.0	*10*
Lin⁻ CD34⁺ CD45RA⁻ CD71⁻ BM	5–10	*23*
Lin⁻ CD34⁺ CD38⁺ BM	2–8	*23*
Lin⁻ CD34⁺ CD38⁻ BM	15–30	*23, 24*
Lin⁻ CD34⁺ HLA⁻ DR⁺ BM	1–3	*9, 21*
Light-density CB	0.002–0.06	*14, 19, 25*
Lin⁻ CD34⁺ CB	0.2–1.0	*26*
Lin⁻ CD34⁺ CD38⁻ CB	20–50	*25, 27*
G-CSF MPB	0.03	*14*
G-CSF CD34⁺ MPB	1–3	*16*
Lin⁻ CD34⁺ fetal liver	0.5–1.2	*17, 18*

[a] LTC-IC assayed on irradiated human marrow, M2–10B4 feeder layers, or M2–10B4:Sl/Sl engineered feeder layers. BM = Bone Marrow; CB = Cord Blood; MPB = Mobilized Peripheral Blood.

tion is highly variable, and the mean CFC generated per LTC-IC may also vary according to the ontological source of cell population assayed (e.g., adult bone marrow (BM), cord blood (CB), fetal liver, blood, or mobilized peripheral blood (MPB) *(10,14,16–18)* and the type of feeder layer used and other culture conditions used *(14,19,20)*. The latter method of LTC-IC quantitation is much simpler, but can only be used if the average CFC/LTC-IC has been predetermined by LDA for a given hematopoietic cell source and previously validated culture conditions.

Human and murine LTC-IC are enriched in fractions of hematopoetic cells that do not express (or express at low levels) cell surface markers associated with differentiation along the various myeloid or lymphoid lineages (lin). Human LTC-IC are present within the CD34⁺ subset of this lin⁻ fraction. Further enrichment is achieved by the isolation of subsets of these lin⁻ CD34⁺ cells defined according to their differential surface expression of other antigens, including CD45RA, CD71, HLA-DR, Thy-1, and CD38 (*see* **Table 1**). The majority of murine LTC-IC are present in the lin⁻Sca-1⁺ cell fraction of hematopoietic cells (*see* **Table 2**).

Although LTC-IC represent a subset of primitive hematopoietic cells that share phenotypic and functional properties with long-term in vivo repopulating cells (Competitive Repopulating Unit [CRU] assay, *see* Chapter 12), it is important to emphasize that the cells detected by both of these assays are functionally heterogeneous. For example, both LTC-IC and cells able to generate

Table 2
Frequency of LTC-IC in Murine Hematopoietic Cell Populations

Cell population	LTC-IC (%)[a]	References
Adult BM	0.002–0.005	*11,12,28*
Lin⁻ Sca-1⁺ WGA⁺ BM	~2%	*12*
Lin⁻ Sca-1⁺ day 14.5 fetal liver	~2%	*29*

[a]LTC-IC assayed on irradiated murine marrow feeders.

lymphoid and myeloid progeny in xenogeneic recipients (immunodeficient mice or sheep) are found in both the CD34⁺CD38⁺ and CD34⁺CD38⁻ populations *(25)*, although those with more sustained proliferative activity appear to be CD34⁺CD38⁻ *(30–32)*. Thus, extension of the LTC period beyond 5 wk has been used as a strategy to select for a more primitive subset of human LTC-IC *(30)*.

The original LTC-IC assays for both murine and human cells used irradiated primary marrow adherent feeder layers of the same species as the test cells. Subsequent studies have shown that a number of pre-adipocyte fibroblast cells can perform the same function. Stromal cell lines that have been investigated most extensively for their ability to support human and murine hematopoetic progenitors in LTC include M2-10B4 *(13)*, MS-5 *(20,33)*, AFT204 *(34,35)*, and S17 *(36)*. The murine fibroblast cell line, M2-10B4 detects human LTC-IC at frequencies comparable to those determined in assays that contain primary human marrow feeders *(13,14)*. The sensitivity of LTC-IC detection (particularly more primitive LTC-IC) is enhanced using a mixed feeder layer of M2-10B4 and Sl/Sl fibroblasts engineered to produce interleukin-3 (IL-3), granulocyte-macrophage colony-stimulating factor (GM-CSF) and steel factor (SF, also known as stem cell factor [SCF]) and a 6-wk interval before their progeny CFC are assessed *(14)*. Note however, that these feeders greatly enhance the reactivation in vitro of latently Epstein-Barr virus (EBV)-infected B cells which occurs much less frequently when normal marrow or parental M2-10B4 cells are used *(37)*. To avoid this problem, either the T or B cells in the test-cell suspension must be removed.

The LTC-IC assays described here detect primitive hematopoietic cells capable of in vitro myeloid differentiation. The identification of conditions that allow both myeloid and lymphoid cells (natural killer (NK) and B cells) to be produced in LTC *(38–41)* has led to the development of derivative LTC-IC assays for the quantitation of primitive cells with both myeloid and lymphoid potential, (LTC-IC$_{ML}$)*(12)* or Myeloid-Lymphoid Initiating Cell (ML-IC)*(42)*.

In this chapter, we describe methodologies for the quantitation of human LTC-IC by LDA or in bulk LTC, using either the original, unmanipulated M2–

10B4 murine fibroblast cell line and a 5-wk assay or the combination of M2-10B4 and Sl/Sl cells (engineered to produce IL-3, G-CSF, and SF, [*14*]) using a 6-wk assay. For quantitation of murine LTC-IC, an LDA procedure using primary murine marrow feeders and a 4-wk endpoint is described.

2. Materials

2.1. LTC-IC Assay for Human Cells

1. Hydrocortisone 21-hemisuccinate sodium salt (StemCell Technologies, Vancouver, BC, Sigma Chemicals, St. Louis, MO). Store powder desiccated at $-20°C$. Dissolve hydrocortisone powder in α-MEM to a final concentration of 10^{-4} M, filter-sterilize using a 0.22-μ-syringe filter, and store at 4°C. As hydrocortisone has a relatively short half-life in solution, it is necessary to prepare a fresh stock solution within 1 wk of use.
2. hLTCM: long-term culture medium for human cells with 10^{-6} M hydrocortisone. (MyeloCult™ 05100; StemCell). This medium can be stored at $-20°C$ for up to 1 y or at 4°C for up to 1 mo. Prepare for use within 1–2 days by adding 1 mL of 10^{-4} M hydrocortisone stock solution to 99 mL MyeloCult™. Composition of hLTCM: 12.5% horse serum (HS), 12.5% fetal bovine serum (FBS), 0.2 mM i-inositol, 20 mM folic acid, 10^{-4} M 2-mercaptoethanol, 2 mM L-glutamine, 10^{-6} M hydrocortisone, Alpha Modification of Eagle's Minimum Essential Medium. Investigators choosing to prepare their own LTC medium are advised to prescreen batches of FBS and HS and test them in combination with other components for their suitability to support hematopoiesis in human or murine LTC. (Pretested lots of FBS and HS selected for this application are also available from StemCell). The addition of antibiotics is not required if sterile culture conditions are used. If desired, penicillin G (50–100 μ/mL) and streptomycin sulfate (100 g/mL) can be added to hLTC medium and mLTC medium. Antibiotics are available from various suppliers (Gibco BRL, Sigma, StemCell, and others).
3. M2-10B4 murine fibroblast cell line. (American Tissue Culture Company, catalog number—CRL1972). If the use of hIL-3/G-CSF/SF-producing M2–10B4 and Sl/Sl fibroblasts (*14*) is preferred, these can be accessed by writing to Dr. D. Hogge, Terry Fox Laboratory, Vancouver, BC, or to StemCell Technologies. In either case, these fibroblasts should not be continuously passaged in vitro for more than 6 mo. Therefore, it is important to establish a large number of vials with early-passage cells. In addition, the engineered cells should be checked periodically (by enzyme-linked immunosorbent assay [ELISA] assay of their supernatants) to ensure that the cells are still producing the expected levels of growth factors.
4. RPMI-1640/10% FBS: RPMI-1640 with 10% FBS for culture of M2-10B4 and M2-10B4-producing hG-CSF and hIL-3. Store at 4°C for up to 1 mo.
5. DMEM/10% FBS: Dulbecco's modified Eagle's medium (DMEM) with 10% FBS for culture of Sl/Sl-producing human SF and human IL-3.
6. HBSS: Hanks Balanced Salt Solution, Ca^{++} and Mg^{++}-free. Store at 4°C.

7. IMDM/2% FBS: Iscove's modified Dulbecco's medium with 2% FBS. Store at 4°C for up to 1 mo.

8. G418 sulfate (Calbiochem, La Jolla, CA) and Hygromycin B (Sigma) for selection of M2–10B4 and Sl/Sl-engineered cell lines. Prepare stock solutions of 100 mg/mL. Handle according to manufacturer's instructions.

9. 1–3 mg/mL collagen solution (StemCell). Store at 4°C.

10. 0.25% trypsin-citrate or 0.25% trypsin-ethylenediaminetetraaceticacid (EDTA) Solution (StemCell). Store in aliquots at –20°C.

11. Medium for human CFC assays. Burst-forming unit-erythroid (BFU-E), colony-forming-unit-granulocyte, macrophage (CFU-GM) and CFU-granulocyte, erythroid, megakaryocyte, macrophage (CFU-GEMM) are assayed in methylcellulose cultures containing IMDM, 1.0% methylcellulose, 30% FBS, 1% bovine serum albumin (BSA), 10^{-4} M 2-mercaptoethanol, 20 ng/mL each of recombinant human (rh) IL-3 (rhIL-3), rh GM-CSF, rhIL-6, 50 ng/mL rhSCF, and 3 U/mL erythropoietin (Epo) (MethoCult 04435; StemCell).

12. Sterile cultureware: T25 cm^2 and T75 cm^2 flasks, 35 mm culture dishes, 96-well flat-bottom culture plates, 100 mm Petri dishes, sterile tubes (12×75, 13×100), pipet, 1- and 3-mL syringes and 35 mm Petri dishes and 16-gauge blunt-end needles for CFC assays (StemCell).

13. L-Calc™ software program (StemCell) for calculating LTC-IC frequencies.

2.2. LTC-IC Assay for Murine Cells

1. MLTCM: long-term culture medium for murine cells with 10^{-6} M hydrocortisone (MyeloCult 05200; StemCell). Prepared and stored as described for hLTCM (*see* **Subheading 2.1., item 2**)

2. Medium for murine CFU-GM, BFU-E, and CFU-GEMM assays. Murine CFC are assayed in IMDM, 1.0% methylcellulose, 15% FBS, 10 µg/mL insulin, 200 µg/mL transferrin, 1% BSA, 10^{-4} M 2-mercaptoethanol, 2 mM L-glutamine, and 10 ng/mL each of murine rIL-3 (mrIL-3), hrIL-6, and 50 ng/mL mrSCF and 3 U/mL Epo (03434; StemCell).

3. Additional media, cultureware, and software required are as described in **Subheading 2.1.**

3. Methods

3.1. Maintenance of M2-10B4 and Sl/Sl Cell Lines

1. M2-10B4 and engineered M2-10B4 are cultured in RPMI-1640/10%FBS, and engineered M2-10B4 are cultured with 0.4 mg/mL G418 and 0.06 mg/mL Hygromycin B every second passage. Engineered Sl/Sl are grown in DMEM/ 10% FCS and cultured with 0.8 mg/mL G418 and 0.125 mg/mL Hygromycin B every second passage. Cell lines are cultured at 37°C and 5% CO$_2$ in air in 25 cm^2 or 75 cm^2 culture flasks.

2. When cells reach confluence, remove media carefully by decanting or suctioning.
3. Add 2 mL HBSS. Rotate flask gently to detach loosely adherent cells, and discard medium and nonadherent cells.
4. Add 2 mL (T25) or 4 mL(T75) trypsin solution. Incubate for 2–10 min at 37°C, or until adherent cells start to detach from the surface of the flask. Add 0.2 mL FBS to neutralize the trypsin, and mix with a pipet to disperse clumps and obtain a single-cell suspension.
5. Wash cells once in RPMI-1640/10% FBS or DMEM/10% FBS. Transfer 1/50 to 1/100 vol of one flask to a new culture flask with appropriate culture medium (T25; 8 mL, T75; 25 mL). Cell should again reach confluency 7–10 d later.

3.2. Preparation of Irradiated M2-10B4 Feeder Layers or Engineered M2-10B4:SI/SI

1. Trypsinize the desired feeder cells (*see* **Subheading 3.1.**) and wash the cells recovered twice in RPMI-1640/10% FBS or DMEM/10% FBS.
2. Resuspend cells at 10^6–10^8 cells/mL in hLTCM and irradiate cells with 8000 cGy from an X-ray or γ-irradiation source.
3. Dilute M2-10B4 cells to 1.5×10^5 cells per mL in hLTCM, or combine engineered M2-10B4 and Sl/Sl at 1:1 ratio and dilute to 1.5×10^5 (7.5×10^4 M2-10B4 and 7.5×10^4 Sl/Sl) per mL in hLTCM. Place 2 mL (3×10^5 cells) per collagen-coated 35-mm tissue-culture dishes (*see* **Note 1**) for LTC-IC assays in bulk culture, or 0.1 mL (1.5×10^4 cells) per well in 96-well flat-bottom culture plates for LTC-IC LDA assays.
4. Incubate at 37°C in 5% CO_2 in air in a humidified incubator. Incubate cultures for a minimum of 24-h prior to the addition of test cells. Irradiated feeders can be used for up to 10 d later, but if delays of >7 d are anticipated, the medium should be changed after the first 7 d.

3.3. Preparation of Test Cells for Human LTC-IC Assays

1. Human LTC-IC are present in a variety of hematopoietic sources, including normal adult marrow, cord blood, peripheral blood, and fetal liver. Although unseparated hematopoietic cell suspensions can be used to perform LTC-IC assay from the first two sources, marrow from patients may be different and require preliminary enrichment of the LTC-IC. In the case of normal blood or mobilized blood obtained from individuals who have not been treated with chemotherapy, the risk of EBV-transformants taking over the LTC, or at least obscuring the CFC assays, is high and either B or T cells should be removed. Human fetal liver cannot be assessed unless the large numbers of macrophage precursors present are first removed by depletion of lin+ cells. Procedures for the isolation of hematopoietic cells from various tissue sources and the preparation of enriched cell fractions are discussed in Chapters 3 and 4 (*see* **Table 1** and Chapters 3 and 4).

3.4. Assay of Human LTC-IC by LDA

The frequencies of LTC-IC in a hematopoietic cell population can be determined using mini-LTC and LDA (**Fig. 1**). Varying doses of test cells are seeded into replicate wells containing irradiated M2-10B4, and cultures are maintained for 5 wk with weekly one-half-medium changes. Alternatively, use of the engineered IL-3, G-CSF, and SF-producing M2-10B4 and Sl/Sl feeder combination (50% each) and maintenance of the cultures for 6 wk prior to harvest, allows more primitive LTC-IC to be detected *(14)*. At the end of the 5- or 6-wk period, the adherent and nonadherent cells are harvested from each individual well, combined, and assayed in methylcellulose cultures for CFC (*see* **Note 2**). Eight to 24 replicates of 3–4 cell doses that bracket the LTC-IC frequency are generally sufficient to provide data with reasonable 95% confidence intervals. The appropriate cell doses may be estimated from the anticipated frequency of LTC-IC in the test-cell suspension. For example, the expected frequency of LTC-IC in suspensions of lin^-CD34^+ normal marrow cells is ~1/100 to 1/500 (**Table 1**). Therefore, LDA analysis using aliquots of 30, 100, 300, and 900 lin^-CD34^+ normal marrow cells per well with 12 replicates per dose should yield an accurate estimation of their LTC-IC content.

1. Prepare dilutions of test cells in hLTCM.
2. Carefully remove ~90% hLTCM from each well already containing the irradiated feeder cells desired, using a multichannel pipetter with sterile tips and discard. Care should be taken not to disturb the adherent feeder layer.
3. Add test cells in 0.1 mL hLTCM to the appropriate wells using a multichannel pipetter with sterile tips.
4. Place 96-well plates in a loosely covered container (e.g., a 20-cm square bacterial plate) with 2–3 uncovered Petri dishes containing sterile water to maintain high humidity and place in a humidified 37°C incubator with 5% CO_2 in air. Incubate cultures for 5–6 wk.
5. Perform one-half media changes at 1, 2, 3, 4 (parental M2-10B4 feeders), and 5 wk (M2–10B4:Sl/Sl engineered feeders) after initiating the cultures by removing 50 µL (including one-half the nonadherent cells) and adding 55 µL of freshly prepared hLTCM. A multichannel pipetter and sterile tips can be used to manipulate 3–6 wells at a time. To avoid contamination, care must be taken not to touch tips to the exterior of the wells. New tips should be used each time cells and/or media are removed to avoid spreading any possible contamination from one replicate to another. Care must also be taken to avoid touching or disturbing the adherent layer.
6. At the end of the 5- or 6-wk culture period, remove hLTCM and nonadherent cells from each well (~0.1 mL), and transfer the cells to a labeled 12 × 75 mm tube. These should be placed in a similar arrangement in a rack that holds 72 tubes closely aligned (e.g., Nalgene 5970_16). A multichannel pipetter can then be used to harvest the nonadherent cells from three wells at a time. It is advisable

to harvest the cells in batches of 48 or less to ensure that wells do not dry out or become overexposed to trypsin.

7. Add 0.1 mL HBSS to each well, and then remove with remaining loosely attached cells and add this to the appropriate tube already containing the nonadherent cells from the same well.

8. Add 0.1 mL 0.25% trypsin solution to each well and incubate at 37°C. After 3–5 min, scan the plate using an inverted microscope to determine if the adherent layer has started to detach from the surface of the well. If necessary, continue incubating up to a maximum of 10 min until the adherent cells are loosened. Then add 10 μL of FBS to each well to neutralize the trypsin.

9. Mix the contents of each well gently to obtain a single-cell suspension and add the suspended cells to the tubes containing the cells previously removed from the same wells.

10. Rinse each well once with IMDM/2% FBS and transfer again to the same tube.

11. Fill the tubes with IMDM/2% FBS and centrifuge at 350*g* for 7–10 min. Carefully decant or suction off the supernatants without disturbing cell pellets, leaving ~0.1 mL media behind.

12. Gently vortex the tube to resuspend the cells, add 1 mL human methylcellulose medium, and vortex vigorously.

13. Draw up the entire contents of each tube (individually), using a 1-cc tuberculin syringe (without the needle attached) and then eject into a 35-mm Petri dish. Rotate dishes to ensure methylcellulose is spread evenly over surface of 35-mm dish. Place 2 dishes in a 100-mm Petri dish containing a third open 35-mm Petri dish with sterile water.

14. Incubate for 16–18 d and record the number of colonies present in each methylcellulose culture. Record the well as negative if no CFC is present, and as positive if ≥1 CFC is present.

3.5. Analysis of Human LTC-IC by LDA

LTC-IC frequencies in the starting cell suspension are determined by application of Poisson statistics and the method of maximum likelihood assuming "single-hit kinetics," i.e., each LTC-IC will produce ≥1 CFC (detectable after ≥5 wk) independent of the other cells seeded. A well is thus scored as negative when no CFC are detected in it. The LTC-IC frequency is given by the reciprocal of the concentration of test cells that gives 37% negative wells. Interpolation of this value is best done using a software program to perform the calculation (i.e., L-Calc™). It is advisable to consult a qualified statistician to confirm the appropriate methodology used to compare LTC-IC frequencies from different test populations.

3.6. Analysis of Human LTC-IC by Bulk LTC

LTC-IC numbers can also be determined from CFC assays of "bulk cultures" (**Fig. 2**), i.e., cultures initiated with large numbers of LTC-IC if the average

Table 3
Numbers of Human Cell Populations for Initiation of LTC-IC
on M2-10B4 or M2-10B4:Sl/Sl-Engineered Feeders

Cell population	Cells per LTC-IC culture in 35-mm dishes[a]
Ammonium-chloride treated BM	$4 \times 10^5 - 2 \times 10^6$
Light-density BM	$2 \times 10^5 - 1 \times 10^6$
Light-density CB	$1 \times 10^5 - 5 \times 10^5$
Lin⁻CD34⁺ BM, CB, MPB, or FL	1000–5000
Lin⁻CD34⁺CD38⁻ BM,CB, MPB, or FL	100–500

[a]The numbers of LTC-IC in different hematopoietic cell populations can vary significantly; therefore, these are suggested values only. It is advisable to initiate bulk LTC-IC at two or more different cell doses.

number of CFC per LTC-IC for the population being tested is known (*see* **Subheading 1.** and **Note 3**). To ensure a representative sampling, such cultures should be initiated with at least 10 and preferably 20 LTC-IC (**Table 1** and **Table 3**). Following 5–6 wk of culture, the total number of CFC present is determined. The number of LTC-IC present in the initial test cell suspension is then calculated by dividing the total number of CFC present by the average output of CFC per LTC-IC (*see* **Note 3**). Alternatively, values can be expressed as LTC-IC-derived CFC for a given number of test cells.

1. Prepare test cells at the appropriate density in hLTCM (*see* **Table 3**).
2. Carefully remove the hLTCM from the 35-mm culture dishes containing irradiated M2-10B4 or engineered M2-10B4:Sl/Sl feeder cells.
3. Add test cells in 2.0 mL volumes, taking care not to disturb adherent layer. Place the dishes in 100-mm Petri dishes containing an additional uncovered 35-mm dish containing sterile water and incubate in a humidified incubator at 37°C in 5% CO_2 in air for 5–6 wk.
4. Perform one-half media exchanges after 1, 2, 3, 4 (parental M2-10B4 feeders), and 5 wk (M2-10B4:Sl/Sl engineered feeders) by first gently swirling the cultures to detach loosely adherent cells and then drawing up half the contents of the culture (medium and cells) into a sterile pipet. Replace the vol removed (i.e., 1.0 mL for 2.0 mL culture) with an equal vol of freshly prepared hLTCM.
5. After 5–6 wk, all the cells are harvested (adherent and nonadherent cells) by first placing all hLTM and nonadherent cells into a sterile 15-mL tube.
6. Rinse the adherent layer twice with 1 mL HBSS, and add all cells and medium to the tube.
7. Add 1 mL of trypsin solution and place at 37°C for 10 min. At intervals, gently swirl cultures and examine using an inverted microscope for evidence of detachment of the adherent layer cells. Once this starts, add 0.2 mL FBS to the dish to neutralize the proteolytic activity of the trypsin.

8. Using a sterile pipet, repeatedly pipet the trypsin/FBS solution over the surface of the dish to ensure that all adherent cells are detached and form a single-cell suspension. Add all cells and medium to the tube. Alternatively, a culture cell scraper can be used to dislodge remaining adherent cells.

9. Rinse the culture dish twice with IMDM/2% FBS, and add all cells and media to the tube in which the nonadherent cells have already been placed.

10. Wash cells twice in IMDM/2% FBS and resuspend in 1–2 mL IMDM/2% FBS. Record the vol and perform a nucleated cell count. To exclude dead cells, if present, cell counts performed using a dye-exclusion viability stain (i.e., trypan blue) and a nucleated cell count (3% acetic acid) can be compared. Hematopoietic cells appear as round, uniform, refractile cells compared to the larger fibroblast cells with dye-exclusion viability stains, and have more compact nuclei when using 3% acetic acid. If desired, a "stroma only" control well can be included to provide an example of how fibroblast cells differ in terms of morphology.

11. Dilute cells to $2–5 \times 10^5$ cells/mL in IMDM/2% FBS (or plate a predetermined fraction of the culture according to the number of CFC expected).

12. Add 0.3 mL of cells to 3 mL of human methylcellulose media (for duplicate assays), or 0.5 mL of cells to 5 mL of methylcellulose (for quadruplicate assays) and vortex. Let stand for 5 min to allow bubbles to rise.

13. Plate 1.1 mL per 35-mm Petri dish, using a 3-cc or 5-cc syringe with an attached 16-gauge blunt-end needle. Incubate dishes as described (*see* **Subheading 3.4.**) for 16–18 d at 37°C.

14. Score total numbers of colonies, and then calculate the number of input LTC-IC per number of cells assayed (*see* **Note 3**).

Example calculation: Quantitation of LTC-IC in a sample of low-density normal adult marrow cells assayed on irradiated M2-10B4 feeders for 5 wk.

Number of test cells initiated per 35-mm dish:	10^6 low-density bone marrow cells.
Total cells harvested at wk 5:	4×10^5
Number of cells plated per methylcellulose culture:	5×10^4
Average number of CFC per methylcellulose culture:	50
Average CFC per LTC-IC *(14)*:	8
Total CFC per LTC culture:	400 CFC per LTC-IC culture (50 times 4×10^5 divided by $5 \times 10^4 = 400$).
LTC-IC numbers:	400 LTC-IC-derived CFC per 10^6 low-density marrow cells = 1 LTC-IC per 2×10^4 low-density marrow cells.

3.7. Assay of Murine LTC-IC by LDA

Assessment of murine LTC-IC involves the same procedures as for human LTC-IC. The only difference is the type of feeder used and the duration and temperature the cultures are kept before CFC assays are performed. The reader should therefore examine the described procedure for human LTC-IC assays for other technical details. Generation of primary murine marrow feeders and LTC containing irradiated marrow feeders or nonirradiated S17 cell line **(29,36)** are maintained at 33°C. Many cell lines suitable for human LTC-IC assays including M2-10B4, are not suitable for feeders in murine LTC-IC assays, likely due to murine M-CSF produced. In addition, since published data for CFC outputs per murine LTC-IC are unavailable, only the LDA strategy is outlined here.

3.7.1. Establishing Murine Marrow Feeder Layers

1. Sacrifice a minimum of two adult C57BL/6 mice, 6–12 wk old, using protocols approved by the host institution.
2. Remove the femurs, cut off both ends with a sharp surgical scissors, and flush the marrow plugs into 1–2 mL cold IMDM/2% FCS, using a sterile 21-gauge needle attached to a 3-cc syringe. Prepare a single-cell suspension by drawing the media and cells up and down once or twice using the same syringe and needle. α-MEM, DMEM, or HBSS supplemented with 2% FBS are also suitable for the isolation of marrow cells.
3. Determine the concentration of nucleated cells in the suspension (should be ~ 1–2×10^7 per femur). Washing of marrow cells is not required if marrow-cell numbers are high ($\geq 10^7$ cells per mL).
4. Dilute marrow cells to 2×10^5/mL in mLTCM. Place 0.15 mL of the cell suspension into each well of a 96-well flat-bottom culture plate (3×10^4 cells per well) using a multichannel pipetter and sterile tips.
5. Incubate at 33°C in 5% CO_2 in air and 1 wk later, feed by removing 75 µL of cells and media and adding 80 µL of freshly prepared mLTCM (*see* **Subheading 3.4, step 5.**).
6. Incubate these cultures for a total of 10–14 d or until the adherent layer has reached ~80% confluency. Irradiate the 96–well plates (without subculturing) with 1500 cGy from a γ-irradiation or X-ray source. Incubate cultures for a minimum of 24 h prior to the addition of test cells. Irradiated murine marrow feeders can be used for up to 14 d, but if delays of >7 d are anticipated, the mLTCM should be changed after the first 7 d.

3.7.2. Initiation of Murine LTC-IC LDA Cultures

Assessment of LTC-IC in different populations of murine cells is subject to many of the same problems that can affect the determination of human LTC-IC values (*see* **Subheading 3.3.**). For example, insert assays of unseparated murine fetal liver on irradiated murine marrow feeders can also result in an outgrowth of macrophages from the input-cell suspension which inhibits all further hematopoietic activity *(29)*. However, this problem can be avoided by prior depletion of the lin$^+$ cells in the suspension to be analyzed and other purification strategies (*see* Chapters 1 and 2). The frequencies of LTC-IC in unseparated bone marrow and purified populations of murine hematopoietic cells shown in **Table 3** can be used to estimate appropriate cell doses. For example, the expected frequency of LTC-IC in murine bone marrow is ~1/20,000 to 1/50,000. Therefore, LDA analysis using aliquots of 6×10^4, 3×10^4, 1.5×10^4, and 7.5×10^3 marrow cells per well with 12 replicates per dose should yield an accurate estimation of their LTC-IC content.

1. Prepare test cells in mLTCM.
2. Remove ~90% of mLTCM from the wells of the 96-well culture plate using a multichannel pipetter and sterile tips.
3. Add test cells in a 0.15-mL vol. to the wells and place the 96-well plate in a loosely covered container (i.e., 20 cm square bacterial plates) with 2–3 uncovered 35-mm dishes containing sterile water. Incubate in a humidified incubator at 33°C in an atmosphere of 5% CO_2 in air.
4. Perform weekly one-half media changes with freshly prepared mLTCM after 1, 2, and 3 wk.
5. At the end of the 4-wk culture period, harvest adherent and nonadherent cells from each individual well, as described in **Subheading 3.4.**
6. Plate cells in methylcellulose media for murine cells as described in **Subheading 3.4.**
7. Incubate murine CFC assays for 12 d and record the number of colonies present in each methylcellulose culture. Record well as negative if no CFC is present, and as positive if ≥1 CFC is present.
8. The frequency of LTC-IC is established using Poisson distribution and the method of maximum likelihood (*see* **Subheading 3.5.**).

4. Notes

1. Collagen-coating of tissue culture dishes promotes and prolongs the adherence to tissue-culture dishes of cell lines such as the M2-10B4 and Sl/Sl lines used as feeders, particularly after they are irradiated. To coat dishes, add 1–2 mL of sterile collagen solution (~1 mg/mL of Type 1 from bovine, rat, or human sources), and spread evenly; then remove excess collagen and allow the surface to dry in biosafety hood. Store tightly wrapped at 4°C for up to 1 mo. The precoated dishes can be rinsed once with sterile phosphate buffered saline (PBS) or culture medium to neutralize the acidity of the thin collagen coating prior to use.
2. A variation of methodology used for quantitation of LTC-IC is one that measures the maturing progeny of the CFC produced in LTC, directly *in situ*, where they tend to form areas that resemble patches of cobblestones—hence the term "cobble-

stone-area-forming cells" (CAFC) (*see* Chapter 9). This procedure avoids the labor and materials required to undertake CFC assays, but it is time-consuming and more subjective to evaluate, since a cobblestone must be distinguished against a background of other cells. The conditions prevailing in LTC are typically suboptimal for stimulating terminal granulopoiesis, whereas these are optimized in CFC assays.

3. The proliferative ability exhibited by individual human LTC-IC in a given tissue has been found to vary over a wide range. In addition, the average proliferative ability of LTC-IC depends on the ontological tissue source of the cells and the LTC-IC assay conditions. The average number of CFC per human bone marrow LTC-IC cultured for 5 wk on irradiated primary marrow or M2-10B4 cells and assayed in methylcellulose media containing 20 ng/mL each of IL-3, IL-6, GM-CSF, and G-CSF and 50 ng/mL SCF is 7 ± 3 *(14)*. The average number of CFC per LTC-IC, assayed using a mixture of M2–10B4:Sl/Sl engineered feeder layers and a 6-wk culture period, is 18 ± 6 for adult bone marrow, 25 ± 5 for G-CSF mobilized blood, 28 ± 2 for cord blood *(14)*, and 72 ± 18 for human fetal liver *(18)*.

References

1. Dexter, T. M., Allen, T. D., and Lajtha, L. G. (1977) Conditions controlling the proliferation of hemopoietic stem cells in vitro. *J. Cell. Physiol.* **91,** 335–344.
2. Dexter, T. M., Spooncer, E., Toksoz, D., and Lajtha, L. G. (1980) The role of cells and their products in the regulation of in vitro stem cell proliferation and granulocyte development. *J. Supramol. Struc.* **13,** 513–524.
3. Gartner, S. and Kaplan, H.S. (1980) Long-term culture of human bone marrow cells. *Proc. Natl. Acad. Sci. USA* **77,** 4756–4759.
4. Whitlock, C. A. and Witte, O. N. (1982) Long-term culture of B lymphocytes and their precursors from murine bone marrow. *Proc. Natl. Acad. Sci. USA* **79,** 3608–3612.
5. van den Brink, M. R., Boggs, S. S., Herberman, R. B., and Hiserodt, J. C. (1990) The generation of natural killer (NK) cells from NK precursor cells in rat long-term bone marrow cultures. *J. Exp. Med.* **172,** 303–313.
6. Miller, J. S., Verfaillie, C., and McGlave, P. (1992) The generation of human natural killer cells from CD34⁺/DR⁻ primitive progenitors in long-term bone marrow culture. *Blood* **80,** 2182–2187.
7. Rawlings, D. J., Quan, S. G., Kato, R. M., and Witte, O. N. (1995). Long-term culture system for selective growth of human B-cell progenitors. *Proc. Natl. Acad. Sci. USA* **92,** 1570–1574.
8. Greenberger, J.S. (1978) Sensitivity of corticosteroid-dependent insulin-resistant lipogenesis in marrow preadipocytes of obese-diabetic (db/db) mice. *Nature* **275,** 752–754.
9. Sutherland, H. J. Eaves, C. J, Eaves, A. C., Dragowska, W., and Lansdorp, P. M (1989) Characterization and partial purification of human marrow cells capable of initiating long-term hematopoiesis in vitro. *Blood* **74,** 1563–1570.
10. Sutherland, H. J., Lansdorp, P. M., Henkelman, D. H., Eaves, A. C., and Eaves, C.

J. (1990). Functional characterization of individual human hematopoietic stem cells cultured at limiting dilution on supportive marrow stromal layers. *Proc. Natl. Acad. Sci. USA* **87,** 3584–3588.

11. Ploemacher, R. E., van der Sluijs, J. P., Voerman, J. S. A., and Brons, N. H. C. (1989) An in vitro limiting-dilution assay of long-term repopulating hematopoietic stem cells in the mouse. *Blood* **74,** 2755–2763.

12. Lemieux, M. E., Rebel, V. I., Lansdorp, P. M., and Eaves, C. J. (1995) Characterization and purification of a primitive hematopoietic cell type in adult mouse marrow capable of lymphomyeloid differentiation in long-term marrow "switch" cultures. *Blood* **86,** 1339–1347.

13. Sutherland, H. J., Eaves, C. J., Lansdorp, P. M., Thacker, J. D., and Hogge, D. E. (1991) Differential regulation of primitive human hematopoietic cells in long-term cultures maintained on genetically engineered murine stromal cells. *Blood* **78,** 666–672.

14. Hogge, D. E., Lansdorp, P. M., Reid, D., Gerhard, B., and Eaves, C. J. (1996) Enhanced detection, maintenance, and differentiation of primitive human hematopoietic cells in cultures containing murine fibroblasts engineered to produce human steel factor, interleukin-3, and granulocyte colony-stimulating factor. *Blood* **88,** 3765–3773.

15. Fazekas de St. Groth, S. (1982) The evaluation of limiting dilution assays. *J. Immunol. Methods* **49,** R11.

16. Prosper, F., Stroncek, D., and Verfaillie, C. M. (1996). Phenotypic and functional characterization of long-term culture-initiating cells present in peripheral blood progenitor collections of normal donors treated with granulocyte colony-stimulating factor. *Blood* **88,** 2033–2042.

17. Roy, V., Miller, J. S., and Verfaillie, C. M. (1997) Phenotypic and functional characterization of committed and primitive myeloid and lymphoid hematopoietic precursors in human fetal liver. *Exp. Hematol.* **25,** 387–394.

18. Nicolini, F. E., Holyoake, T. L., Cashman, J. D., Chu, P. P. Y., Lambie, K., and Eaves, C. J. (1999) Unique differentiation programs of human fetal liver stem cells revealed both in vitro and in vivo in NOD/SCID mice. *Blood* **94,** 2686–2695.

19. Punzel, M., Moore, K. A., Lemischka, I. R., and Verfaillie, C. M. (1999) The type of stromal feeder used in limiting dilution assays influences frequency and maintenance assessment of human long-term culture initiating cells. *Leukemia* **13,** 92–97.

20. Croisille, L., Auffray, I., Katz, A., Izac, B., Vainchenker, W., and Coulombel, L. (1994) Hydrocortisone differentially affects the ability of murine stromal cells and human marrow-derived adherent cells to promote the differentiation of CD34^{++}/CD38$^-$ long-term culture initiating cells. *Blood* **84,** 4116–4124.

21. Verfaille, C. (1992) Direct contact between human primitive hematopoietic progenitors and bone marrow stroma is not required for long-term *in vitro* hematopoiesis. *Blood* **79,** 2821–2826.

22. Pettengell, R., Luft, T., Henschler, R., Hows, J. M., Dexter, M., Ryder, D., and Testa, N. G. (1994) Direct comparison by limiting dilution analysis of long-term

culture-initiating cells in bone marrow, umbilical cord blood and blood stem cells. *Blood* **84,** 3653–3659.

23. Sauvageau, G., Lansdorp, P. M., Eaves, C. J., Hogge, D. E., Dragowska, W. H., Reid, D. S., et al. (1994) Differential expression of homeobox genes in functionally distinct CD34+ subpopulations of human bone marrow cells. *Proc. Natl. Acad. Sci. USA* **91,** 12,223–12,227.

24. Petzer, A., Hogge, D. E., Lansdorp, P. M., Reid, D. S., and Eaves, C. J. (1996) Self-renewal of primitive human hematopoietic cells (long-term-culture-initiating cells) *in vitro* and their expansion in defined medium. *Proc. Natl. Acad. Sci. USA* **93,** 1470–1474.

25. Conneally, E., Cashman, J., Petzer, A., and Eaves, C. (1997) Expansion in vitro of transplantable human cord blood stem cells demonstrated using a quantitative assay of their lympho-myeloid repopulating activity in nonobese diabetic-*scid/scid* mice. *Proc. Natl. Acad. Sci. USA* **94,** 9836–9841.

26. Kogler, G., Callejas, J., Sorg, R. V., and Wernet, P. (1998) An eight-fold *ex vivo* expansion of long-term culture-initiating cells from umbilical cord blood in stirred suspension cultures. *Bone Marrow Transplant* **21(Suppl. 3),** S48–S53.

27. Zandstra, P. W., Conneally, E., Piret, J. M., and Eaves, C. J. (1998) Ontogeny-associated changes in the cytokine responses of primitive human haemopoietic cells. *Br. J. Haematol.* **101,** 770–778

28. Miller, C. L., Rebel, V. I., Lemieux, M. E., Helgason, C. D., Lansdorp, P. M., and Eaves, C. J. (1996) Studies of *W* mutant mice provide evidence for alternate mechanisms capable of activating hematopoietic stem cells. *Exp. Hematol.* **24,** 185–194.

29. Miller, C. L., Rebel, V. I., Helgason, C. D., Lansdorp, P. M., and Eaves, C. J. (1997) Impaired steel factor responsiveness differentially affects the detection and long-term maintenance of fetal liver hematopoietic stem cells in vivo. *Blood* **89,** 1214–1223.

30. Hao, Q-L., Shah, A. J., Thiemann, F. T., Smogorzewska, E. M., and Crooks, G. M. (1995) A functional comparison of CD34+CD38− cells in cord blood and bone marrow. *Blood* **86,** 3745–3753.

31. Civin, C. I., Almeida-Porada, G., Lee, M. J., Olweus, J., Terstappen, L. W., and Zanjani, E. D. (1996) Sustained, retransplantable, multilineage engraftment of highly purified adult human bone marrow stem cells in vivo. *Blood* **88,** 4102–4109.

32. Bhatia, M., Wang, J. C. Y., Kapp, U., Bonnet, D., and Dick J. E. (1997) Purification of primitive human hematopoietic cells capable of repopulating immune-deficient mice. *Proc. Natl. Acad. Sci. USA* **94,** 5320–5325

33. Itoh, K., Tezuka, H., Sakoda, H., Konno, M., Nagata, K., Uchiyama, T., et al. (1989) Reproducible establishment of hemopoietic supportive stromal cell lines from murine bone marrow. *Exp. Hematol.* **17,** 145–153.

34. Wineman, J., Moore, K., Lemischka, I., and Müller-Sieberg, C. (1996) Functional heterogeneity of the hematopoietic microenvironment: rare stromal elements maintain long-term repopulating stem cells. *Blood* **87,** 4082–4090.

35. Thiemann, F. T., Moore, K. A., Smogorzewska, E. M., Lemischka, I. R. and Crooks, G. M. (1996) The murine stromal cell line AFT204 acts specifically on human CD34⁺CD38⁻ progenitors to maintain primitive function and immunophenotype in vitro. Exp. Hematol. **26,** 612–619.

36. Collins, L. S. and Dorshkind, K. (1987) A stromal cell line from myeloid long term bone marrow cultures can support myelopoiesis and B lymphopoiesis. *J. Immunol.* **138,** 1082–1087.

37. Ponchio, L., Conneally, E., and Eaves, C. (1995) Quantitation of the quiescent fraction of long-term culture-initiating cells in normal human blood and marrow and the kinetics of their growth factor-stimulated entry into S-phase in vitro. *Blood* **86,** 3314–3321.

38. Hunt, P., Robertson, D., Weiss, D., Rennick, D., Lee, F., and Witte, O. N. (1987) A single bone marrow-derived stromal cell types supports the *in vitro* growth of early myeloid and lymphoid cells. *Cell* **48,** 997–1007.

39. Berardi, A. C., Meffre, E., Pflumio, F., Katz, A., Vainchenker, W., Schiff, C., and Coulombel, L. (1997) Individual CD34⁺CD38^low^CD19⁻CD10⁻progenitor cells from human cord blood generate B lymphocytes and granulocytes. *Blood* **89,** 3554–3564.

40. Hao, Q-L., Smogorzewska, E. M., Barsky, L. W., and Crooks, G. M. (1998) In vitro identification of single CD34⁺CD38⁻ cells with both lymphoid and mycloid potential. *Blood* **91,** 4145–4151.

41. Miller, J. S., McCullar, V., Punzel, M., Lemischka, I. R., and Moore, K. A. (1999). Single adult human CD34⁺/Lin⁻ CD38⁻ progenitors give rise to natural killer cells, B-lineage cells, dendritic cells and myeloid cells. *Blood* **93,** 96–101.

42. Punzel, M., Wissink, S. D., Miller, J. S., Moore, K. A., Lemischka, I. R., and Verfaillie, C. M. (1999) The myeloid-lymphoid initiating cell (ML-IC) assay assesses the fate of multipotent human progenitors in vitro. *Blood* **93,** 3750–3756.

9

The Cobblestone-Area-Forming Cell Assay

Gerald de Haan and Rob Ploemacher

1. Introduction

Hematopoietic stem cell (HSC) subsets are defined by the capacity to which their offspring can contribute to the various mature blood-cell lineages. However, the proliferative potential of stem cells is highly dependent on the environment in which they reside, and it is only in retrospect that the characteristics of a stem cell can be identified. Partly because of these elusive properties of stem cells, various functional assays to measure their frequency have been developed, both in vivo and in vitro. Various chapters in this volume each describe one of these assays. All these assays have the ability to quantify stem cells with certain properties, but not others. Therefore, the determination of which stem-cell assay will be most appropriate to use is highly dependent on a particular experimental setting. This chapter describes the cobblestone-area-forming cell (CAFC) assay *(1)*.

The CAFC assay is a miniaturized long-term bone-marrow culture set up in 96-well plates in which a stromal cell layer is first allowed to grow to confluency. Because of reproducibility and other practical considerations, it is easiest to use a defined stromal-cell line for this purpose. Stromal-cell lines exhibit great variation in their methods of sustaining such long-term bone-marrow cultures, and therefore it is of crucial importance to select one that has been demonstrated to be a good "supporter." Few single-lab published studies have compared the various cell lines that have been described, but two excellent papers from Muller-Sieburg et al. may be useful for for this purpose *(2,3)*. Some lines with reasonable-to-good supportive activity include S17 *(4)* (originating from the Dorshkind lab), CFC034, 2012, AFT024 *(5,6)* (from the

From: *Methods in Molecular Medicine, vol. 63: Hematopoietic Stem Cell Protocols*
Edited by: C. A. Klug and C. T. Jordan © Humana Press Inc., Totowa, NJ

Lemishka lab), and Flask Bone Marrow Dexter-1 (FBMD-1), the cell line we routinely use *(7)* (from the Neben lab).

When the stromal cells have grown confluent, the layer is seeded by the cell suspension to be tested in a limiting-dilution analysis (LDA). For unknown reasons, primitive cells present in the inoculated cell sample migrate through the stromal layer, where they begin to proliferate at time-points defined by their primitiveness. At sequential time-points after initiation of the assay individual wells are microscopically screened for the presence or absence of "cobblestone areas," which we define as colonies of at least five small, nonrefractile cells that grow underneath the stromal layer. The frequency of more committed progenitor subsets is evaluated by scoring the plates at d 7 (mouse) or d 14 (human), whereas colonies that appear later in time are derived from more primitive cell subsets. In the mouse, we routinely evaluate our cultures for 5 wk, and for human measurements we extend the period to wk 8.

As with any technique, there are advantages and disadvantages in using this assay. Many mouse studies have shown that CAFC subsets measured over a 5-wk period correlate very well with stem-cell frequencies obtained by in vivo colony-forming unit-spleen (CFU-S) or competitive repopulation assays *(8–11)*. Clearly, for these in vivo assays, large numbers of animals are needed, compared to several 96-wells plates for a CAFC assay. Thus, an important consideration for using this assay is its extreme cost reduction. In addition, the CAFC assay evaluated at multiple time-points measures the entire spectrum of hematopoietic progenitor- and stem-cell frequencies in one single-assay system (2–4 96-well plates), which compares favorably with the unavoidable separate analysis of CFU-S d-8, CFU-S d-12, and long-term repopulating ability/competitive repopulating unit (LTRA/CRU) frequencies.

As the most strict definition of a pluripotent HSC states that such a cell should be able to fully reconstitute all the blood-cell lineages of a properly conditioned recipient, the most important weakness of the CAFC (and any in vitro) assay is that it will always remain a surrogate method to quantify stem cells. It is likely that conditions exist in which stem cells will flourish upon in vivo transplantation, but will fail to thrive in a CAFC assay. Conversely, stem cells may be detected in the CAFC assay, although their existence cannot be confirmed in an in vivo setting. In such situations, it is important to remember that a stem cell may reveal its presence in only one environment (in vitro or in vivo)—not in the other.

2. Materials

1. Stromal-cell line with proven capacity to support in vitro growth of stem cells.
2. 96-well plates, tissue-culture-treated, low evaporation lid (Costar #3595).
3. 14-mL plastic tubes for preparing cell dilutions (Greiner #191180).

4. Iscove's modified Dulbecco's medium (IMDM) supplemented with L-glutamine (Gibco-BRL #10099–141).
5. Horse serum (HS)(Gibco-BRL #16050–098) and fetal calf serum (FCS) (Gibco-BRL *10099–141), pretested batches.
6. Hydrocortison hemisuccinate (Sigma #H4881).
7. Penicillin/streptomycin (Gibco-BRL #15140–114).
8. β-mercaptoethanol (B-ME) (Merck #805740).
9. 0.05% trypsin/EDTA (ethylenediaminetetraaceticacid).
10. Phosphate-buffered saline (PBS).
11. Gelatin (Sigma # G2500).
12. Multichanel pipettor.
13. Eppendorf varipette.
14. Vacuum line/system with sucking device.
15. Inverted (phase-contrast) microscope (×100).

3. Methods

3.1. Stromal-Cell Lines

Several investigators have described stromal-cell lines that can be used in a CAFC assay. Some of these cell lines, like AFT024, require irradiation of the confluent layer before the CAFC assay is initiated, to prevent continuous cell proliferation. Others, like FBMD-1, are contact-inhibited and will stop dividing upon reaching confluency. Before 96-well plates are inoculated with stromal cells, great care should be taken to handle the cells, each according to its own specific demands. For FBMD-1 cells this implies regular passaging (2–3 times per wk), and ensuing that the cells never grow confluent. To passage the FBMD-1 cells, we culture them in Dulbecco's modified Eagle's medium (DMEM), 15% FCS, 5 HS, 10^{-5} M hydrocortisone, 80 U/mL penicillin, 80 µg/mL streptomycin, and 10^{-4} M β-mercaptoethanol (B-ME) in an incubator at 33°C, flushed with 5% CO_2 in air.

3.2. Mouse CAFC Assay

FBMD-1 cells are harvested 10–14 d prior to an experiment using a standard trypsinization protocol and seeded in 96-well plates at a frequency of ~1000 cells/well (in 200 µL). To avoid evaporation and contamination only the inner 60 wells of each plate are used. The outer wells of the plate can be filled with sterile water if evaporation of the inner wells is a problem. Within 1 wk a confluent monolayer of cells will form. In the mouse system we have used the CAFC assay to measure stem cells in the bone marrow, spleen, peripheral blood, and liver. Great care should be taken to harvest these test cells in conditions as sterile as possible, because the risk of contamination is substantially higher than with short-term CFU assays. The CAFC assay is a limit-

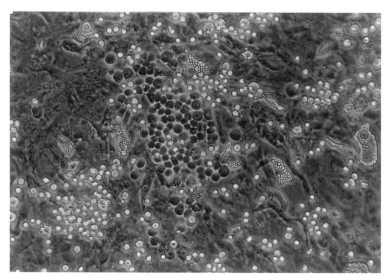

Fig. 1. A cobblestone area. The distinction between phase-dim cells proliferating underneath the FBMD-1 stromal layer (true cobblestone areas) and phase-bright cells that settle on top of the stroma is clearly visible. Also note fat accumulation in FMBD-1 cells, which may sometimes confound analysis.

ing-dilution type assay, and therefore the test cells are inoculated onto the stroma in various dilutions. We always use six dilutions per sample, with each dilution threefold apart. Using normal bone-marrow cells, we start with a cell concentration of 81,000 cells/well, going down to 333 cells/well. Because of the low frequency of stem cells in the normal spleen we start our spleen assay with 729,000 cells/well, going down in six steps to 3000 cells/well. However, experimental conditions may result in much higher or lower stem-cell numbers than normal, and the dilutions to be tested should then be adjusted accordingly. When test cells are introduced in the assay, the medium is switched from 15% FCS/5% HS to 20% HS. Most of the medium is taken from the wells, with a multichannel pipet or a sucking device that can be flame-sterilized. Test samples are inoculated in a vol of 200 µL. For each cell dilution, 20–30 replicate wells are tested. Early-appearing cobblestone areas (d 7) correspond to colony-forming unit-granulocyte, macrophage (CFU-GM), and their frequency is relatively high in normal marrow. Therefore, cell dilutions with low cell numbers (typically 3000–333) are scored at this time. With increasing culturing time wells that were seeded with higher cell doses are evaluated. Only dilutions containing both negative and positive wells are informative for the frequency analysis. Thus, only three of the six dilutions are typically scored at a given time. To assay the entire stem-cell spectrum, the appearance of cobblestone areas is evaluated at weekly intervals, for 5 wk. It is important to emphasize that only colonies growing underneath the stromal layer—consisting of at least five small nonrefractile cells are counted—at × 100 magnification and phase-contrast illumination on an inverted microscope. A photograph of a cobblestone area is shown in **Fig. 1**. It is important to note that because of light deflection in a 96-well plate, the dim appearance of true cobblestones illuminated by phase-contrast is somewhat lost. For those unfamiliar with the appearance of cobblestone areas, it may be worthwhile to set up a culture in a tissue-culture flask where the colonies are much easier to detect. Once a week one-half of the medium (~100 µL) in a well is replaced with fresh medium. There are various ways to do this; one can use a multichannel pipet or a sucking device. Inevitably some nonadherent cells may be removed as well, but since immature cells will reside underneath the stroma, this will not affect frequency analysis. The actual volume of medium in the well may change over time because of the repeated removal and adding of medium. As long as there is no excessive evaporation (which we have never encountered), this is no problem, since the frequency analysis is based on the number of cells that have initiated the culture, and not the volume in which they were suspended.

3.3. Human CAFC Assay

The human CAFC assay exploits a visual end point for multiple enumeration of a series of stem-cell subsets differing in their sensitivity to e.g. chemotherapeutic agents as 5-fluorouracil (5-FU) and busulphan, expression of various cell-surface markers (CD34, HLA-DR) or dyes that relate to intracellular organels or parameters (rhodamine 123, calcein, FURA-2), and their ability for transient and long-term engraftment of stromal layers *(12)*. Technically, this assay is performed according to the method outlined in **Subheading 3.2.** for mouse cells. However, addition of low concentrations of human IL-3 and G-CSF may be considered, since this will result in larger cobblestone areas. The striking and overlapping characteristics of human and murine CAFC subsets strongly suggest that the human CAFC wk 1–2 subset is analogous to the murine spleen colony forming CFU-S, whereas the human CAFC wk 6–12 enumerates primitive stem cells that are responsible for the sustained maintenance of blood-cell production or for stable in vivo engraftment of hematopoiesis following cytotoxic treatment. In fact, the CAFC wk 12s are most indicative for the NOD/SCID repopulating ability *(13,14)*. The validation of the human CAFC/long-term culture-initiating cell (LTC-IC) wk 6–12 as an assay detecting in vivo engrafting potential awaits long-term follow-up of sufficient numbers of patients (co)engrafted with genetically marked stem cells, which include the phenotypic criteria described for these primitive stem cells.

Stroma-supported long-term cultures (LTC) allow estimation of stem-cell quality by simultaneous enumeration of HSC frequencies in a graft using the

Table 1
CAFC Frequencies per 10⁵ Cells in Bone Marrow and Peripheral Blood in Mice and Humans

	wk 1	wk 2	wk 3	wk 4	wk 5	wk 6
C57BL/6 BM	100 (63–142)	18 (14–19)	5 (4–12)	2.3 (2–6)	1.1 (0.8–2.6)	nd
DBA/2 BM	125 (88–200)	77 (45–85)	18 (5–38)	7.6 (8–10)	3.7 (3–4)	nd
BDF1 BM	111 (79–127)	30 (25–42)	8 (7–11)	5 (4–6)	3.1 (2.6–4.1)	nd
Human BM	47 (20–100)	114 (20–330)	110 (30–400)	69 (15–300)	36 (5–120)	23 (3–80)
Human peripheral blood	19 (0.8–210)	31 (0.9–200)	41 (11–230)	21 (0.4–200)	15 (0.4–100)	10 (0.4–57)

Data are presented as mean values +/- range. nd = not determined.

CAFC assay, and the ability of the graft to generate progenitors in flask long-term culture-colony-forming cells (LTC-CFC). Thus, we have recently observed that the number and quality of mobilized peripheral-blood (MPB) stem cells was low in patients who received multiple rounds of chemotherapy *(15)*. Moreover, grafts with low numbers of HSC and poor HSC quality had a high probability of graft failure upon their autologous infusion. Similarly, our data have indicated that, although CAFC wk-2 *qualities* differ little (1-log ranges), the CAFC wk-6 *frequencies* are within 2-log ranges in bone marrow and umbilical-cord blood (UCB), and a 3-log range in MPB. In addition, CAFC quality varied little between the bone-marrow grafts (1-log range) and more between peripheral blood grafts (3-log), and ranges of CAFC quality differed even 4-log in UCB grafts. There was little difference in variability when the data were plotted per nucleated cells, or per CD34+ cells. These data suggest that some UCB grafts will be associated with poor engraftment.

3.4. Frequency Estimation, Limiting-Dilution Analysis

As a reference **Table 1** provides CAFC frequencies that can be observed in normal tissues. Typically, within inbred strains of mice, the CAFC frequencies measured in bone marrow are very consistent, whereas human CAFC frequencies vary much more. Between inbred strains of mice, however, significant variation is observed *(16–19)*.

4. Notes

1. Over time, many cells will accumulate in wells that at one time contain a stem- or progenitor cell. Counting cells on top of the stroma (cells that appear phase-bright) will result in a gross overestimation of the number of stem cells present. Experiments in which the entire content of a well was replated in a methylcellulose assay have revealed that only wells containing true cobblestone areas, growing underneath the stroma, will produce CFU-GM (varying from a few to several dozens per positive well), indicating that primitive hematopoietic cells can only be found in wells containing cobblestone areas.

2. One of the major problems with the CAFC assay is that the stromal layer may detach from the surface of the 96-well plate. This is particularly evident when human cells are used, because these cultures must be maintained significantly longer than for the mouse system. Obviously, if the entire stromal layer has disappeared, no reliable quantification is possible. To avoid detachment several steps may be considered. First, the choice of the 96-well plates may need to be re-evaluated. Be sure to use flat-bottom, tissue-culture-treated plates. Second, detachment is most frequently observed in wells that were inoculated with a high cell number. Therefore, it is important to reduce the cell dose as much as possible. Third, the 96-well plates may be precoated with gelatin. For this purpose, use a 0.3% gelatin solution (add 1.5 g to 500 mL distilled water and autoclave). Add

200 µL to each well and incubate the plates for 4 h at 37°C, or overnight at room temperature. After coating, the entire content of the wells is removed, and plates are ready for use. Plates can be dried after coating by placing them on one side and slightly opened in a laminar flow hood. After drying, plates can be stored at 4°C for weeks when packed in aluminum foil.

3. Since CAFC cultures must be maintained for extended periods of time, during which the cells are repeatedly fed, contamination can be a major problem of the CAFC assay. If this occurs the best solution is to add 1 M NaOH to the contaminated well plus the surrounding wells, remove the entire contents from the wells, and fill the wells completely with 1 M NaOH. It is advisable to change the lid of the plate as well. Check for spreading of the contamination during the next few days, and repeat the procedure if needed.

References

1. Ploemacher, R. E., van der Sluijs, J. P., van Beurden, C. A., Baert, M. R., and Chan, P. L. (1991) Use of limiting-dilution type long-term marrow cultures in frequency analysis of marrow-repopulating and spleen colony-forming hematopoietic stem cells in the mouse. *Blood* **78,** 2527–2533.
2. Deryugina, E. I. and Muller-Sieburg, C. E. (1993) Stromal cells in long-term cultures: keys to the elucidation of hematopoietic development? *Crit. Rev. Immunol.* **13,** 115–150.
3. Muller-Sieburg, C. E. and Deryugina, E. (1995) The stromal cells' guide to the stem cell universe. *Stem Cells* (Dayton) **13,** 477–486.
4. Collins, L. S. and Dorshkind, K. (1987) A stromal cell line from myeloid long-term bone marrow cultures can support myelopoiesis and B lymphopoiesis. *J. Immunol.* **138,** 1082–1087.
5. Moore, K. A., Ema, H., and Lemischka, I. R. (1997) In vitro maintenance of highly purified, transplantable hematopoietic stem cells. *Blood* **89,** 4337–4347.
6. Wineman, J., Moore, K., Lemischka, I., and Muller-Sieburg, C. (1996) Functional heterogeneity of the hematopoietic microenvironment: rare stromal elements maintain long-term repopulating stem cells. *Blood* **87,** 4082–4090.
7. Neben, S., Anklesaria, P., Greenberger, J., and Mauch, P. (1993) Quantitation of murine hematopoietic stem cells in vitro by limiting dilution analysis of cobblestone area formation on a clonal stromal cell line. *Exp. Hematol.* **21,** 438–443.
8. Down, J. D. and Ploemacher, R. E. (1993) Transient and permanent engraftment potential of murine hematopoietic stem cell subsets: differential effects of host conditioning with gamma radiation and cytotoxic drugs. *Exp. Hematol.* **21,** 913–921.
9. Down, J. D., Boudewijn, A., Vanos, R., Thames, H. D., and Ploemacher, R. E. (1995) Variations in radiation sensitivity and repair among different hematopoietic stem cell subsets following fractionated irradiation. *Blood* **86,** 122–127.
10. Ploemacher, R. E., van der Loo, J. C., van Beurden, C. A., and Baert, M. R. (1993) Wheat germ agglutinin affinity of murine hemopoietic stem cell subpopulations is an inverse function of their long-term repopulating ability in vitro and in vivo. *Leukemia* **7,** 120–130.

11. Down, J. D., de Haan, G., Dillingh, J. H., Dontje, B., and Nijhof, W. (1997) Stem cell factor has contrasting effects in combination with 5–fluorouracil or total-body irradiation on frequencies of different hemopoietic cell subsets and engraftment of transplanted bone marrow. *Radiat. Res.* **147,** 680–685.
12. Breems, D. A., Blokland, E. A., Neben, S., and Ploemacher, R. E. (1994) Frequency analysis of human primitive haematopoietic stem cell subsets using a cobblestone area forming cell assay. *Leukemia* **8,** 1095–1104.
13. van Hennik, P. B., Verstegen, M. M., Bierhuizen, M. F., Limon, A., Wognum, A. W., Cancelas, J. A., et al. (1998) Highly efficient transduction of the green fluorescent protein gene in human umbilical cord blood stem cells capable of cobblestone formation in long-term cultures and multilineage engraftment of immunodeficient mice. *Blood* **92,** 4013–4022.
14. Verstegen, M. M., van Hennik, P. B., Terpstra ,W., van den Bos, C., Wielenga, J. J., van Rooijen, N., et al. (1998) Transplantation of human umbilical cord blood cells in macrophage- depleted SCID mice: evidence for accessory cell involvement in expansion of immature CD34+CD38– cells. *Blood* **91,** 1966–1976.
15. Breems, D. A., van Hennik, P. B., Kusadasi, N., Boudewijn, A., Cornelissen, J. J., Sonneveld, P., et al. (1996) Individual stem cell quality in leukapheresis products is related to the number of mobilized stem cells. *Blood* **87,** 5370–5378.
16. de Haan, G., Nijhof, W., and Van Zant, G. (1997) Mouse strain-dependent changes in frequency and proliferation of hematopoietic stem cells during aging: correlation between lifespan and cycling activity. *Blood* **89,** 1543–1550.
17. de Haan, G. and Van Zant, G. (1999) Dynamic changes in mouse hematopoietic stem cell numbers during aging. *Blood* **93,** 3294–3301.
18. de Haan, G. and Van Zant, G. (1997) Intrinsic and extrinsic control of hemopoietic stem cell numbers: mapping of a stem cell gene. *J. Exp. Med.* **186,** 529–536.
19. de Haan, G. and Van Zant, G. (1999) Genetic analysis of hemopoietic cell cycling in mice suggests its involvement in organismal life span. *FASEB J.* **13,** 707–713.

10

CFU-S

An Assay for Pluripotent Myelopoietic Stem Cells

Ernest A. McCulloch

1. Introduction

The functional cells of the blood are short-lived; they are replaced continuously by proliferation and differentiation of hematopoietic precursors. Since cell division is required, exposure to agents that destroy proliferative potential is followed by loss or reduction in blood-cell production, and often death. Ionizing radiation and certain chemotherapeutic drugs are examples of agents that are toxic to stem-cell proliferation. Death after irradiation can be prevented by transplanting hematopoietic cells from healthy donors. In the injured host, these are capable of initiating and maintaining the blood-cell production required for survival.

Hematopoietic cells are arranged as an hierarchy, headed by stem cells that can either make new cells like themselves (self-renewal) or pass through a process called determination. After determination, the cells lose their self-renewing capacity, but are able to undergo limited terminal divisions associated with the appearance of differentiated features, such as hemoglobin in red blood cells (RBC) and the specific organelles of granulocytes or platelets. Research on hematopoietic regulation, function, and response to damage requires assays for cells at different stages in the hierarchy. Measurements of stem cells—the origins of the hierarchy—are important because these cells are required to maintain hematopoiesis. The assay must be selective because the stem-cell population is small—approximately one stem cell is hidden in a thousand mature or maturing progeny. The spleen-colony assay measures hematopoietic

From: *Methods in Molecular Medicine, vol. 63: Hematopoietic Stem Cell Protocols*
Edited by: C. A. Klug and C. T. Jordan © Humana Press Inc., Totowa, NJ

stem cells (HSC) because it selects for cells with extensive proliferative capacity. The assay depends upon the observation that murine myelopoietic stem cells transplanted into suitable recipients lodge in the spleen, where they grow and differentiate locally, forming macroscopic colonies of hematopoietic cells.

The linear relationship observed between the number of bone-marrow cells transplanted and the spleen-colony count has provided statistical evidence that a single entity is responsible for each spleen colony. This single entity has a functional name: colony-forming unit (CFU). Cytological evidence has provided convincing proof that each spleen colony is a clone derived from a single cell *(1)*. The nomenclature has been retained, however, since it remains possible that a second accessory cell contributes to the CFU. Later, as clonogenic hematopoietic cells were identified by culture methods, the designation of the cells forming spleen colonies was expanded to CFU-spleen, or CFU-S.

The composition of spleen colonies provides the evidence that CFU-S are HSC. First, spleen colonies regularly contain more than 10^6 cells; thus, CFU-S have extensive proliferative capacity. Second, the three lineages of myelopoiesis, erythropoietic, granulocytic, and megakaryocytic cells are regularly found in spleen colonies. Thus, CFU-S have the potential for multilineage differentiation. Third, CFU-S are found readily in spleen colonies by transplantation of cells from individual colonies into new hosts. Evidence indicating that expansion of a single cell into a colony includes the generation of new clonogenic cells has shown that CFU-S can differentiate and give rise to cells like themselves. The ability to undergo self-renewal is the most important evidence of the stem-cell nature of CFU-S *(2–4)* *(see* **Note 1**).

2. Materials

1. The most important requirement for the spleen-colony assay is a clean colony of healthy mice that can survive 900–1000 rads of irradiation for 2 wk, while CFU-S form macroscopic colonies (*see* **Note 2**). The mice are inbred, and are usually specific-pathogen-free. They are used for experiments at age 8–10 wk. It is useful if the colony also supports mutant mice of interest, such as animals of genotypes W/W^v and Sl/Sl^d.

2. A convenient and well-calibrated irradiation source is required. Careful measurement of the radiation dose is important. The dose must be large enough to suppress endogenous spleen colony-formation—but not greater, because excess radiation increases mortality. The source of radiation is not crucial; the photons must be sufficiently energetic to provide a uniformly high whole-body dose to the test animals. A convenient radiation source is the mouse irradiator supplied by Nordion International, Inc. (Canada).

3. The other materials are commonly found in laboratories; syringes, needles of various gauges, pipets, test tubes, hemocytometers, counting fluids, and balanced

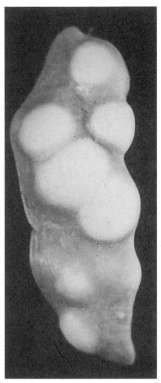

Fig. 1. A mouse spleen showing spleen colonies. The animal was heavily irradiated and injected intravenously with 8×10^4 nucleated marrow cells. Twelve days later, the animal was killed, and the spleens were removed and fixed in Bouin's solution. Reprinted with permission from: McCulloch, E. A. (1996) The origin of the cells of the blood, in *the Physiological Basis of Medical Practice* (Best, C. H. and Taylor, N. B., eds.) 8th ed., pp. 568–584, Williams and Wilkins, Baltimore.

salt solutions and fixatives such as Bouin's solution. To immobilize mice for tail-vein injections, it is useful to cut the tapered end from acrylic centrifuge tubes of sufficient size so that each can hold a mouse. The tail of the mouse is then threaded through a hole in an appropriately sized stopper. The mouse is immobilized, but can breathe through the hole in the tube.

3. Methods

3.1. Transplantation Assay for CFU-S

Waves of hematopoietic repopulation are seen in the spleens of irradiated recipients after transplantation of normal bone-marrow cells. At low transplant-cell numbers, each wave can be identified as macroscopic colonies. Six to seven d after transplantation, small colonies can be seen. These transient colonies are entirely erythropoietic, are characteristic of fetal or rapidly regenerating hematopoiesis, and are under the genetic control of the *f/f* locus *(5,6)*. These early colonies disappear with time, and are replaced by d 9–11 after transplantation by larger colonies that contain the three myelopoietic lineages. These also disappear and by d 12–14 trilineage colonies are seen, with hematopoietic stem-cell progenitors (**Fig. 1**)*(7)*. Assays of colonies of the first two waves are seldom used, since their progenitors may be studied more effectively by tissue-culture methods. However, the capacity to form spleen colonies from d 12–14 remains an important criterion for the identification of myelopoietic stem cells.

1. The CFU-S assay has four components. First, the recipient animals are irradiated; second, the donor marrow suspension is prepared and injected. The irradiation procedure requires preliminary work to ensure appropriate conditions and dose. It is useful to irradiate animals with doses increasing from 700–1000 rads, and to examine their spleens after 12–14 d for macroscopic colonies. This pretest allows the choice of conditions that both suppress endogenous colony formation and permit animal survival (*see* **Note 3**). At the time of experiment, however, the irradiation should be routine; the time between irradiation and bone-marrow injection should be as short as possible (usually no longer than 1 h).

2. The preparation of the bone-marrow suspension should be as aseptic as possible. All instruments, syringes, and test tubes should be sterile at the start of the procedure. If the experimental design calls for culture of the marrow suspension, in addition to CFU-S assay, rigid aseptic conditions may be needed. However, routine clean handling is sufficient.

   a. Femurs are easily removed at the acetabulum, with attached soft tissues. The bones are cleaned by rubbing them gently with aseptic gauze. Then the ends are cut and a 19– or 20-gauge needle, attached to a 5-cc syringe containing Hanks' balanced salt solution (HBSS), is inserted into one end.

   b. The bone-marrow contents are easily flushed into a small test-tube containing HBSS. This tube should be stored in ice water at all times when it is not in use. A single mouse femur usually yields about 10^7 nucleated bone-marrow cells. This value can be used to determine the number of donor mice needed for the cell injections specified in the design.

   c. When marrow collection is completed, the nucleated cell content should be determined by counting the cells in a hemocytometer, after suitable dilution in an acidic counting fluid that lyses erythrocytes. The counts are then used to prepare suspensions for injection as specified in the experimental design. These suspensions are also kept in ice water when not in use.

3. The test suspensions are injected intravenously, usually into the tail vein. Injections of 0.5 mL of cell suspensions are made using a 25-gauge needle and a 1.0-mL tuberculin-type syringe. Injection of a carefully measured volume is required to obtain quantitative measurements of CFU-S (*see* **Notes 4–6**). Once mastered, the injection procedure is easy. It is very useful to observe a proficient person and to learn as part of a working team.

4. The final phases of the method include the housing of the experimental animals, harvesting of spleens after a time specified in the experimental design, and counting the spleen colonies. The mouse colony is protected if the experimental animals are housed in a separate room, because the compromised animals are subject to infection. The cages should inspected at least daily; dead animals should be recorded and removed. To collect the spleens, surviving animals are killed using a protocol approved by the local animal-care committee. The spleens are removed through a left lateral incision and immediately fixed in Bouin's solution or a comparable fixative. The colonies quickly become visible, and can be counted with the naked eye, although some investigators prefer to use a two- to threefold magnifying glass. When the counts are completed, the data is ready for analysis. The results of control and experimental groups are usually expressed as colony-forming efficiency—the number of colonies observed for a fixed number of injected cells (i.e., colonies per 10^5 cells).

3.2. The "F-Factor" for CFU-S

Like other clonogenic assays, the spleen-colony method has a plating efficiency. A component of the plating efficiency can be determined by measuring the fraction "F" of injected CFU-S that reach the spleen (*see* **Note 7**)*(8)*.

1. Aliquots of a marrow suspension are injected into two groups of mice; in the first group of 10 irradiated mice, the cell number is small (8×10^4 cells per mouse) in order to measure the CFU-S concentration in the suspension. The largest possible cell number is injected (approaching 10^7 per animal) into the second group of 5 irradiated mice.
2. 1 h after injection, the mice of the second group are killed, their spleens are removed, and a cell suspension is prepared and counted. The cell count is a measure of the cellular content of the spleens, and is also used to prepare a number of dilutions, ranging from 10^6 to 10^7 cells per mL. These spleen cells are then injected into groups of irradiated recipients.
3. After 12–14 d, mice of groups 1 and the recipients of spleen cells from group 2 are killed, and spleen colonies are enumerated. The first group, together with the cell count, provides a measurement of the number of CFU-S injected into each mouse of group 2. At least one of the groups of recipients of the spleen cells from group 2 will contain an adequate number of colonies. This number is combined with the number of cells recovered per spleen to calculate the number of CFU-S in the spleens of the mice of group 2. These CFU-S will all arrive at the spleen following marrow injection, since the endogenous CFU-S will be inactivated by the high dose of irradiation given to the recipients. Thus, both the number of CFU-S injected and the number recovered from recipient spleens are determined. From these numbers, the fraction of injected cells reaching the spleens can be calculated.

3.3. Mice of Genotype w/wᵛ as Recipients

Mice of genotype *w/wᵛ* are anemic because they have defective CFU-S. When transplanted into irradiated co-isogenic recipients, their marrow fails to form spleen colonies. When normal marrow is injected into intact mice of genotype *w/wᵛ*, spleen colonies are observed, although the recipients have not been irradiated *(9)*. It follows that mice of genotype *w/wᵛ* can be used as recipients in the assay for CFU-S. They are particularly useful when an experimental procedure yields only enough cells for injection into a single animal, since with mice of genotype *w/wᵛ* there is no mortality during the time required for colony formation. Although irradiation is not needed, a small dose (200 rads) makes the colonies more distinct and improves counting, without introducing mortality into the procedure.

3.4. The Endogenous Spleen-Colony Assay

The successive waves of spleen colonies seen in irradiated recipients of normal marrow was described in **Subheading 3.1.** Similar events occur in mice irradiated with sublethal radiation doses. From 10–14 d after such irradiation, mouse spleens contain macroscopic colonies that resemble, grossly and microscopically, the colonies seen after transplantation (*see* **Note 8**). The number of such endogenous spleen colonies decreases exponentially with increasing radiation doses over a range of 750–1000 rads. Endogenous colonies can be used in assays; the procedure is indicated where a need is identified to exclude manipulations of donor cells and transplantation as potential sources of error. For example, the radiation survival curve for CFU-S as measured by the standard spleen-colony assay can be confirmed using the endogenous method. The endogenous method is also useful for preliminary experiments designed to examine the influence of drugs or regulators, since these agents can be administered after radiation and their effects on endogenous colonies can be observed.

4. Notes

1. In the discussion, the identification of CFU-S as a pluripotent HSC was based on three properties, with self-renewal capacity considered the most significant. The observations do not require that CFU-S be the only HSC, or even the most primitive. Experiments either support or deny the possibility that a more primitive stem cell is required for long-term hematopoietic reconstitution after marrow ablation, while CFU-S supplies the short-term reconstitution required for survival. The issue remains controversial *(10–12)*.
2. Survival of a large percentage of mice in each experimental group (>50%) is needed. A higher mortality rate increases the possibility of erroneous results because of selection; the increased number of mice required per group if mortality is high makes the assay very expensive. Survival is improved if the mice are housed

in small, sterile cages with no more than three animals per cage. Drinking water should be sterile, but the addition of antibiotics has not been proven to be helpful.

3. Treatment of mice with a number of substances such as endotoxin prior to irradiation will increase endogenous colony formation. Thus, it is important to ensure adequate irradiation doses when an experimental design includes treatment of recipients before transplantation. Control groups should be included, consisting of mice that received the experimental treatment and radiation but no hematopoietic cells after irradiation. The spleens of these controls should be blank.

4. It is important that the experimental design specify cell numbers to be injected that yield an average from 2–12 colonies per spleen. Small numbers of colonies, while useful, yield small data sets with which to calculate the CFU-S content of the suspensions. Spleens with 1–3 colonies are needed if the design calls for dissection of individual colonies to determine their composition. Spleens with large colony numbers are difficult to count because of overlap. If previous experience with the design is not adequate for establishing the cell number to be injected, it is useful to measure each point by transplanting cell suspensions with two or more different cell concentrations. Then, the linear portion of the curve relating cell number injected to colonies enumerated can be used to describe the CFU-S concentration in the test suspension.

5. It is possible to simplify the injection procedure by loading several doses in a single syringe. This eliminates the need to reload the syringe between injections, but this temptation should be avoided. Cell settling occurs in a syringe loaded with more that 0.5 mL. The results of such settling is wide variation in the number of colonies in the spleens of animals belonging to a single group; the precision of the quantitation is decreased as the error of the mean number of colonies per spleen increases. It is useful to examine the distribution of spleen colonies within a single group. If a striking divergence from Poisson is seen, the mixing of the test sample between injections may have been inadequate.

6. The number of cells injected into each irradiated recipient is a critical part of each experimental design. If sufficient preliminary information is available, it is possible to adjust the injected cell number so that the colony number in the spleens from each experimental group is very similar. For example, in a radiation-dose-response experiment, if a radiation dose is expected to reduce survival of colony-forming capacity to 10% of control, then the cell number injected should be increased 10-fold. This process greatly increases the range of a CFU-S dose-response curve that can be measured; the statistical analysis of the data is also improved. Alternatively, if the expectation is that CFU-S will be greatly reduced, as with some cell separation experiments,the maximum cell number should be injected. At very high cell numbers ($>10^7$ cells/mL), animals may convulse and die during or after injection. This adverse effect can be lessened if small amounts of heparin (1 U/mL) are added to the cell suspension.

7. The measurement of "F" is important in comparisons of the frequency of CFU-S in various suspensions. For example, "F" is higher for fetal liver and lower for spleen compared to adult marrow. "F" also influences the sensitivity of the assay

at low CFU-S frequencies. This may become important in cell-separation experiments, in which some fractions may not lead to spleen colonies and may not be truly negative.

8. Endogenous colonies are much more variable than those seen after marrow transplantation. With a given experimental group of mice receiving the same radiation dose, a wide variation is seen which may be approximated by a log-normal distribution. A similar variation in colony size is also evident. These features limit the quantitative accuracy of the endogenous method.

References

1. Becker, A. J., McCulloch, E. A., and Till, J. E. (1963) Cytological demonstration of the clonal nature of spleen colonies derived from transplanted mouse marrow cells. *Nature* **197,** 452.
2. Till, J. .E and McCulloch, E. A. (1961) A direct measurement of the radiation sensitivity of normal mouse bone marrow cells. *Radiat. Res.* **14,** 213–222.
3. Siminovitch, L., McCulloch E. A., and Till, J. E. (1963) The distribution of colony-forming cells among spleen colonies. *J. Cell. Comp. Physiol.* **62,** 327–336.
4. Till, J. E. and McCulloch, E. A. (1980) Hematopoietic stem cell differentiation. *Biochem. Biophys. Acta* **605,** 431–459.
5. Fowler, J. H., Till, J. E., McCulloch, E. A., and Siminovitch, L. (1967) The cellular basis for the defect in haemopoiesis in flexed-tailed mice. II. The specificity of the defect for erythropoiesis. *Br. J. Haematol.* **13,** 256–264.
6. Gregory, C. J., McCulloch, E. A., and Till, J. E. (1975) The cellular basis for the defect in flexed-tailed mice. III. Restriction of the defect to erythropoietic progenitors capable of transient colony formation in vivo. *Br. J. Haematol.* **30,** 401–410.
7. Magli, M. C., Iscove, N. N., and Odartchenko, N. (1982) Transient nature of early haematopoietic spleen colonies. *Nature* **295,** 527–529.
8. Till, J. E. and McCulloch, E. A. (1972) The "F-factor" of the spleen colony assay for hematopoietic stem cells. *Ser. Haematol.* **5,** 15–21.
9. McCulloch, E. A., Siminovitch, L., and Till, J. E. (1964) Spleen colony formation in anemic mice of genotype *W/W^v*. *Science* **144,** 844–846.
10. Spangrude, G. J, Heimfeld, S., and Weissman, I. L. (1988) Purification and characterization of mouse hematopoietic stem cells. *Science* **241,** 58–62.
11. Spangrude, G. J., Smith, L., Uchida, N., Ikuta, K., Heimfeld, S., Friedman, J., et al. (1991) Mouse hematopoietic stem cells. *Blood* **78,** 1395–1402.
12. Jones, R. I., Wagner, J. E., Celano, P., Zicha, M. S., Sharkis, S. J. (1990) Separation of pluripotent haematopoietic stem cells from spleen colony-forming cells. *Nature* **347,** 188–189.

11

Intrathymic Injection for Analysis of T-Cell Progenitor Activity

Libuse Jerabek and Irving L. Weissman

1. Introduction

Within our field, improvement in fluorescence-activated cell sorting (FACS) and molecular technologies has led to various types of correlative studies that imply the developmental sequence and subsequent emigration of thymic-lymphocyte subsets. Unfortunately, the implied conclusions are often accepted unequivocally by most of the immunology community. In fact, direct demonstration of precursor progeny relationships by specific cell marking within the thymus, or specific delivery of purified cells at a particular stage of isolation back into the thymus, are the only methods that reproducibly identify cell stages and intermediates *(1–11)*.

Radioactive or fluorescent labels can be infused directly into the thymus. If reutilization does not occur or is prevented, the movement of the labeled cells from one stage of maturation to the next, and the emergence of thymus-cell migrants can be quantitated. The use of fluorescent markers allows the retrieval of such populations for further biological and immunological testing. The injection of cells, ranging from purified hematopoietic stem cells (HSC) *(12–14)* to progenitor cells *(15)* to intrathymic intermediate stages, can result in their redistribution to the appropriate thymic subregions *(16)* and subsequent maturation and migration. Although it may seem to the uninitiated that the surgery is complex and highly invasive, it is actually a simple procedure that can be carried out by the experienced technician or investigator in less than 10 min per mouse. A simple description of the technique as currently practiced in our laboratory is outlined here.

From: *Methods in Molecular Medicine, vol. 63: Hematopoietic Stem Cell Protocols*
Edited by: C. A. Klug and C. T. Jordan © Humana Press Inc., Totowa, NJ

2. Materials

1. Sterile latex surgical gloves.
2. 70% ethanol.
3. Betadine solution (povidone-iodine 10%) (The Purdue Frederich Co., Norwalk, CT 06856).
4. Surgical board, three rubber bands 3-mm wide, push-pins.
5. Sterile Q tips.
6. Sterile gauze sponge 2" × 2".
7. Sterile microdissecting scissors, 4" straight, blunt (Biomedical Research Instruments [BRI], cat. #11–3000).
8. Two sterile microdissecting forceps, 4", curved (BRI cat. #10–2675).
9. Autoclip Wound Clip Applier, for 9-mm clips (Roboz Surgical Instruments, cat. #RS9260).
10. Autoclip 9-mm stainless-steel wound clip, for Applier in **step 9** (Roboz Surg. Instr. Cat. #RS9262).
11. Hamilton syringe with removable needle 17ORN (Hamilton Co., cat. #80230).
12. Removable needle-30-gauge, 1", 45°-pt (Hamilton Co., cat. #79630).
13. Heated pad: Deltaphase Isothermal Pad (Braintree Scientific, Model 39DP).
14. Anesthetics:
  a. Avertin or ketamine and xylazine.
  b. Avertin: 100% stock—10 g of tribromoethyl alcohol (Aldrich) mix with 10 mL of tertiary amyl alcohol (Aldrich) Working stock: dilute to 2.5% in isotonic saline; wrap both stocks in foil and keep at 4°C.
  c. The dose of avertin can vary slightly with every preparation, and should be tested each time a new 100% stock is made. The usual dosage is 0.015–0.017mL/1 g of body wt. Ketamine/xylazine mixture: Ketamine HCl injection: order (Ketalar-100mg/ml, Parke-Davis, 5-mL vial); Xylazine: order (Rompun 20 mg/mL, Bayer, 20-mL bottle).
  Mix: 1 part of Ketalar + 1 part of Rompun + 10 parts of saline.
  Dosage: 0.01 mL/1 g of body wt.

3. Methods

1. Anesthetize the mouse (*see* **Note 1**).
2. Fill the syringe with the cell suspension/dye (*see* **Note 2**) to be injected..
3. Immobilize the mouse in a supine position on the surgical board, with its head towards you. Slip its feet under the rubber bands, and loosely stretch an additional rubber band over the mouth (**Fig. 1**).
4. Swab the chest area with 70% ethanol and then with betadine solution.
5. Make a midline incision in the lower cervical and upper thoracic region—about 2 cm long, loosen the skin by gently inserting a forceps jaw underneath the skin, and gently lift up the salivary gland to expose the sternum (*see* **Note 3**).
6. Insert one blunt blade of the microdissecting scissors about 3 mm underneath the

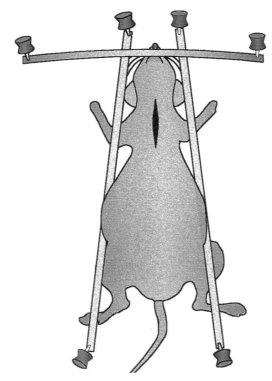

Fig. 1. Immobilization of mouse in preparation for surgery.

sternum and split the bone in the middle, about 3 mm in length. Spread the halves gently sideways to expose the thymus.

7. Remove the membrane on the top of the thymus if necessary to completely expose the thymus.
8. Inject 5–10 µL of cell suspension or injectate per thymic lobe. Slowly withdraw the needle to minimize the leakage (*see* **Note 4**).
9. Dry the area with a Q tip if necessary.
10. Free the mouse of rubber bands, return the salivary gland to its original position, press the incision together, and with your fingers squeeze the chest cavity gently to release as much air as possible from the cavity.
11. Close the incision by stapling the skin tightly together using three 9-mm autoclips.
12. Place the mouse on the heated pad until it recovers (*see* **Note 5**).

4. Notes

1. Anesthetic is administered by intraperitoneal injection. The mouse will stay unconscious for 30–40 min, depending on the mouse strain used.

2. Injected volume should not exceed 10 µL/lobe; a larger volume causes more destruction of the thymic architecture.
3. Salivary gland is a tan-pink, opaque gland that lies directly below the skin between the larynx and sternal notch.
4. Try to inject close to the middle of the lobe, 2–3 mm deep, depending on the age of the mouse. The technique can be practiced by injecting a dye (e.g., India ink) followed by removal and dissection of the thymus to observe the site of injection.
5. The success of this procedure is dependent on rapid performance. The same surgical procedure can be used to perform a complete thymectomy. Instead of injection into the thymus (**step 8**), both lobes of the thymus are removed by gently separating them from the connective tissue and pulling them out. Then continue from **step 9** to finish.

References

1. Weissman, I. L. (1967) Thymus cell migration. *J. Exp. Med.* **126,** 291–304.
2. Weissman, I. L. (1973) Thymus cell maturation: studies on the origin of cortisone-resistant thymic lymphocytes. *J. Exp. Med.* **137,** 504–510.
3. Scollay, R., Kochen, M., Butcher, E., and Weissman, I. L. (1978) Lyt markers on thymus cell migrants. *Nature* **276,** 79–80.
4. Scollay, R., Butcher, E., and Weissman, I. L. (1980) Thymus cell migration. Quantitative aspects of cellular traffic from the thymus to the periphery in mice. *Eur. J. Immunol.* **10,** 210–218.
5. Scollay, R., Jacobs, S., Jerabek, L., Butcher, E., and Weissman, I. L. (1980) T cell maturation: thymocyte and thymus migrant subpopulations defined with monoclonal antibodies to MHC region antigens. *J. Immunol.* **124,** 2845–2853.
6. Scollay, R. and Weissman, I. L. (1980) T cell maturation: thymocyte and thymus migrant subpopulations defined with monoclonal antibodies to the antigens Lyt-1, Lyt-2 and ThB. *J. Immunol.* **124,** 2841–2844.
7. Butcher, E. C., Scollay, R. G., and Weissman, I. L. (1980) Direct fluorescent labeling of cells with fluorescein or rhodamine isothiocyanate: II. Potential application to studies of lymphocyte migration and maturation. *J. Immunol. Methods* **37,** 109–121.
8. Guidos, C. J., Danska, J. S., Fathman, C. G., and Weissman, I. L. (1990) TCR-mediated negative selection of autoreactive T lymphcyte precursors occurs after commitment to the CD4 or CD8 lineages. *J. Exp. Med.* **172,** 835–845.
9. Akashi, K. and Weissman, I. L. (1996) The c-kit positive maturation pathway in mouse thymic T cell development: lineages and selection. *Immunity* **5,** 147–161.
10. Akashi, K., Kondo, M., and Weissman, I. L. (1998) Two distinct pathways of positive selection for thymocytes. *PNAS* **95,** 2486–2491.
11. Akashi, K., Richie, L. I., Miyamoto, T., Carr, W. H., and Weissman, I. L. B (2000) lymphopoiesis in the thymus. *J. Immunol.* **164,** 5221–5226.
12. Spangrude, G. J., Muller-Sieburg, C. E., Heimfeld, S., and Weissman, I. L. (1988) Two rare populations of mouse Thy-1^{lo} bone marrow cells repopulate the thymus. *J. Exp. Med.* **167,** 1671–1683.

13. Spangrude, G. J., Heimfeld, S., and Weissman, I. L. (1988) Purification and characterization of mouse hematopoietic stem cells. *Science* **241,** 58–62.
14. Spangrude, G. J. and Weissman, I. L. (1988) Mature T cells generated from single thymic clones are phenotypically and functionally heterogeneous. *J. Immunol.* **141,** 1877–1890.
15. Kondo, M., Weissman, I. L., and Akashi, K. (1997) Identification of clonogenic common lymphoid progenitor in mouse bone marrow. *Cell* **91,** 661–672.
16. Adkins, B., Mueller, C., Okada, C. Y., Reichert, R. A., Weissman, I. L., and Spangrude, G. J. (1987) Early events in T-cell maturation. *Annu. Rev. Immunol.* **5,** 325–365.

12

Quantitation of Murine and Human Hematopoietic Stem Cells by Limiting-Dilution Analysis in Competitively Repopulated Hosts

Stephen J. Szilvassy, Franck E. Nicolini, Connie J. Eaves, and Cindy L. Miller

1. Introduction

In designing functional assays for the various classes of hematopoietic cells described in this book, one needs to consider the properties of the cell to be measured which must be incorporated into the assay design, and the end points to allow its specific detection. The most primitive hematopoietic stem cells (HSC) in mouse and man are characterized by two cardinal properties that distinguish them from more mature clonogenic cells and their terminally differentiated progeny. Firstly, HSCs are *pluripotent*: they are characterized by the potential to differentiate into all of the eight major lineages of lymphoid, myeloid, and erythroid cells in vivo *(1–3)*. Secondly, HSCs are able to *self-renew*, or generate daughter stem cells in vivo and in vitro that are functionally identical to the stem cell that gave rise to them *(3–5)*. These hallmark properties of HSCs are measured empirically by their potential to regenerate and maintain lymphocytes, granulocytes, and erythrocytes upon transplantation into lethally irradiated or immunocompromised primary and secondary hosts. However, functional assays for primitive HSCs must also consider the fact that differentiated cells present in the hematopoietic organs at different times after bone marrow transplantation are derived from different types of precursors *(6)*, and particularly at later times, cannot be assumed to be of donor origin *(7)*. Support for this concept derives from the relatively recent demonstration in mice that most, if not all, spleen colonies detectable ~2 wk after transplantation originate

From: *Methods in Molecular Medicine, vol. 63: Hematopoietic Stem Cell Protocols*
Edited by: C. A. Klug and C. T. Jordan © Humana Press Inc., Totowa, NJ

from progenitors (colony-forming unit-spleen [CFU-S]) *(8)* that are phenotypically and functionally separable from more primitive HSCs capable of long-term reconstitution *(7,9,10)*.

Just as increasingly longer assay times are required to detect the most primitive classes of cobblestone area-forming cells (CAFC) in vitro (*see* Chapter 9), in vivo assays for precursors of CFU-S must also incorporate delayed end points. Two approaches to the development of long-term assays have been used. The first—and technically simplest—has been to measure the number of cells required to promote the survival, usually for 30 d, of mice exposed to a lethal dose of radiation *(11)*. The radioprotection assay has the advantage of being quantitative, but the exclusive use of survival as the assay end point fails to consider the possibility that death may result from the absence in the graft of adequate numbers of progenitors capable of rapid—although transient—hematopoiesis, even in the presence of more primitive stem cells whose differentiated progeny are not detectable until later times. An alternative approach to extending the time of hematopoietic reconstitution assays has been to use a double-transplant procedure to measure the number of CFU-S in the marrow of mice transplanted 2 wk previously with the test cells under consideration *(12)*. However, this so-called pre-CFU-S assay is technically complex, and potential limitations in its sensitivity complicate derivation of stem cell frequencies by limiting-dilution analysis (LDA).

The need for a practical assay that allowed the specific identification—and more importantly, quantitation—of stem cells with long-term lymphomyeloid repopulating ability led to the development in 1990 of an in vivo assay for murine HSCs called "competitive repopulating units" (CRU) *(13)*. The CRU assay was an outgrowth of a competitive repopulation assay originally developed by David Harrison. In its simplest form, the Harrison assay provides a relative measure of "repopulating activity," usually compared to a reference standard of normal bone marrow cells *(14)*. However, analysis of covariance in the degree of donor lymphocyte and erythrocyte engraftment between recipients injected with a single dose of test cells (together with competitors) can also be used to provide an absolute measure of stem cell concentration *(15)*. The murine CRU assay incorporates two new features. The first is the use of competitor cells that have been subjected to two previous cycles of marrow transplantation to reduce or "compromise" their competitive long-term repopulating ability without altering the frequency of more mature clonogenic cells *(14,16)*. Their coinjection ensures the survival of lethally irradiated mice independent of the stem cell content of the test population being assayed, and allows the assay to be performed on small numbers of highly enriched stem cells, which may not be radioprotective on their own. In addition, because competitor cells can contribute to long-term hematopoietic regeneration under appropriate circumstances *(13)*, they provide a "selective pressure" that increases the specificity of the assay for totipotent stem cells with high competitive long-term repopulating potential. This conclusion is supported by the finding that even in mice injected with limiting numbers of test cells, engraftment is almost always associated with the presence of lymphoid and myeloid progeny that can be shown by retroviral-marking to be derived from a common multipotent precursor *(3,17)*.

The second, more significant modification from early competitive repopulation assays is the use of a limiting-dilution experimental design to allow stem cell quantitation. This approach had been used previously to measure HSCs by their potential to cure the macrocytic anemia of unirradiated *W/W^v* mice *(18)*. The CRU assay involves transplanting decreasing numbers of "test" cells into lethally irradiated and histocompatible, but genetically distinguishable, mice together with a radioprotective dose of compromised bone marrow cells syngeneic to the recipient strain. The proportion of animals whose regenerated hematopoietic tissues are determined 5–10 wk later to contain ≥5% lymphoid *and* myeloid cells of test cell origin is then used to calculate the frequency of CRU in the original test suspension by Poisson statistics *(13,19)*. Originally, transplants were sex-mismatched so that male donor cells could be distinguished from those of female host or competitor cell origin by Southern blot analysis, using a Y-chromosome specific probe *(13,20)*. Because this method could not uniquely type cells of different lineages, the specificity of the CRU assay for pluripotent stem cells was achieved by analysis of the marrow and thymus from individual mice. Selectivity of the CRU assay for a stem cell with dual lymphoid and myeloid potential was demonstrated by the high concordance (83%) of repopulation of these organs, even when mice were retrospectively determined to have been transplanted with no more than one CRU *(13)*. However, this technique had several major disadvantages; it was labor-intensive and required 1–2 wk before an answer could be obtained. Recipient analysis was also a fatal process, and thus could only be performed at one time after transplantation. This warranted a modification of the CRU assay design, implemented in 1993, using Ly-5 congenic C57BL/6 mouse strains whose white blood cells (WBC) could be distinguished by their expression of the "a" (Ly-5.1) or "b" (Ly-5.2) forms of the alloantigen *ptprc* (*p*rotein *t*yrosine *p*hosphatase *r*eceptor type *c* polypeptide) *(21,22)*. Donor cell contribution to lymphocytes and myeloid cells could now be quantitated in real time by two-color flow cytometric analysis of peripheral blood cells stained with appropriate combinations of anti-Ly-5.1 or -5.2, and lineage-specific antibodies. Congenic mouse strains bearing allelic differences in hemoglobin or glucose phosphate isomerase (GPI) genes *(23,24)* can also be used to distinguish donor from recipient red blood cells (RBC) and to monitor erythroid engraftment. With these modifications, blood could now be sampled at multiple times after transplantation, allowing the demonstration that calculated stem cell frequencies did not vary significantly when recipients were analyzed between 10 wk and 1 y *(22)*.

Application of similar theoretical and technical considerations that defined the murine CRU assay have led to the recent development of quantitative in vivo assays for human CRU *(25–27)*. During the past decade, several laboratories have developed in vivo model systems that support the engraftment of human hematopoietic cells transplanted into immunodeficient xenogeneic hosts including fetal sheep *(28)* and certain strains of mutant mice *(29–31)*. In the latter case, the highest overall levels of human hematopoiesis were obtained in sublethally irradiated *nonobese diabetic severe combined immunodeficiency scid/scid* (NOD/SCID) mice *(30,32)*. The high degree of amplification, multilineage composition, durability, and retransplantability of the human cell populations regenerated in these mice suggested that they had originated from a transplantable human cell that met the criteria for a HSC as described previously.

In the human CRU assay, sublethally irradiated NOD/SCID animals are injected intravenously with limiting numbers of human test cells together with irradiated human bone marrow carrier cells to promote engraftment. In early studies, the presence of human CRU in the test population was defined by the presence of human B lymphocytes (≥ 5 CD34$^-$CD19$^+$ cells per 2×10^4 cells) and myeloid progenitors (≥ 1 CD34$^+$ colony-forming cells [CFC] per 10^6 cells) in the host marrow 6–8 wk later *(25)*. However, the requirement for cell sorting and in vitro progenitor assays hampered the rapid assessment of large numbers of mice. Recently, the human CRU assay has been modified to allow identification of positive mice (i.e., detection of both human B lymphoid and myeloid cells in the same recipient) by staining with monoclonal antibodies (MAb) against selected human cell surface antigens and flow cytometric analysis *(27)*. The frequency of human CRU in the test cell population is then calculated from the proportions of negative mice within each test cell dose group, using Poisson statistics and the method of maximum likelihood.

The human CRU assay *(25,27)*, and the comparable assay for SCID-repopulating cells (SRC) *(26,33)*, have been used to quantitate and characterize human repopulating cells from various hematopoietic tissues including fetal liver, umbilical-cord blood (UCB), bone marrow, and cytokine-mobilized peripheral blood. These assays are invaluable to studies of the molecular and cellular processes that regulate the proliferation and differentiation of normal and leukemic hematopoietic stem cells.

The aim of this chapter is to offer a technical description of how to perform the murine and human CRU assays, and to provide insight into some of the variables that must be considered in quantitating hematopoietic stem cells in vivo. Alternative procedures for measuring stem cell activity have been reported, and the present methodologies should not be interpreted as exclusive. Nevertheless, these assays serve as useful tools in any hematological studies requiring an absolute measure of long-term repopulating (LTR) HSC numbers.

2. Materials

2.1. Preparation of Competitor Bone Marrow Cells

1. B6.SJL (Ly-5.1) mice, 6–12 wk old. Commercial suppliers include Jackson Laboratories, Bar Harbor, MA; Taconic, Germantown, NY; and Charles River Laboratories, Wilmington, MA (*see* **Note 1**).
2. DMEM/2% FBS: Dulbecco's modified Eagle's medium containing 2% (v/v) fetal bovine serum (FBS). Filter-sterilize and store at 4°C.

2.2. LDA of Murine CRU

1. Lethally irradiated B6.SJL (Ly-5.1) mice, 6–12 wk old, for use as CRU assay recipients (*see* **Note 1**).
2. Compromised B6.SJL (Ly-5.1) mice for use as a source of competitor bone marrow cells (*see* **Notes 1** and **2**).
3. Source of murine test cells derived from C57BL/6 (Ly-5.2) strain (*see* **Notes 1** and **2**).
4. DMEM/2% FBS.
5. Ethylenediaminetetraacetic acid (EDTA)-coated Microtainer® tubes (Becton Dickinson, #365973).
6. 1-mm diameter heparinized glass microcapillary tubes (Fisher Scientific, Pittsburgh, PA).
7. Red cell removal buffer (RCRB): 0.16 M NH$_4$Cl, 0.13 mM EDTA, 12 mM NaHCO$_3$. Filter-sterilize and store at 4°C.
8. HF buffer: Hank's balanced salt solution (HBSS) containing 2% (v/v) FBS. Filter-sterilize and store at 4°C.
9. Fluorochrome-conjugated MAb: Anti-mouse Ly-5.2~FITC (clones ALI4A2 or 104; IgG$_{2a}$), CD45R/B220~PE (clone RA3-6B2; IgG$_{2a}$), Thy-1.2~PE (clone 30H12; IgG$_{2b}$), Ly6G/Gr-1~PE (clone RB6-8C5; IgG$_{2b}$), CD11b/Mac-1~PE (clone M1/70; IgG$_{2b}$), and IgG~FITC, and IgG~PE isotype controls. All are available from Pharmingen/Becton Dickinson.
10. HF/PI: Propidium iodide (PI) prepared at 2–5 µg/mL in HF buffer.

2.3. LDA of Human CRU

1. NOD/LtSz-*scid/scid* (NOD/SCID) recipients, 6–8 wk old (Jackson Laboratories).
2. Human bone marrow cells irradiated with 1500 cGy for use as carrier cells (*see* **Note 3**).

3. Human test cells to be assayed for CRU.
4. Human cytokines (optional, *see* **Note 4**).
5. IMDM/2% FBS: Iscove's modified Dulbecco's medium with 2% (v/v) FBS. Filter-sterilize and store at 4°C.
6. RCRB.
7. HF buffer.
8. Normal human serum; heat-inactivated at 56°C for 40 min.
9. HF/5% human serum: HF with 5% (v/v) human serum.
10. Murine anti-F_c receptor γ antibody; either purified material (F_c Block, Pharmingen) or hybridoma-conditioned medium (from clone 2.4G2; American Type Culture Collection).
11. Fluorochrome-conjugated MAb: Anti-human CD34~FITC (clone 8G12, IgG_1), CD15~FITC (clone MMA, IgM), CD66b~FITC (clone 80H3, IgG_1), CD19~PE (clone 4G7, IgG_1), CD20~PE (clone L27, IgG_1), CD71~PE (clone M-A712, IgG_{2a}), CD45~PE (clone HI30, IgG_1), and FITC- and PE-conjugated mouse isotype controls. Commercial suppliers include Becton Dickinson/Pharmingen, and Immunotech/Beckman Coulter.
12. HF/PI.

3. Methods

The general design of the murine CRU assay is depicted in **Fig. 1**. The first step in the procedure, which requires 10 wk to complete, is the generation of "compromised" mice to be used as the source of competitor bone marrow cells. However, since this step demands considerable advance planning which is not always possible, many investigators elect instead to use either normal bone marrow competitor cells or employ assay recipients containing stem cells that can provide endogenous competition (*see* **Note 2** for details).

3.1. Preparation of Competitor Bone Marrow Cells

1. Harvest and pool bone marrow cells from two mice that are syngeneic to the recipient strain to be used in the competitive repopulation assay. If donor cells will be detected by flow cytometry, it is simplest to use C57BL/6 test cells (Ly-5.2^+) and Ly-5 congenic B6.SJL recipients. Competitor cells must therefore also be generated from B6.SJL mice. If Y-chromosome typing is to be used to assess test (male) cell engraftment, as is advantageous in retroviral marking studies *(3,17)*, compromised bone marrow cells and recipients must be female. Flush marrow plugs from femoral shafts into ~ 2 mL of cold DMEM/2% FBS using a sterile 21-gauge needle and a 3-mL syringe.
2. Dilute B6.SJL bone marrow cells to 4×10^6 c/mL in cold DMEM/2% FBS and intravenously inject 0.25 mL (10^6 cells) into each of two B6.SJL mice that have been lethally irradiated as described in **Subheading 3.2., step 1**.
3. After 5 wk, harvest the regenerated bone marrow cells from both primary animals as in **step 1** and repeat **step 2** by transplanting 10^6 cells into a second group

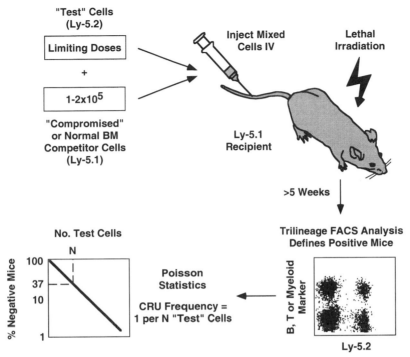

Fig. 1. Schematic representation of the murine CRU assay. Lethally irradiated Ly-5.1 (B6.SJL) mice are injected with limiting numbers of Ly-5.2 (C57BL/6) test cells together with $1–2 \times 10^5$ Ly-5.1 (B6.SJL) "compromised" or normal bone marrow cells. The proportion of Ly-5.2$^+$ cells in hematopoietic tissues of the competitively repopulated recipients ≥5 wk later is determined by two-color flow cytometry using Ly-5.2–specific and lymphoid or myeloid-specific MAbs. The variation in the proportion of positive animals (>5% test cells detectable in lymphoid *and* myeloid compartments) with test cell dose is analyzed by Poisson statistics to provide an absolute measure of CRU frequency in the test graft.

of lethally irradiated B6.SJL mice. These secondary recipients will be used after reconstitution as the source of "compromised" bone marrow cells for competitive repopulation assays. Sufficient numbers of mice should therefore be generated to support all anticipated experiments for ~10–12 wk (*see* **Note 5**).

4. Beginning 5 wk after secondary transplantation, repopulated mice may be used as a source of "compromised" bone marrow cells for competitive repopulation assays. Typically, one animal will provide sufficient cells for each assay using $1–2 \times 10^5$ cells per mouse (*see* **Note 6**).

3.2. LDA of Murine CRU

Once "compromised" mice have been generated to provide a source of competitor cells, or alternative measures have been taken to eliminate their requirement for radioprotection (*see* **Note 2**), performing the CRU assay is simply a matter of transplanting varying numbers of test cells together with a fixed number of competitors such that the ultimate proportion of repopulated animals in each group yields data which can be analyzed by Poisson statistics. From a practical perspective, this means that test cells should be transplanted at three or four doses, and separated by two- or threefold dilutions. *See* **Subheading 3.4.** for further discussion.

1. Lethally irradiate B6.SJL (Ly-5.1) recipient mice by exposure to a dose of γ-irradiation (900–1200 cGy) sufficient to kill all nontransplanted animals in 10–14 d. Radiation can be administered in a single dose, or in two equal doses ~3 h apart to minimize gut-cell damage, and ideally at a rate not exceeding ~250 cGy per min. Sufficient recipients should be prepared to accommodate the suspensions to be assayed in **step 3**, with 4–8 mice per group being typical.

2. Harvest femoral bone marrow cells from one "compromised" mouse into 2 mL of cold DMEM/2% FBS using a sterile 21-gauge needle and a 3-mL syringe. Count viable nucleated bone marrow cells.

3. Prepare three or four cell mixtures such that 0.25 mL contains the various desired doses of test cells and 2×10^5 compromised bone marrow cells. *See* **Table 1** as a guide for selecting appropriate test cell doses for various hematopoietic cell types. Keep cells cold and inject intravenously into the lateral tail vein of B6.SJL mice (4–8 per group) irradiated in **step 1**. Maintain recipient animals on acidified water with or without antibiotics (*see* **Note 7**).

4. Hematopoietic reconstitution may be analyzed at any time at least 5 wk after transplantation. Collect 3–4 drops of peripheral blood from the retroorbital sinus into an EDTA-coated Microtainer® tube by puncturing the venous plexus with a 1-mm diameter heparinized glass microcapillary tube cut to 1-cm lengths using a diamond scribe. Alternatively, blood can be collected by gently warming mice for 3–5 min using a heat lamp, and then either making a shallow nick in a lateral tail vein at a position one-third from the end of the tail or removing 0.5 cm from the end of the tail using a sharp scalpel blade. Blood should also be collected from normal B6 and B6.SJL mice to serve as positive and negative controls, respectively.

5. Aliquot ~50 μL of each "test" blood sample into three polystyrene FACS tubes (Falcon #2008, Becton Dickinson). Lyse RBC by adding ~3 mL of warmed RCRB and incubate 5 min at room temperature. Pellet cells and repeat lysis once more. Wash cells for a third time in ~2 mL of cold HF buffer, then decant the supernatant, leaving the pelleted cells in the ~100 μL of HF which remains behind in the tube. Shake the tubes in a rack to disaggregate the pelleted leukocytes.

6. To each triplicate set of blood cells, add saturating amounts of:
   a. anti-Ly-5.2~fluorescein-5-isothiocyanate (FITC) and anti-B220~phycoerythrin (PE) MAbs.
   b. anti-Ly-5.2~FITC and Thy-1.2~PE MAbs.

Table 1
Frequency of CRU in Murine Hematopoietic Tissue

Cell source	Phenotype	CRU frequencies[a]	Ref
Adult bone marrow	Unseparated	1 per $1–2 \times 10^4$	*13,34*
Adult bone marrow	Sca-1$^+$Lin$^-$WGA$^+$	1 per 40	*34*
	Sca-1$^+$Lin$^{lo/-}$Thy-1^{lo}	1 per 30–40	*21,35*
	Sca-1$^+$Lin$^-$c-kit$^+$	1 per 15	*36*
	Rh-123^{lo}Ho^{lo}Lin$^{-/lo}$ [b]	1 per 10–20	*37*
	Sca-1$^+$Lin$^{lo/-}$Thy-1^{lo}Mac- 1$^-$CD4$^-$	1 per 10	*38*
Post-5–FU marrow[c]	Unseparated	1 per 2,000	*13,39*
Day 14.5 fetal liver	Unseparated	1 per 15,000	*40,41*
Day 14.5 fetal liver	Sca-1 $^+$[Lin^d]$^-$Mac-l$^+$	1 per 40	*40*
	Sca-1$^+$[Lin^d]$^-$Thy-1^{lo}Mac-1$^+$CD4$^-$	1 per 6	*41*

[a] This Table (and Table 2) aim to assist researchers in selecting suitable cell dose ranges for quantitation of CRU in various hematopoietic tissues. As the stem cell phenotypes listed are not comprehensive, the reader is advised to consult additional published literature describing strategies for the isolation of enriched HSC populations.

[b] Rh-123; Rhodamine-123, Ho; Hoechst 33342 (Hst).

[c] Mice are injected with 150 mg/kg 5–Fluorouracil (5-FU) and bone marrow cells are isolated 4 d later.

[d] HSCs from d 14.5 post-coitum fetal liver express CD11b/Mac-1, so this Mab should not be included in strategies for isolation of lineage negative (Lin$^-$) cells.

   c. anti-Ly-5.2~FITC, Gr-1~PE and Mac-1~PE MAbs.
   Samples containing unstained cells, cells stained only with PE-conjugated antibody, FITC-conjugated antibody or FITC- and PE-conjugated isotype control antibodies should also be prepared for establishing threshold and compensation settings on the FACS instrument.

7. Protect from light and incubate for 30 min on ice.

8. Add ~3 mL HF buffer and pellet cells. Decant the supernatant and repeat this wash step once more. Finally resuspend cells in 0.2 mL of HF/PI buffer for flow cytometric analysis.

9. In each group of mice transplanted with different numbers of test cells, determine the proportion of recipients exhibiting at least 5% viable (PI$^-$) Ly-5.2$^+$ leukocytes. Score as positive only those animals in which donor-derived (test) cells are detectable among B220$^+$ (B lymphoid), Thy-1.2$^+$ (T lymphoid) *and* Gr-1/Mac-1$^+$ (myeloid) compartments. **Fig.2** shows an example of this trilineage FACS analysis, as well as an alternative method of determining the contribution of donor-derived cells to lymphoid and myeloid compartments based on the unique light-scattering properties of these cell types (*see* **Note 8**).

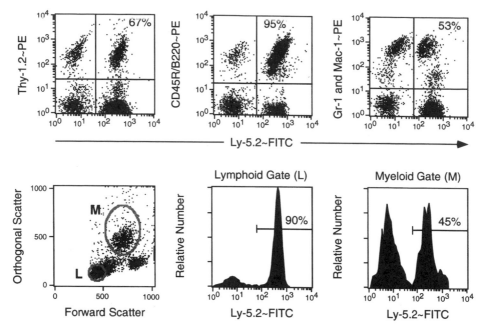

Fig. 2. Example of flow cytometric analysis to evaluate recipient mice in the murine CRU assay. A lethally irradiated Ly-5.1 mouse was transplanted with 100 Sca-1$^+$c-kit$^+$Lin$^-$ (Ly-5.2$^+$) marrow cells together with 10^5 Ly-5.1 compromised bone marrow cells and analyzed 10 wk later. The upper panels depict the use of lineage antibodies to ascertain the contribution of Ly-5.2$^+$ stem cells to circulating B (CD45R/B220$^+$) and T (Thy-1.2$^+$) lymphocytes, and granulocytes (Gr-1$^+$) and monocytes (Mac-1$^+$). In the lower panels, the contribution of test stem cells to lymphoid (L) and myeloid (M) compartments is determined instead by their unique forward and orthogonal light-scattering properties. The concordance of these two methods of analysis is confirmed by the similar proportion of Ly-5.2$^+$ cells among CD45/B220$^+$ B cells (95%) and lymphocytes in gate "L" (90%), and Gr-1$^+$/Mac-1$^+$ granulocytes/monocytes (53%) and myeloid cells in gate "M" (45%).

3.3. LDA of Human CRU

A schematic representation of the human CRU assay is shown in **Fig. 3**. It is very similar in design and principle to the murine CRU assay, but because it is a xenogeneic system, some modifications are needed:

1. Acidified water (pH 3.0) containing antibiotics should be provided to NOD/SCID mice, *ad libitum* 2–7 d prior to irradiation and for 4–6 wk following transplantation *(see* **Note 7**).
2. Sublethally irradiate NOD/SCID recipients by exposure to 350 cGy of total body γ-irradiation administered in a single dose at <250 cGy/min. Irradiate sufficient animals to allow 3–4 groups of 4–8 animals per group.

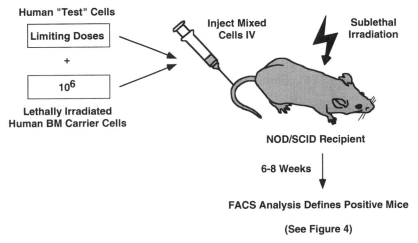

Fig. 3. Schematic representation of the human CRU assay. Sublethally irradiated NOD/SCID mice are injected with limiting numbers of human test cells and 10^6 lethally irradiated human bone marrow cells as carriers. The proportion of human cells in hematopoietic tissues is determined 6–8 wk later by two-color flow cytometry using cocktails of monoclonal anti-human antibodies against CD15, CD19, CD20, CD34, CD45, CD66b and CD71. Positive recipients are defined as mice containing ≥ 5 CD34$^-$ CD19/20$^+$ human B cells and ≥ 5 CD45/71$^+$CD15/66b$^+$ granulocytes per 2×10^4 viable cells analyzed (*see* **Fig. 4**). The variation in the proportion of positive animals with the number of transplanted human cells is analyzed by Poisson statistics to provide an absolute measure of CRU frequency in the human graft.

3. Irradiate normal human bone marrow cells with 1500 cGy for use as carrier cells (*see* **Note 3**).
4. Prepare cell mixtures in IMDM/2% FBS, so that 0.25 mL contains the desired dose of test cells and 10^6 carrier cells. *See* **Table 2** as a guide for selecting appropriate test cell doses for LDA.
5. Inject 0.25 mL of each cell mixture intravenously into the tail veins of irradiated NOD/SCID mice. Recipients should be injected within 24 h following irradiation.
6. Hematopoietic reconstitution is typically analyzed 6–8 wk after transplantation. Collect bone marrow cells from both femora into 2 mL of cold HF/5% HS using the method described in **step 2** of the murine CRU assay protocol (*see* **Note 9**).
7. Pellet bone marrow cells. Lyse erythrocytes by resuspending cells in ~3 mL of RCRB and incubate 5 min on ice. Wash cells once with cold HF buffer and decant supernatant. Finally, resuspend cells in 2 mL HF/5% HS. Note that lysis of RBC is not required if they are excluded by gating during FACS analysis (*see* **Fig. 4**).
8. Dispense 0.2 mL cells into each of five FACS tubes and add 2.4G2 MAb to a final concentration of 3 µg/mL. This facilitates blocking of F_c receptors and pre-

Table 2
**Frequency of CRU in Human Hematopoietic Tissues Assayed
in Irradiated NOD/SCID Recipients**

Cell source	Phenotype	CRU frequencies	References
Adult bone marrow	Mononuclear Cells	1 per $3-4 \times 10^6$	*26,42*
	CD34+	1 per $2-1 \times 10^5$	*26,27*
G-CSF MPB	Mononuclear Cells[a]	1 per 6×10^6	*26*
	CD34+	1 per 2×10^6	*43*
Cord blood	Mononuclear Cells	1 per $6-9 \times 10^5$	*25,26*
	CD34+	1 per $2-3 \times 10^4$	*27*
	CD34+CD38−	1 per $6-9 \times 10^2$	*25,44*
Fetal liver	CD34+	1 per $1-2 \times 10^4$	*27*

[a] G-CSF MPB was obtained from normal donors on d 4 or 5, following administration of 5–10 µg G-CSF/kg on d 1–4.

vents nonspecific binding of subsequent antibodies. Incubate cells for 10 min at 4°C. It is unnecessary to wash cells before proceeding to **step 9**.

9. Add the following antibodies to the five sample tubes:
   a. Nothing; cells in HF/PI only (unstained control).
   b. IgG~FITC and IgG~PE (isotype controls).
   c. IgM~FITC and IgG~PE (isotype controls).
   d. CD34~FITC, CD-19~PE and CD20~PE.
   e. CD15~FITC, CD66b~FITC, CD71~PE and CD45~PE.
   Tubes a, b, and c are used to establish threshold settings (*see* **Note 10**).
10. Protect all tubes from light and incubate for 30 min on ice.
11. Wash all samples twice with ~3 mL HF and finally resuspend cells in 0.2 mL HF/PI for flow cytometric analysis.
12. Establish quadrant or region parameters for negative cells based on the background levels of fluorescence observed with PI− cells stained with FITC- and PE-labeled isotype-matched control antibodies. Positive cells are defined as those exhibiting a fluorescence that exceeds 99.98% of that obtained with isotype controls labeled with the same fluorochromes. Score mice as positive if there are ≥5 CD34−CD19/20+ human B cells *and* ≥5 CD45/71+CD15/66b+ human granulocytes per 2×10^4 viable (PI−) cells analyzed (*see* **Note 10**).

3.4. Statistical Analysis of Limiting-Dilution Data: Important Considerations

CRU frequencies are determined by maximum likelihood analysis of the proportions of negative recipients, measured as described in **Subheadings 3.2.** and **3.3.**, in groups of mice transplanted with different numbers of test cells. Statistical analysis software are widely available for this application (e.g.,

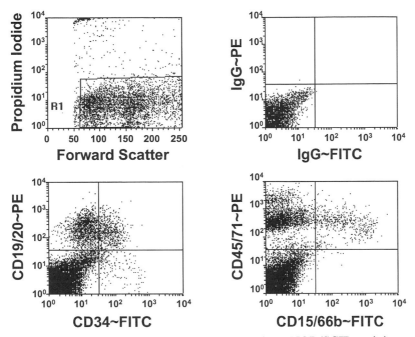

Fig. 4. Example of flow cytometric analysis to evaluate NOD/SCID recipients transplanted with human cells. A sublethally irradiated NOD/SCID mouse was injected with 1.5×10^5 human CD34$^+$ CB cells and 10^6 irradiated human bone marrow cells. Marrow cells were immunostained and analyzed by two-color flow cytometry 6 wk later. The upper left panel depicts the gates used to exclude PI$^+$ cells and the majority of murine erythroid cells. The upper right panel shows cells stained with FITC- or PE-conjugated isotype controls with quadrant settings to define positive cells (excludes 99.98% of cells). In the lower left panel, lymphoid engraftment is defined by the presence of ≥ 5 CD34$^-$CD19/20$^+$ human B cells per 2×10^4 events analyzed. In the lower right panel, myeloid engraftment is confirmed by the presence of ≥ 5 CD45/71$^+$CD15/66b$^+$ human granulocytes per 2×10^4 viable cells.

L-Calc™, StemCell Technologies, Vancouver), and are generally designed to accept three key pieces of data: the number of test cells transplanted per mouse (i.e., the test cell dose), the total number of mice in each dose group, and the number of animals that scored negative at each dose tested. Clearly, the last piece of information—and hence the calculated CRU frequency—is subject to some variation depending on how a positive response is defined and when it is measured. Positive mice are defined as those which exhibit *any level* of engraftment above the background observed with untransplanted negative control animals; i.e., ≥ 5% Ly-5.2$^+$ cells detectable in B (B220$^+$) and T (Thy-1$^+$) lymphoid *and* (Gr-1$^+$/Mac-1$^+$) myeloid lineages for murine CRU assays, or ≥ 5

human B lymphoid cells (CD34⁻CD19/20⁺) *and* ≥5 human granulocytes (CD45/71⁺CD15/66b⁺) per 2×10^4 viable bone marrow cells for human CRU assays. Arguably, these thresholds do allow inclusion of assay recipients with relatively low levels of engraftment, which can lead to overestimation of CRU frequency. In practice, however, low engraftment is rare when test cell doses are selected correctly (*see* **Tables 1** and **2**). A higher level of chimerism may arbitrarily be defined that must be achieved for an animal to score as positive. However, in murine CRU assays, this is complicated by the fact that the ratio of competitor to test cells—and hence the competitive pressure—can vary 100-fold over a range of test cell doses being evaluated. Increased competition at the low end of the test cell range may therefore decrease the absolute contribution of donor CRU to end cell compartments, although such stem cells may compete very effectively in other transplant settings. To circumvent this potential complicating factor, successful engraftment is defined simply as the minimum discernible above background, and the actual *level* of chimerism is irrelevant to the LDA.

When should transplanted animals be evaluated to determine whether they are positive or negative? The issue of timing is critical to ensure that the progeny of primitive stem cells with sustained hematopoietic potential are being measured, and that such clones have expanded sufficiently to allow detection. For murine CRU assays, calculated stem cell frequencies do not vary significantly when recipients of highly enriched HSCs are evaluated between ~10 wk and 1 y after competitive repopulation *(22)*. Therefore, there appears to be no advantage to waiting many months to quantitate the progeny of CRU in this setting. In contrast, recipients of heterogeneous (i.e., unfractionated) cell populations that contain large numbers of more mature progenitors as well as CRU are generally assessed later (>4 mo), when hematopoiesis has stabilized and transiently repopulating clones have been exhausted *(2)*. In NOD/SCID recipients of human CRU, human hematopoietic cells generally reach maximal levels from 6–8 wk after transplantation, thus animals are typically scored after this time *(32)*. If animals die prior to 10 wk for murine CRU assays and 6–8 wk for human CRU assays, they should **not** be included in the analysis as negative responses, but simply omitted from consideration. Such animals should be rare if appropriate numbers of compromised cells are used for murine CRU assays, and if irradiation of NOD/SCID mice is sublethal.

Once the required data is entered into the statistical analysis program of choice, a line-of-best-fit is generated, using the maximum likelihood method of analysis by relating the number of test cells transplanted to the log-percent negative animals at each dose *(19)*. It is advisable to consult a qualified statistician to confirm the validity of the data analysis program used. The CRU frequency is calculated as the reciprocal of the number of test cells that yields a

37% negative response. This calculation assumes single-hit kinetics, i.e., that a single HSC is sufficient to generate the response observed, an assumption that has been validated by CRU assays performed with retrovirally-marked HSCs *(3,17)*. The CRU frequency is derived from so-called "informative" groups in the linear portion of the limiting-dilution "curve." Test cell doses that yield either all negative or all positive responses are not informative, and statistical software developed for LDA often does not even accept data from these latter groups. Investigators are therefore reminded to design experiments to ensure that sufficient partial-response dose groups are available for analysis. Even so, moderate interexperimental variation and relatively large error limits on CRU measurements are typical. It is therefore suggested that each test cell population be assayed at least three times and data pooled for CRU calculations.

As a final point, investigators should appreciate that as with any in vivo system, the murine and human CRU assays by necessity provide only minimal estimates of stem cell frequency that differ from the true values by a factor, f, corresponding to the "seeding fraction" of the cell type being measured. The f value for CRU is currently unknown, but is almost certain to be <1. If one assumes that CRU are subject to similar nonspecific losses in highly perfused, nonhematopoietic organs as CFU-S, then it is likely that the true number of HSCs with competitive LTR potential may be 10- to 20-fold higher than estimated.

4. Notes

1. The use of congenic mouse strains with allelic differences at the Ly-5 locus facilitates the rapid and simple determination of donor-derived lymphoid and myeloid cells in hematopoietic tissues of recipients by flow cytometry. For researchers who also desire to monitor erythroid engraftment, test cells can be derived from B6.SJL (GPI[b], Ly-5.1) donors, and B6.CAST (GPI[a], Ly-5.2) mice (Jackson Laboratories) used as the source of helper cells (either normal or compromised bone marrow cells) *(see* **Note 2**) and recipients. In this case, the proportions of lymphoid and monocytic/granulocytic cells can be quantitated either by FACS analysis or GPI assay, and erythroid engraftment monitored by GPI analysis (Cindy Miller, unpublished observations).

2. The use of serially transplanted "compromised" bone marrow cells is highly recommended when murine CRU are assayed in myeloablated recipients, because of their diminished competitive LTR ability. However, since their preparation requires considerable advance planning that is not always feasible, two other approaches may be taken to circumvent the need for these cells. The first and simplest alternative is to use normal bone marrow cells as competitors instead. Investigators should be aware that this may result in a lower overall level of engraftment by limiting numbers of "test" stem cells and, if the threshold defined for positivity in the assay is not reduced, calculated CRU frequencies may be

lower than if "compromised" bone marrow cells were used. It is also advisable to perform radioprotection assays using normal bone marrow cells, and then use the minimal number required to promote the long-term survival of >90% of transplanted recipients in the CRU assay. A dose of 10^5 normal or 2×10^5 compromised bone marrow cells is usually sufficient to ensure survival *(13,34,39)*.

An alternative approach is to omit the use of transplanted competitor cells altogether and rely on the selective pressure provided by endogenous stem cells in W-series (c-kit mutant) mice. Mice of the W^{41}/W^{41} strain are particularly attractive for use as CRU assay recipients because they contain 17-fold fewer CRU, but near normal numbers of d 9 and d 12 CFU-S, and marrow progenitors able to generate mixed and lineage-restricted myeloid colonies in vitro *(45)*. Sublethal conditioning of W^{41}/W^{41} recipients prior to transplantation with 400 cGy of γ-irradiation is sufficient to achieve CRU frequencies and levels of engraftment comparable to lethally irradiated C57BL/6 mice cotransplanted with 10^5 helper marrow cells *(5,46)*. Note that since the W^{41}/W^{41} mutation exists on a uniform C57BL/6 genetic background (i.e., is Ly-5.2), test cells must be derived from B6.SJL (Ly-5.1) mice if they are to be identified using Ly-5 allotyping.

3. Carrier cells are useful to facilitate handling and to minimize cell loss in grafts containing $<10^6$ human test cells. Carriers may also promote engraftment of small numbers of purified human cells through their production of human cytokines *(47)*. Because carrier cells have been functionally inactivated by irradiation, cell suspensions with low progenitor numbers (i.e., low CD34+ content) may be used.

4. Both retroviral marking studies *(31)* and LDA *(25,27)* indicate that human CRU can engraft NOD/SCID mice in the absence of exogenous cytokines. Although injection of human cytokines does not alter engraftment kinetics of UCB stem cells, administration of interleukin (IL)-3, granulocyte-macrophage colony-stimulating factor (GM-CSF), stem-cell factor (SCF), and erythropoietin three times per wk for 2 wk immediately prior to sacrifice increased CRU numbers in primary recipients *(48,49)*. Recent studies also suggest that cotransplantation of irradiated human hematopoietic cells or cytokine treatment of recipients early after transplantation promotes engraftment in assays of low numbers of purified stem cells *(47,50)*.

5. Empirical experience indicates that long-term stem cell function will eventually recover after secondary transplantation. Therefore, compromised mice do have a "use-by" date that expires ~12 wk after production (i.e., 17 wk after the date of secondary transplant). Animals not used by this time should be discarded and a new cohort should be generated. Alternatively, it is possible to sacrifice all secondary mice at **step 4** of **Subheading 3.1.** and freeze "compromised" bone marrow cells in 10% dimethyl sulfoxide (DMSO)/90% FBS for future use. This ensures a uniform population of competitors for subsequent assays.

6. Investigators are advised to test the quality of each compromised cell population before use in CRU assays, particularly if cells have been previously frozen (*see* **Note 5**). A small-scale radioprotection assay performed by transplanting two groups of lethally irradiated mice with 10^5 or 2×10^5 cells is usually sufficient to

establish the dose required to promote the long-term survival of >90% of animals. Perhaps not surprisingly, this dose corresponds to the number of "compromised" bone marrow cells that contains 1–2 CRU (**22**).

7. The use of a radioprotective dose of competitor cells (*see* **Note 6**) and a clean animal facility should preclude the need to maintain mice on antibiotics during hematopoietic reconstitution. However, investigators may wish to decrease gut microbial flora and minimize radiation-induced mortality by providing assay recipients with acidified (pH 3.0) drinking water containing 0.5–1 mg/mL neomycin sulfate (No. N1876; Sigma Chemical Co., St. Louis, MO) and 500 U/mL polymyxin B sulfate (No. P1004; Sigma) for 2–14 d prior to and for 4–6 wk following transplantation. This applies for both B6.SJL and NOD/SCID mice in murine and human CRU assays, respectively.

8. It is possible to omit the use of lineage antibodies in the flow cytometric determination of hematopoietic reconstitution. Instead, the presence of test cell derived (Ly-5.2$^+$) cells including both lymphoid and myeloid elements can be established by their distinct forward and orthogonal light-scattering characteristics as shown in **Fig. 2**. This approach is more subjective than immunostaining, especially in recipients with <10% donor-derived cells, and is not generally recommended.

9. It is possible to perform FACS analyses on blood from NOD/SCID mice reconstituted with human cells. However, because the levels of human cells circulating in the periphery is often lower than detectable in the bone marrow, the latter tissue is preferable for LDA. Engraftment can also still be monitored over time by aspiration of marrow cells from anesthetized mice (*51,52*).

10. The combination of MAbs used for recipient analysis in the human CRU assay has been selected to enable bright and specific staining of human B cells and granulocytes. All anti-human MAbs must be titrated using human cells, and tested for nonreactivity against bone marrow cells from naive NOD/SCID mice. Because the threshold of engraftment used to define positive animals is very close to the limit of sensitivity of FACS analysis, it is critical that isotype controls are employed each time an experiment is performed. Gates established to define B cells (CD34$^-$CD19/20$^+$) and granulocytes (CD45/71$^+$CD15/66b$^+$) should be set to exclude or minimize the number of isotype-stained events (i.e., <0.02% of PI$^-$ events). If technical limitations or proficiency with flow-cytometric analysis compromise these criteria, investigators are advised to analyze mice using alternative techniques (*see* **ref. 25**).

References

1. Abramson, S., Miller, R.G., and Phillips, R.A. (1977) The identification in adult bone marrow of pluripotent and restricted stem cells of the myeloid and lymphoid systems. *J. Exp. Med.* **145**, 1567–1579.
2. Jordan, C. T. and Lemischka, I. R. (1990) Clonal and systemic analysis of long-term hematopoiesis in the mouse. *Genes Dev.* **4**, 220–232.
3. Szilvassy, S. J. and Cory, S. (1994) Efficient retroviral gene transfer to purified long-term repopulating hematopoietic stem cells. *Blood* **84**, 74–83.

4. Fraser, C. C., Eaves, C. J., Szilvassy, S. J., and Humphries, R. K. (1990) Expansion *in vitro* of retrovirally marked totipotent hematopoietic stem cells. *Blood* **76,** 1071–1076.

5. Miller, C. L. and Eaves, C. J. (1997) Expansion *in vitro* of adult murine hematopoietic stem cells with transplantable lympho-myeloid reconstituting ability. *Proc. Natl. Acad. Sci. USA* **94,** 13,648–13.653.

6. Magli, M. C., Iscove, N. N., and Odartchenko, N. (1982) Transient nature of early haematopoietic spleen colonies. *Nature* **295,** 527–529.

7. Jones, R. J., Celano, P., Sharkis, S. J., and Sensenbrenner, L. L. (1989) Two phases of engraftment established by serial bone marrow transplantation in mice. *Blood* **73,** 397–401.

8. Till, J. E. and McCulloch, E. A. (1961) A direct measurement of the radiation sensitivity of normal mouse bone marrow cells. *Radiat. Res.* **14,** 213–222.

9. Ploemacher, R. E. and Brons, R. H. C. (1989) Separation of CFU-S from primitive cells responsible for reconstitution of the bone marrow hemopoietic stem cell compartment following irradiation: evidence for a pre-CFU-S cell. *Exp. Hematol.* **17,** 263–266.

10. Jones, R. J., Wagner, J. E., Celano, P., Zicha, M. S., and Sharkis, S. J. (1990) Separation of pluripotent haematopoietic stem cells from spleen colony-forming cells. *Nature* **347,** 188–189.

11. McCulloch, E. A. and Till, J. E. (1960) The radiation sensitivity of normal mouse bone marrow cells, determined by quantitative marrow transplantation into irradiated mice. *Radiat. Res.* **13,** 115–125.

12. Hodgson, G. S., Bradley, T. R., and Radley, J. M. (1982) The organization of hemopoietic tissue as inferred from the effects of 5–fluorouracil. *Exp. Hematol.* **10,** 26–35.

13. Szilvassy, S. J., Humphries, R. K., Lansdorp, P. M., Eaves, A.C., and Eaves, C. J. (1990) Quantitative assay for totipotent reconstituting hematopoietic stem cells by a competitive repopulation strategy. *Proc. Natl. Acad. Sci. USA* **87,** 8736–8740.

14. Harrison, D. E., Astle, C. M., and Delaittre, J. A. (1978) Loss of proliferative capacity in immunohemopoietic stem cells caused by serial transplantation rather than aging. *J. Exp. Med.* **147,** 1526–1531.

15. Harrison, D. E., Jordan, C. T., Zhong, R. K., and Astle, C. M. (1993) Primitive hemopoietic stem cells: direct assay of most productive populations by competitive repopulation with simple binomial, correlation and covariance calculations. *Exp. Hematol.* **21,** 206–219.

16. Harrison, D. E. and Astle, C. M. (1982) Loss of stem cell repopulating ability upon transplantation: effects of donor age, cell number, and transplantation procedure. *J. Exp. Med.* **156,** 1767–1779.

17. Szilvassy, S. J., Fraser, C. C., Eaves, C. J., Lansdorp, P. M., Eaves, A. C., and Humphries, R. K. (1989) Retrovirus-mediated gene transfer to purified hemopoietic stem cells with long-term lympho-myelopoietic repopulating ability. *Proc. Natl. Acad. Sci. USA* **86,** 8798–8802.

18. Boggs, D. R., Boggs, S. S., Saxe, D. F., Gress, L. A., and Canfield D. R. (1982) Hematopoietic stem cells with high proliferative potential. Assay of their concentration in marrow by the frequency and duration of cure of W/W^v mice. *J. Clin. Investig.* **70**, 242–253.
19. Taswell, C. (1980) Limiting dilution assays for the determination of immunocompetent cell frequencies. I. Data analysis. *J. Immunol.* **126**, 1614–1619.
20. Lamar, E. E. and Palmer, E. (1984) Y-encoded, species-specific DNA in mice: evidence that the Y chromosome exists in two polymorphic forms in inbred strains. *Cell* **37**, 171–177.
21. Spangrude, G. J., Heimfeld, S., and Weissman, I. L. (1988) Purification and characterization of mouse hematopoietic stem cells. *Science* **241**, 58–62.
22. Szilvassy, S. J. and Cory, S. (1993) Phenotypic and functional characterization of competitive long-term repopulating hematopoietic stem cells enriched from 5–fluorouracil-treated murine marrow. *Blood* **81**, 2310–2320.
23. Eppig, J. J., Kozak, L. P., Eicher, E. M., and Stevens, L. C. (1977) Ovarian teratomas in mice are derived from oocytes that have completed the first meiotic division. *Nature* **269**, 517–518.
24. Harrison, D. E., Astle, C. M., and Lerner, C. (1988) Number and continuous proliferative pattern of transplanted primitive immunohematopoietic stem cells. *Proc. Natl. Acad. Sci. USA* **85**, 822–826.
25. Conneally, E., Cashman, J., Petzer, A., and Eaves, C. (1997) Expansion *in vitro* of transplantable human cord blood stem cells demonstrated using a quantitative assay of their lympho-myeloid repopulating activity in nonobese diabetic-*scid/scid* mice. *Proc. Natl. Acad. Sci. USA* **94**, 9836–9841.
26. Wang, J. C. Y., Doedens, M., and Dick, J. E. (1997) Primitive human hematopoeitic cells are enriched in cord blood compared to adult bone marrow or mobilized peripheral blood as measured by the quantitative *in vivo* SCID-repopulating cell (SRC) assay. *Blood* **89**, 3919–3925.
27. Holyoake, T. L., Nicolini, F. E., and Eaves, C. J. (1999) Functional differences between transplantable human hematopoeitic stem cells from fetal liver, cord blood and adult marrow. *Exp. Hematol.* **27**, 1418–1427.
28. Zanjani, E. D., Flake, A. W., Rice, H., Hedrick, M., and Tavassoli, M. (1994) Long-term repopulating ability of xenogeneic transplanted human fetal liver hematopoietic stem cells in sheep. *J. Clin. Investig.* **93**, 1051–1055.
29. Kamel-Reid, S. and Dick, J. E. (1988) Engraftment of immune-deficient mice with human hematopoietic stem cells. *Science* **242**, 1706–1709.
30. Pflumio, F., Izac, B., Katz, A., Shultz, L. D., Vainchenker, W., and Coulombel, L. (1996) Phenotype and function of human hematopoietic cells engrafting immune-deficient CB17–severe combined immunodeficiency mice and nonobese diabetic-severe combined immunodeficiency mice after transplantation of human cord blood mononuclear cells. *Blood* **88**, 3731–3740.
31. Nolta, J. A., Dao, M. A., Wells, S., Smogorzewska, E. M., and Kohn, D. B. (1996) Transduction of pluripotent human hematopoietic stem cells demonstrated by

clonal analysis after engraftment in immune-deficient mice. *Proc. Natl. Acad. Sci. USA* **93**, 2414–2419.

32. Cashman, J. D., Lapidot, T., Wang, J. C., Doedens, M., Shultz, L. D., Lansdorp, P., et al. (1997) Kinetic evidence of the regeneration of multilineage hematopoiesis from primitive cells in normal human bone marrow transplanted into immunodeficient mice. *Blood* **89**, 4307–4316.

33. Larochelle, A., Vormoor, J., Hanenberg, H., Wang, J. C., Bhatia, M., Lapidot, T., et al. (1996) Identification of primitive human hematopoietic cells capable of repopulating NOD/SCID mouse bone marrow: implications for gene therapy. *Nat. Med.* **2**, 1329–1337.

34. Rebel, V. I., Dragowska, W. H., Eaves C. J., Humphries, R. K. and Lansdorp, P. M. (1994) Amplification of Sca-1⁺Lin⁻WGA⁺ cells in serum-free cultures containing Steel factor, interleukin-6 and erythropoietin with maintenance of cells with long-term *in vivo* reconstituting potential. *Blood* **83**, 128–136.

35. Szilvassy, S. J., Weller, K. P., Chen, B., Tsukamoto, A., and Hoffman, R. (1996) Partially differentiated *ex vivo* expanded cells accelerate hematologic recovery in myeloablated mice cotransplanted with highly enriched long-term repopulating hematopoietic stem cells. *Blood* **88**, 3642–3653.

36. Szilvassy, S. J., Bass, M. J., Van Zant, G., and Grimes, B. (1999) Organ-selective homing defines engraftment kinetics of murine hematopoietic stem cells and is compromised by *ex vivo* expansion. *Blood* **93**, 1557–1566.

37. Wolf, N.S., Kone, A., Priestley, G.V., and Bartelmez, S.H. (1993) *In vivo* and *in vitro* characterization of long-term repopulating primitive hematopoietic cells isolated by sequential Hoechst 33342–rhodamine 123 FACS selection. *Exp. Hematol.* **21**, 614–622.

38. Morrison, S. J. and Weissman, I. L. (1994) The long-term repopulating subset of hematopoietic stem cells is deterministic and isolatable by phenotype. *Immunity* **1**, 661–673.

39. Szilvassy, S. J., Lansdorp, P. M., Humphries, R. K., Eaves, A. C., and Eaves, C. J. (1989) Isolation in a single step of a highly enriched murine hematopoietic stem cell population with competitive long-term repopulating ability. *Blood* **74**, 930–939.

40. Rebel, V. I., Miller, C. L., Thornbury, G. L., Dragowska, W. H., Eaves C. J. and Lansdorp, P. M. (1996) A comparison of long-term repopulating stem cells in fetal liver and adult bone marrow from the mouse. *Exp. Hematol.* **24**, 638–648.

41. Morrisson, S. J., Hemmati, H. D., Wandycz, A. M. and Weissman, I. L. (1995) The purification and characterization of fetal liver hematopoietic stem cells. *Proc. Natl. Acad. Sci. USA* **92**, 10,302–10,306.

42. Holyoake, T. L., Nicolini, F., Cashman, J., and Eaves, C. J. (1997) Development and validation of an improved *in vivo* assay for quantitating human hematopoietic stem cells. *Blood* **90**, 159a (Abstract).

43. Van der Loo, J. C. M., Hanenberg, H., Cooper, R. J., Luo, F.-Y., Lazaridis, E. N., and Williams, D. A. (1998) Nonobese diabetic/severe combined immunodeficiency (NOD/SCID) mouse as a model system to study the engraftment and mobilization of human peripheral blood stem cells. *Blood* **92**, 2556–2570.

44. Bhatia, M., Wang, J. C., Kapp, U., Bonnet, D., and Dick, J. E. (1997) Purification of primitive human hematopoietic cells capable of repopulating immune deficient mice. *Proc. Natl. Acad. Sci. USA* **94,** 5320–5325.

45. Miller, C. L., Rebel, V. I., Lemieux, M. E., Helgason, C. D., Lansdorp, P. M., and Eaves, C. J. (1996) Studies of *W* mutant mice provide evidence for alternate mechanisms capable of activating hematopoietic stem cells. *Exp. Hematol.* **24,** 185–194.

46. Trevisan, M., Yan, X-Q., and Iscove, N. N. (1996) Cycle initiation and colony formation in culture by murine marrow cells with long-term reconstituting potential *in vivo. Blood* **88,** 4149–4158.

47. Bonnet, D., Bhatia, M., Wang, J. C., Kapp, U., and Dick, J. E. (1999) Cytokine treatment or accessory cells are required to initiate engraftment of purified human hematopoietic cells transplanted at limiting dose into NOD/SCID mice. *Bone Marrow Transplant.* **23,** 203–209.

48. Cashman, J., Bockhold, K., Hogge, D. E., Eaves, A. C., and Eaves, C. J. (1997) Sustained proliferation, multi-lineage differentiation and maintenance of primitive human haemopoietic cells in NOD/SCID mice transplanted with human cord blood. *Br. J. Haematol.* **98,** 1026–1036.

49. Cashman, J. D. and Eaves, C. J. (1999) Human growth factor-enhanced regeneration of transplantable human hematopoietic stem cells in non-obese diabetic/severe combined immunodeficient mice. *Blood* **93,** 481–487.

50. Verstegen, M.A.A., van Hennik, P.B., Terpstra, W., van den Bos, C., Wielenga, J.J., van Rooijen N., et al. (1998) Transplantion of human umbilical cord blood cells in macrophage-depleted SCID mice: evidence for accessory cell involvement in expansion of immature CD34$^+$CD38$^-$ cells. *Blood* **91,** 1966–1976.

51. Drize, N. J., Keller, J. R., and Chertkov, J. L. (1996) Local clonal analysis of the hematopoietic system shows that multiple small short living clones maintain lifelong hematopoiesis in recostituted mice. *Blood* **88,** 2927–2938.

52. Verlinden, S. F. F, van Es, H. H. G., and van Bekkum, D. W. (1998) Serial bone marrow sampling for long-term follow up of human hematopoiesis in NOD/SCID mice. *Exp. Hematol.* **26,** 627–630.

13

Ex Vivo Expansion of Human and Murine Hematopoietic Stem Cells

Cindy L. Miller, Julie Audet, and Connie J. Eaves

1. Introduction

The last decade has seen major advances in our knowledge of the molecular control of hematopoiesis, widespread access to cytokines, and the development of practical assays for quantitating highly primitive hematopoietic cells. This progress has now made feasible the predictable manipulation of hematopoietic stem cells (HSC) and progenitors for a variety of experimental and clinical applications. Nevertheless, our understanding of events that induce and/ or block the differentiation of primitive hematopoietic cells is still very limited. Therefore, it is not surprising that procedures for expanding HSC populations ex vivo are based largely on a small set of empirical observations. The incentive to improve this situation is provided by many clinical situations in which the number of stem cells available for particular types of transplants is inadequate, or where HSC amplification may be useful as part of a purging strategy to reduce the potential burden of malignant cells in an autograft. Cell division with retention of stem cell integrity could also facilitate the generation in vitro of many specific types of differentiated cells (e.g., dendritic cells) and is a requirement for retroviral-mediated gene therapy. Progress in each of these rapidly evolving areas has recently been reviewed in greater depth elsewhere *(1–5)*.

In adult humans, mature blood cells of all hematopoietic lineages are produced continuously as a result of the balanced proliferation and differentiation of a small self-sustaining pool of stem cells. These are located primarily within the extravascular space of the bone marrow. Proliferation, commitment, and survival of HSC and progenitors is regulated in vivo by their interaction with

From: *Methods in Molecular Medicine, vol. 63: Hematopoietic Stem Cell Protocols*
Edited by: C. A. Klug and C. T. Jordan © Humana Press Inc., Totowa, NJ

local gradients within hematopoietic tissues of both inhibitory and stimulatory molecules as well as by direct cell-cell interactions mediated by adhesion molecules. Amplification of genetically marked repopulating cells has been demonstrated to occur both after their transplantation in vivo *(6–9)* and in vitro in the presence of an adherent stromal layer prior to transplanting the cells in vivo *(10)*. These two types of studies provided the first formal evidence that murine stem cells are capable of self-renewal. More recently, studies of cells initially labeled with fluorescent dyes such as PKH26 *(11)* or carboxyfluorescein diacetate succinimidyl ester (CFSE) *(12,13)*, which then showed reduced fluorescence postculture, have demonstrated the ability of stem cells to undergo self-renewal divisions in cytokine-supplemented suspension cultures. Many investigators have documented net increases in vitro of various types of hematopoietic progenitors, including colony-forming cells (CFC) and even long-term culture-initiating cells (LTC-IC). However, only recently have net expansions of both murine *(14,15)* and human stem cell populations *(16–17)* been conclusively demonstrated. The procedures described in **Subheading 1.1.** are drawn from the latter studies in which stem cell-enriched sources of cells are cultured in suspension (in the absence of stroma) in medium containing high concentrations of recombinant cytokines.

1.1. Quantitation of HSC

HSC are normally concentrated in different tissues at different stages of ontogeny: in the liver of the fetus, in the blood at birth, and in the bone marrow of the adult. Nevertheless, in all of these tissues, the HSC population is present at very low frequencies. Numerous techniques have been used to obtain enriched populations of HSC (and progenitors) based on differences in cell size and density, surface antigen expression, dye uptake, and sensitivity to cytotoxic drugs. Currently, there is no purification strategy that allows the reproducible isolation of a biologically homogeneous population of either murine or human HSC. Therefore, the definitive identification and quantitation of HSC continues to rely on the detection of their differentiated progeny produced in engrafted recipients.

The competitive repopulating unit (CRU) assay, first developed for the quantitation of murine HSC *(18)* provides a reproducible and specific method for determining the frequency of transplantable cells with long-term in vivo lympho-myeloid repopulating activity. To perform the CRU assay, different numbers of test cells are injected into cohorts of irradiated congenic recipients whose survival is assured independently. Poisson statistics and the method of maximum likelihood are then used to calculate the frequency of CRU in the test-cell suspension from the measured proportions of recipients in each test-cell-dose group in which >1% of the regenerated myeloid *and* lymphoid populations are found to be derived from the injected test cells four or more months later (*see* Chapter 12). Recently, the same principles have been applied to allow the quantitation of human HSC in sublethally irradiated immunodeficient nonobese diabetic/severe combined immunodeficient (NOD/SCID) mice *(17,19,20)*.

Measurements of the expansion activity of HSC populations are therefore critically dependent on several experimental design parameters. These include the use of adequate sample sizes, accurate measurements of input (or output) CRU numbers, and the use of correct assumptions in calculating total CRU outputs from data obtained when using a portion of the original culture. Recent findings suggest that the ability of primitive hematopoietic cells to engraft may be an additional variable parameter *(21,22)* subject to reversible changes that are not necessarily linked to a loss of pluripotentiality or self-maintenance *(23)*. It should also be emphasized that the expansion either in vivo *(24)* or in vitro *(25)* of cells expressing surface markers ascribed to HSC does not necessarily correlate with retention of long-term in vivo repopulating activity.

1.2. Cytokine Supplements

Numerous cytokines have been identified as important extracellular regulators of hematopoiesis, and have become useful reagents for the stimulation of these cells in vitro. To obtain a net expansion in vitro of human umbilical cord blood (UCB) or adult mouse bone marrow, CRU appears to require a combination of synergistic cytokines. These include steel factor (SF, also known as stem cell factor [SCF]) Flt-3 ligand (FL), and cytokines from the family that signal through gp130 (**Table 1**). The combination of interleukin-11 (IL-11), SF, and FL, has been found to stimulate an amplification in vitro of adult murine marrow CRU *(14)*, and IL-6 in concert with FL, SF, IL-3, and granulocyte-colony-stimulating factor (G-CSF) can support the expansion in vitro of human cord blood CRU *(16,17)*.

Other cytokines, or cytokine combinations, can have a negative effect on the ability of HSC to maintain their activity in vitro. For example, Yonemura et al. *(27,28)* and others *(26)* have reported that the addition of IL-3 or IL-1 to cytokine combinations that can maintain murine stem cell in vivo repopulating potential will eliminate this activity. Excessive IL-3 concentrations have also been found to have a negative impact on the expansion of human LTC-IC in cultures of CD34$^+$CD38$^-$ cells isolated from normal adult marrow *(31)*, although some IL-3, together with high concentrations of FL and SF, is required to maximize the expansion of human LTC-IC in such cultures *(31,32)*. Among the various combinations of cytokines tested on purified human CD34$^+$ UCB

Table 1
Ex Vivo Expansion of Human and Murine In Vivo Repopulating Cells (CRU)

Input cell populations	Culture time (days)	Cytokine combination	In vivo repopulating ability (relative to input)	Ref
Human CD34+CD38− cord blood	5–8	FL, SF, IL-3, IL-6, G-CSF	Expansion (2×)	17
Human CD34+CD38− cord blood	4	FL, SF, IL-3, IL-6, G-CSF	Expansion (2–4×)	16
Murine Lin−Sca-1+ adult marrow	10	IL-11, SF, FL	Expansion (3×)	14
Murine Lin−Sca-1+WGA+ adult marrow	14	SF, IL-6, Epo	Maintenance	25
Murine adult marrow	4	SF, IL-11, IL-1, IL-6	Maintenance	26
Murine Sca-1+c-kit+lin− adult marrow	7	SF, IL-6, IL-11, Epo	Maintenance	27
Murine Sca-1+c-kit+lin− 5-FU adult marrow	7, 14, 21	IL-11, FL IL-11, SF	Maintenance Maintenance	28
Murine adult marrow	6	IL-11 and SF	Increased survival after 30 d	29
Murine lin−Sca-1+c-kit+ 5-FU adult marrow	7	TPO alone IL-6 and FL	Maintenance	30

cells, FL plus thrombopoietin (TPO) was found to maintain hematopoiesis in vitro for up to 6 mo *(33)*. In experiments with murine cells, the ability of TPO in combination with other cytokines to stimulate the proliferation and differentiation of long-term repopulating (LTR) stem cells was shown to be directly mediated *(34)*. As a single factor, TPO stimulated a small net increase in LTC-IC numbers in 10 d cultures of adult human CD34$^+$CD38$^-$ marrow cells *(32,35)*, and promoted the survival in vitro of murine in vivo repopulating cells *(30)*.

Early progenitor functions can be affected by the type of cytokines they are exposed to and by the absolute and relative concentrations of such cytokines in the medium *(31)*. For example, maximal expansion of adult human marrow LTC-IC required the presence of 30 times more FL, SF, IL-3, IL-6, and G-CSF than the amount that concomitantly stimulates the near-maximal expansion of CFC. Similarly, expansion of adult mouse bone-marrow CRU numbers has been found to require a 10 times higher concentration of hyper-IL-6 (H-IL-6, a fusion protein of IL-6 and IL-6R, *[36]*) in combination with SF and FL than the concentration of H-IL-6 that maximizes CFC expansion in the same cultures *(15,37)*.

However, it should be noted that the cytokine combinations and concentrations recommended in **Subheadings 3.3** and **3.6.** for expanding stem cell populations in cultures of human UCB *(16,17)* and murine bone marrow *(14,15)* cells are likely to be suboptimal and may not even be appropriate for other sources of cells. Factorial analysis of the contribution of different cytokines to the yield of LTC-IC in 10 d cultures initiated with adult human CD34$^+$CD38$^-$ marrow cells has shown that a combination of FL, SF, and IL-3 is necessary and sufficient to achieve the greatest effect (among the cytokines evaluated) *(32)*. In contrast, in cultures of human CD34$^+$CD38$^-$ UCB cells, a similar analysis identified FL and IL-6 plus sIL-6R as the most important *(38)*. These results exemplify the changes that occur during ontogeny in the cytokine dependence of proliferative and differentiative responses of functionally analogous human hematopoietic progenitor cells. Similarly, cytokine combinations able to maintain or expand adult murine stem cell populations failed to sustain the long-term repopulating ability of their counterparts in d 14.5 fetal liver *(14,39)*.

1.3. Cell Inoculum and Culture Conditions

The range of concentrations of cells that can be used to initiate a culture and still allow a net expansion of the input stem cell population is quite small. As a "rule of thumb" the output of at least 10–20 CRU must be evaluated in order to ensure representative sampling. This requirement is a result of the heterogeneity in self-renewal responses of individual CRU. In addition, the rapid production of mature hematopoietic cells that accompanies stem cell expansion (since the same cytokines support both stem cell self-renewal and their differentiation) can limit the further expansion of very primitive cells because of an accumulation of inhibitory factors and/or depletion of stimulatory cytokines from the culture medium *(40,41)*. The use of stem cell-enriched populations and low starting-cell densities (<10^3 cells/mL) helps to delay the onset of such problems, and frequent medium exchanges may help to avoid them to some extent. The reader is advised to consult other published studies for a more detailed discussion of how changes in culture conditions can alter the expansion of hematopoietic cells in vitro *(42,43)*.

1.4. Large-Scale Culture Systems

The protocols described in this chapter are designed to support the expansion of small numbers of HSC contained in highly purified cell suspensions and maintained in static cultures with defined cytokines for relatively short periods (10 d). This approach has proven useful to evaluate different cytokines for their ability, either alone or in combination, to stimulate primitive hematopoietic cells, including human *(16,17)* as well as murine *(14,15)* CRU. It should be emphasized, however, that these culture conditions are unlikely to be exclusive or even optimal for the expansion of clinically useful numbers of HSC with the ability to sustain long-term engraftment in autologous or allogeneic transplant recipients.

Nevertheless, numerous investigators have also begun to evaluate the expansion that can be achieved in culture systems designed to handle large numbers of cells. These have included the use of gas-permeable culture bags *(44–49)* and T-flasks *(50)*, as well as various perfusion bioreactor systems *(51–55)*. In most cases, infusion of the cultured cells into myelosuppressed patients has resulted in a hematological reconstitution comparable to historical controls or patients rescued with an aliquot of noncultured cells, but quantitative assessment of in vivo repopulating cells obtained from such large-scale cultures has not yet been reported. However, significant LTC-IC expansion has been documented. For example, Moore and Hoskins *(48)* have reported an 18-fold expansion of human UCB LTC-IC in suspension cultures containing IL-1 and IL-3 maintained in gas-permeable bags. Similarly, Bathia et al. *(49)* measured a five-fold expansion of LTC-IC when adult CD34$^+$HLA-DR$^-$ bone marrow cells from patients with chronic myeloid leukemia were cultured in bags. Expansion of LTC-IC (~10-fold) in cultures of adult human bone marrow *(41,56)* or UCB *(57)* cells maintained in flat-bottomed, constantly stirred, spinner flasks have been described as well. Significant LTC-IC expansion (7.5-fold) was also seen in cultures maintained in a stroma-containing flat-plate perfusion bioreactor using a medium supplemented with IL-3, SF, GM-CSF, and erythropoietin *(51)*.

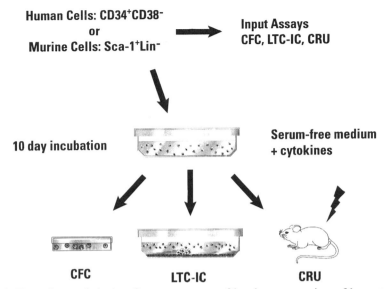

Fig. 1. Experimental design for assessment of in vitro expansion of hematopoeitic cells in 10–d cultures. Aliquots of purified human or murine hematopoietic cells are assayed for their content of CFC, LTC-IC, and CRU. Aliquots of these cell suspensions are also placed in stroma-free suspension cultures in serum-free medium (SFM) supplemented with recombinant cytokines. After 10 d incubation, cultured cells are harvested, pooled, and assayed for CFC, LTC-IC, and CRU content. Expansion potentials can then be determined by relating the content of the target cell population in the cultured cells to the content present in the input inoculum.

2. Materials

A general outline of the steps used to expand and assess the total cells, CFC, LTC-IC, and CRU produced in cultures of $CD34^+CD38^-$ UCB cells or murine lin^-Sca-1^+ adult bone marrow cells is shown in **Fig. 1**. A summary of the expected results from such a protocol is presented in **Tables 2** and **3** for human and murine cells, respectively.

2.1. Ten-Day Suspension Cultures of Human $CD34^+CD38^-$ UCB Cells

1. Serum-free medium (SFM). The SFM has been modified from the formulation originally described by Iscove et al. *(58)*. When preparing SFM, it is critical to use quality-assessed, prescreened components.

   A stock solution of 10% bovine serum albumin (BSA) Fraction V in Iscove's modified Dulbecco's medium (IMDM) prepared according to the method originally described by Worton et al. *(59)*.

   Final concentration of SFM components (in IMDM) are: 1% (10 mg/mL) BSA, 10 μg/mL bovine pancreatic insulin, 200 μg/mL human transferrin (iron-satu-

Table 2
Experimental Details to Assess Stem Cell Expansion in Cultures of Human CD34+CD38− Cord Blood Cells

Assay	Input (d 0) per 2 mL culture (18 cultures)	Number of CD34+CD38− cells assayed at 0	Postulated 10-d expansion (fold)	Total output per culture (10 d)	Proportion of culture assayed at 10
Total cell	500		200–1000	100,000–500,000	
CFC	50	1,000/1.1 mL methylcellulose culture (2–4 replicates)	40–250	2,000–12,500	1–5% of a starting culture equivalent (~1000–25,000 cells) per 1.1 mL methylcellulose culture (2–4 replicates)
LTC-IC	25–100	200/2.5 mL bulk LTC-IC (2–4 replicates)	2–30	50–3,000	Bulk LTC-IC cultures 20% of a culture (~20,000–100,000 cells) per LTC; 5% of a culture (~5,000–25,000 cells) per LTC
CRU	0.83	by LDA (5 recipients each to receive 300 cells, 600 cells, 900 cells)	2	1.7	By LDA 100% of a culture (10^{-5}–5×10^5 cells) per 4 mice; 50% of the culture (5×10^4–2.5×10^5) per 4 mice; 25% of the culture (2.5×10^4–1.25×10^5) per 4 mice

[a]Human CD34+CD38− cord-blood cells are cultured in SFM supplemented with 100 ng/mL human FL, 100 ng/mL human IL-3, 20 ng/mL human IL-6, and 20 ng/mL human G-CSF for 10 d. A minimum of 18 cultures are needed to provide sufficient cells for the assays described.

Table 3
Experimental Details to Assess Stem Cell Expansion in Cultures of Murine Sca-1[+] Lin[−] Bone Marrow Cells

Assay	Input (d 0) per 2 mL culture (5 cultures)	Number of Lin[−]Sca-1[+]cells assayed at d 0	Postulated 10-d expansion (-fold)	Total output per culture (10 d)	Proportion of culture assayed at d 10
Total cell	500		100–1000	50,000–500,000	
CFC	50–150	300–1000/1.1 mL methylcellulose culture (2–4 replicates)	40–100	2,000–15,000	0.7–5% of a starting culture equivalent (~3,000 cells) per 1.1 mL methylcellulose culture) (2–4 replicates)
LTC-IC	5–10	By LDA with 12 wells By LDA with 12 wells, each containing	3–15	15–150	By LDA with 12 wells, each containing 10% (~5000–50000 cells); 3% (~1700–17000 cells); 1% (~500–5000 cells); 0.3% (~170–1700 cells) of a culture
CRU	5–10	By LDA with 6–8 recipients at 25, 50, 100, and 200 cells	1–10	5–100	By LDA with 6–8 mice/ group, each given 10% (~5000–50000 cells); 3% (~1700–17000 cells); 1% (~500–5000 cells); 0.3% (~170–1700 cells) of a culture

[a]Murine Lin[−]Sca-1[+] mouse bone marrow cells are cultured at 500 cells/culture in SFM supplemented with 100 ng/mL human FL, 100 ng/mL human IL-11, and 50 ng/mL murine SF for 10 d. A minimum of five such cultures are needed to provide enough cells to perform the assays described.

rate$_d$), 10^{-4} M 2-mercaptoethanol (2-ME), 2 mM glutamine, and 10–40 μg/mL low-density lipoproteins. Combine components and filter-sterilize using a 0.22-μ filter. Store at –20°C for up to 1 y or at 4°C for up to 1 mo. Add low-density lipoproteins (Sigma, St. Louis, MO) at a final concentration of 10–40 μg/mL and cytokines just prior to use. SFM (StemSpan™ SFEM) is commercially available from StemCell Technologies (Vancouver, BC). Other SFM are also available from other commercial suppliers.

2. Ficoll-Paque (Amersham, Pharmacia, Uppsala, Sweden). Use and store according to the manufacturers' instructions.

3. IMDM/2%FBS: IMDM with 2% fetal bovine serum (FBS). Store at 4°C for up to 1 mo.

4. HF buffer. Phenol red-free Hank's Balanced Salt Solution (HBSS) containing 2% FBS. Filter-sterilize. Can be stored at 4°C for up to 1 mo.

5. HF/5% HS. HF with 5% heat-inactivated human serum.

6. HF/PI: HF with 2 μg/mL propidium iodide (PI)(Sigma).

7. Anti-human fluorochrome-conjugated antibodies: anti human-CD34~Fluorescein-isothiocyanate (FITC), anti-human CD38~PE and FITC- and phycoerythrin-conjugated isotype-control antibodies. Commercial suppliers include Pharmingen, Becton Dickinson and Immunotech, Beckman Coulter.

8. Recombinant cytokines including human FL, human SF, human IL-3, human IL-6, and human G-CSF are available from various commercial sources including StemCell, R&D Systems (Minneapolis, MN), and Peprotech (Rocky Hill, NJ).

9. CFC assays for granulocyte/macrophage (CFU-GM), erythroid burst-forming cells (BFU-E), and multilineage (CFU-GEMM) progenitors. Human CFC are assayed in IMDM containing 1.0% methylcellulose, 30% FBS, 1% BSA, 10^{-4} M 2-ME, 20 ng/mL each of human IL-3, human GM-CSF, human IL-6, and 50 ng/mL human SF (04435; StemCell).

10. Reagents for LTC-IC assay (see Chapter 8).

11. Reagents for human CRU assay (see Chapter 12).

12. Sterile cultureware including 35-mm tissue-culture dishes and 35-mm Petri dishes (StemCell). Petri dishes obtained from other sources should be prescreened and selected for their inability to promote the adherence of fibroblasts.

13. Human CD34+CD38− UCB input cells (see **Note 1**).

2.2. Suspension Cultures of Adult Murine Lin⁻Sca-1⁺ Bone-Marrow Cells

1. SFM. Prepare as described in **Subheading 2.1.**, including addition of LDL at a final concentration of 10–40 μg/mL and desired cytokines (see **step 5**) just prior to use.

2. IMDM/2%FBS. HF and HF/PI. Prepare and store as described in **Subheading 2.1.**

3. Anti-mouse fluorochrome-conjugated antibodies: Ly6A/Sca-1~PE (clone E13-161-7), FITC-labeled CD45R/B220 (clone RA3-6B2), Ly6G/Gr-1 (clone RB6-8C5), CD11b/Mac-1 (clone M1/70), CD5/Ly1(clone 53-7.3, and FITC and

phycoerythrin-labeled isotype controls. Unlabeled mouse anti-Fc receptor antibody (clone 2.4G2) (Pharmingen).

4. Recombinant cytokines including human FL, murine SF, and human IL-11 are available from various commercial sources, including StemCell, R&D Systems, and Peprotech.

5. Assays for CFU-GM, BFU-E, and CFU-GEMM: Murine CFC are assayed in IMDM containing 0.9% methylcellulose, 15% FBS, 10 µg/mL insulin, 200 µg/mL transferrin, 1% BSA, 10^{-4} M 2-ME, 2 mM L-glutamine, and 10 ng/mL each of murine IL-3, murine IL-6, and 50 ng/mL murine SF (03434; StemCell). Culture according to the manufacturers' instructions.

6. Reagents for murine LTC-IC assays (*see* Chapter 8).

7. Reagents for murine CRU assays (*see* Chapter 12).

8. Sterile cultureware including 96-well flat-bottom culture plates, as described in **Subheading 2.1.**

9. Murine lin⁻Sca-1⁺ bone-marrow input cells (*see* **Note 1**).

3. Methods

3.1. Isolation of Human CD34⁺CD38⁻ Cells

To decrease the sorting time required to isolate CD34⁺CD38⁻ cells from light-density UCB cells, lineage marker-positive (lin⁺) cells can first be removed using various bulk-separation strategies, including immunomagnetic cell separation (*see* Chapter 3 and **ref. *60***).

1. Isolate the light-density fraction of the UCB cells (<1.077 g/mL) by centrifugation on Ficoll-Paque according to manufacturers' instructions. Wash the UCB cells twice in HF.

2. Resuspend the light-density UCB cells at ~10^7 cells/mL, and incubate for 15 min at 4°C with HF/5% HS. It is not necessary to wash cells prior to the addition of the fluorochrome-labeled antibodies.

3. Add 10^5 cells to each of four labeled tubes. Add FITC and phycoerythrin-conjugated isotype control antibodies to one tube, anti-CD34~FITC to a second tube, anti-CD38~PE to a third tube, and HF only to the fourth tube. Place the remaining cells in a fifth tube, and add anti-CD34~FITC and anti-CD38~PE. Incubate all tubes for 30 min on ice and protect from light.

4. Add HF to all tubes and centrifuge the cells at 300–350 g for 7–10 min. Discard the supernatants and repeat adding HF/PI to the second wash. Finally, resuspend the cells in HF for flow-cytometric analysis. Tubes containing fluorochrome-conjugated isotype control antibodies, anti-CD34~FITC, anti-CD38~PE, and PI only are used to establish threshold and compensation settings on the FACS instrument. Positive staining is defined as the level of fluorescence that exceeds that of >99% of cells stained with fluorochrome-conjugated isotype control antibodies.

5. Collect viable (PI⁻) cells with a CD34⁺CD38⁻ phenotype into sterile tubes containing SFM.

3.2. Assessment of Frequencies of CFC, LTC-IC, and CRU in the Input (and Cultured) Human CD34⁺CD38⁻ UCB Cells

Remove appropriate cell aliquots and assay for CFC, LTC-IC, and CRU content, using protocols described in Chapters 7, 8 and 12. Note that it may be necessary to partially purify the LTC-IC in the cultured population in order to make their enumeration possible.

3.3. Suspension Cultures of Human CD34⁺CD38⁻ UCB Cells in Cytokine-Supplemented SFM

1. Resuspend the purified human CD34⁺CD38⁻ UCB cells in SFM supplemented with 100 ng/mL each of human FL and human SF and 20 ng/mL each of human IL-3, human IL-6, and human G-CSF.
2. Place 500–2000 cell aliquots in total vol of 2.0 mL in sterile 35-mm Petri dishes and incubate them undisturbed for 10 d in a humidified incubator at 37°C with 5% CO_2 in air. The cell density should not be allowed to exceed $1–2 \times 10^6$ cells/mL at any time during the culture period. Prepare sufficient replicate cultures to allow accurate quantitation of CFC, LTC-IC, and CRU in the cultured-cell suspension present after the 10 d of incubation (*see* **Table 2**).
3. At the end of the incubation period, pool the nonadherent cells from all cultures and place in a sterile 15-mL collection tube. Any adherent cells remaining should also be harvested by rigorous pipetting or by incubation with 0.25% trypsin/ethylenediaminetetraacetic acid (EDTA) at room temperature for 4 min. Rinse the culture dishes once again with IMDM/2% FCS, and wash the combined nonadherent and adherent cells.
4. Count the cells and assay appropriate aliquots for CFC, LTC-IC, and CRU. An illustrative experiment is shown in **Table 2**. Estimates of the numbers of cells to be used in the assays of the input cell suspension and suggested proportions of the completed cultures to be used are based on data derived from **ref. *17***.

3.4. Isolation of Adult Murine Lin⁻Sca-1⁺ Bone Marrow Cells

Note that when the input and cultured cells are to be assayed for their CRU content, the cells must be harvested from a donor mouse genotype which allows specific discrimination of the progeny in a histocompatible, irradiated, or immunocompromised recipient (*see* Chapter 12). To decrease the sorting time required to isolate lin⁻Sca-1⁺ cells from freshly isolated adult mouse bone marrow cells, it is useful to first remove the lin⁺ cells by one of several bulk strategies including immunomagnetic cell separation (*see* Chapter 3).

1. Sacrifice 5–7 mice (8–12 wk of age) according to procedures approved by the institution.

2. Flush the bone marrow cells from the femora into a tube using a sterile 21-gauge needle attached to a 3-cc syringe containing 1–2 mL of cold, sterile HF. Obtain a single-cell suspension by gently aspirating the cells once or twice though the same syringe and needle.

3. Resuspend the cells to ~10^7/mL in HF supplemented with 3 μg/mL anti-Fc antibody (clone 24G2). Incubate the cells on ice for 15 min. It is not necessary to wash the cells prior to addition of the labeled antibodies.

4. Add 10^5 cells to each of four labeled FACS tubes. Add FITC and phycoerthrin-conjugated isotype-control antibodies to a first tube, lin~FITC (anti-Gr-1, anti-Mac-1, anti-Ly-1, anti-B220) to a second tube, anti-Sca-1~PE to the third tube, and HF only to the fourth tube. Place the remaining cells in a fifth tube and add lin~FITC and anti-Sca-1~PE. Incubate all tubes for 30 min on ice and protect from light.

5. Add HF to all tubes and centrifuge the cells at 300–350 *g* for 7–10 min. Discard the supernatants and repeat adding HF/PI to the second wash. Resuspend the cells in HF for flow-cytometric analysis. Tubes containing fluorochrome-conjugated isotype control antibodies, lin~FITC only, anti-Sca-1~PE only, and PI only are used to establish threshold and compensation settings on the FACS instrument. If appropriate conjugated isotype-control antibodies are unavailable, minimum fluorescence thresholds are established using PI-treated unstained cells. Positive staining is defined as the level of fluorescence that exceeds that of >99% of cells stained with conjugated isotype-control antibodies.

6. Viable (PI⁻) cells with low-to-medium forward scattering and low forward scattering properties and a lin⁻Sca-1⁺ phenotype are isolated by FACS into SFM.

3.5. Assessment of the Frequencies of CFC, LTC-IC, and CRU in the Input (and Cultured) Murine Lin⁻Sca-1⁺ Bone Marrow Cells

Remove appropriate cell aliquots and assay for CFC, LTC-IC, and CRU content, using protocols described in Chapters 7, 8 and 12.

3.6. Suspension Cultures of Murine Lin⁻Sca-1⁺ Bone Marrow Cells in Cytokine-Supplemented SFM

1. Resuspend the murine lin⁻Sca-1⁺ bone marrow cells in SFM supplemented with 100 ng/mL each of human FL and human IL-11 and 50 ng/mL of murine SF.

2. Place aliquots of 500–1000 cells in vol of 2 mL into 35-mm Petri dishes and incubate for 10 d at 33°C in a humidified atmosphere of 5% CO_2 in air. The cell density should not be allowed to exceed ~5×10^5/mL at any time during the 10-d culture period.

3. At the end of 10 d, pool the nonadherent cells from all cultures and place into a sterile 15-mL collection tube. Any remaining adherent cells should be harvested by rigorous pipetting or by incubation with 0.25% trypsin/EDTA at room temperature for 4 min. Rinse the culture dishes again with IMDM/2% FCS, and wash the combined nonadherent and adherent cells.

4. Count the cells and assay appropriate aliquots for CFC, LTC-IC and CRU. An illustrative experiment is shown in **Table 3**. Estimations of the numbers of cells to be used in assays of the starting cells and proportions of the completed cultures to be used are based on data derived from **refs.** *14* and *15*.

3.7. Calculations to Estimate the Expansion of Each Human or Murine Hematopoietic Cell Population Measured

As illustrated in **Tables 2** and **3**, it is useful to design experiments and express results based on the frequency of target cells per defined number of input cells (e.g., per 1000 $CD34^+CD38^-$ or lin^-Sca-1^+ cells) or per culture. Expansion of the total cell population usually exceeds the changes in numbers of CFC, LTC-IC, or CRU, and therefore, proportional plating of pooled, harvested cultures is recommended. Estimations of expansion potential are derived by relating the content of the target-cell population in the cultured cells to the content measured in the input-cell population.

Example: Calculation of expansion of murine LTC-IC in cultures of lin^-Sca-1^+ bone-marrow cells. Input cells: 500 lin^-Sca-1^+ cells per culture; frequency of LTC-IC in lin^-Sca-1^+ cells is 1 per 50. Therefore, the LTC-IC content of the input cell population is 10 LTC-IC per culture or 10 LTC-IC per 500 lin^-Sca-1^+ cells. Cultured cells: 7.5×10^4 cells per culture is obtained after a 10-d culture period; LTC-IC LDA analysis shows 1 LTC-IC per 1500 cultured cells. Therefore, the LTC-IC content of the cultured cells is 50 per culture or 50 per 500 input cells. The estimated total expansion of murine LTC-IC in these cultures is 50/10=5.

As a final point, it is advisable to consult a qualified statistician to ensure that appropriate statistical analyses are applied for estimations of ex vivo expansion of HSC and progenitor populations.

4. Notes

1. The published literature contains numerous strategies not described here for the isolation of cell suspensions enriched for their content of in vitro long-term repopulating cells based on the expression of various cell-surface antigens. Many of these strategies are likely to yield cell subsets suitable for expanding human or murine CRU under the conditions described here. For example, the isolation of the lin^- $CD34^+$ cells from normal human bone marrow, UCB, mobilized peripheral blood (MPB), or fetal liver yields a suspension that is highly enriched in CRU *(17,19,20)*. Selection of lin^-CD34^+ subsets expressing Thy-1 *(61,62)* and/or AC133 *(63,64)* further enrich for CRU in a fashion similar to that obtained when the $CD38^-$ subset of $CD34^+$ cells is selected. Recent evidence also indicates that a proportion of human HSC may be lin^-CD34^- *(65,66)*. The majority of murine CRU appears to be contained within the lin^-Sca-1^+ fraction. Antibodies directed against murine Thy-1 *(67)*, CD117/c-kit *(68,69)*, and CD34 *(70,71)* have been

used to obtain more highly enriched suspensions of LTR cells. Detailed descriptions of the isolation of human and murine HSC are provided in Chapters 1–4.

2. If desired, other parameters including total cell numbers, and the concentrations of various cytokines, nutrients, and metabolites may be monitored during the culture period.

References

1. Emerson, S. G. (1996) Ex vivo expansion of hematopoietic precursors, progenitors and stem cells: the next generation of cellular therapeutics. *Blood* **87,** 3082–3088.

2. Williams, D.A. and Smith, F.O. (2000) Progress in the use of gene transfer methods to treat genetic blood diseases. *Hum. Gene. Ther.* **11,** 2059–2066.

3. Aglietta, M., Bertolini, F., Carlo-Stella, C., De Vincentiis, A., Lanata, L., Lemoli, R. M., et al. (1998) Ex vivo expansion of hematopoietic cells and their clinical use. *Haematologica* **83,** 824–848.

4. Hoffman, R. (1999) Progress in the development of systems for *in vitro* expansion of human hematopoietic stem cells. *Curr. Opin. Hematol.* **6,** 184–191.

5. Srour, E. F., Abonour, R., Cornetta, K., and Traycoff, C. M. (1999) Ex vivo expansion of hematopoietic stem and progenitor cells: are we there yet? *J. Hematother.* **8,** 93–102.

6. Wu, A. M., Till, J. E., Siminovitch, L., and McCulloch E.A. (1968) Cytological evidence for a relationship between normal hematopoietic colony-forming cells and cells of the lymphoid system. *J. Exp. Med.* **127,** 455–464.

7. Dick, J. E., Magli, M. C., Huszar, D., Phillips, R. A., and Bernstein, A. (1985) Introduction of a selectable gene into primitive stem cells capable of long-term reconstitution of the hemopoietic system in W/Wv mice. *Cell* **42,** 71–79.

8. Lemischka, I. R., Raulet, D. H., and Mulligan, R. C. (1986) Developmental potential and dynamic behavior of hematopoietic stem cells. *Cell* **45,** 917–927.

9. Keller, G. and Snodgrass, R. (1990) Life span of multipotential hematopoietic stem cells *in vivo*. *J. Exp. Med.* **171,** 1407–1418.

10. Fraser, C. C., Szilvassy, S. J., Eaves, C. J., and Humphries, R. K. (1992) Proliferation of totipotent hematopoietic stem cells *in vitro* with retention of long-term competitive *in vivo* reconstituting ability. *Proc. Natl. Acad. Sci. USA* **89,** 1968–1972.

11. Luens, K. M., Travis, M. A., Chen, B. P., Hill, B. L., Scollay, R., and Murray, L. J. (1998) Thrombopoietin, kit ligand, and flk2/flt3 ligand together induce increased numbers of primitive hematopoietic progenitors from human CD34+Thy-1+Lin⁻ cells with preserved ability to engraft SCID-hu bone. *Blood* **91,** 1206–1215.

12. Oostendorp, R. A. J., Audet, J., Miller, C. M., and Eaves, C. J. (1999) Cell division tracking and expansion of hematopoietic long-term repopulating cells. *Leukemia* **13,** 499–501.

13. Glimm, H. and Eaves, C. J. (1999) Direct evidence for multiple self-renewal divisions of human *in vivo* repopulating cells in short-term culture. *Blood* **94,** 2161–2168.

14. Miller, C. L. and Eaves, C. J. (1997) Expansion *in vitro* of adult murine hematopoietic stem cells with transplantable lympho-myeloid reconstituting ability. *Proc. Natl. Acad. Sci. USA* **94,** 13,648–13,653.
15. Audet, J., Miller, C. L., Rose-John, S., Piret, J., and Eaves, C. J. (2001) Distinct role of gp130 activation in promoting self-renewal divisions by mitogenically stimulated murine hematopoietic stem cells. *Proc. Natl. Acad. Sci. USA* **98,** 1757–1762.
16. Bhatia, M., Bonnet, D., Kapp, U., Wang, J., Murdoch, B., and Dick , J. (1997) Quantitative analysis reveals expansion of human hematopoietic repopulating cells after short-term ex vivo culture. *J. Exp. Med.* **186,** 619–624.
17. Conneally, E., Cashman, J., Petzer, A., and Eaves, C. (1997) Expansion *in vitro* of transplantable human cord blood stem cells demonstrated using a quantitative assay of their lympho-myeloid repopulating activity in nonobese diabetic-scid/scid mice. *Proc. Natl. Acad. Sci. USA* **94,** 9836–9841.
18. Szilvassy, S. J., Humphries, R. K., Lansdorp, P. M., Eaves, A. C., and Eaves, C. J. (1990) Quantitative assay for totipotent reconstituting hematopoietic stem cells by a competitive repopulation strategy. *Proc. Natl. Acad. Sci. USA* **87,** 8736–8740.
19. Wang, J. C. Y., Doesdens, M., and Dick, J. E. (1997) Primitive human hematopoietic cells are enriched in cord blood compared with adult bone marrow or mobilized peripheral blood as measured by the quantitative *in vivo* SCID-repopulating cell assay. *Blood* **89,** 3919–3924.
20. Holyoake, T. L., Nicolini, F. E., and Eaves, C. J. (1999) Functional differences between transplantable human hematopoietic stem cells from fetal liver, cord blood and adult marrow. *Exp. Hematol.* **27,** 1418–1427.
21. Papayannopoulou, T., Craddock, C., Nakamoto, B., Priestley, G. V., and Wolf, N. S. (1995) The VLA4/VCAM-1 adhesion pathway defines contrasting mechanisms of lodgement of transplanted murine hemopoietic progenitors between bone marrow and spleen. *Proc. Natl. Acad. Sci. USA* **92,** 9647–9651.
22. Gothot, A., van der Loo, J. C., Clapp, D. W., and Srour, E. F. (1998) Cell cycle-related changes in repopulating capacity of human mobilized peripheral blood CD34+ cells in non-obese diabetic/severe combined immune-deficient mice. *Blood* **15,** 2641–2649.
23. Habibian, H. K., Peters, S. O., Hsieh, C. C., Wuu, J., Vergilis, K., Grimaldi, C. I., et al.. (1998) The fluctuating phenotype of the lymphohematopoietic stem cell with cell cycle transit. *J. Exp. Med.* **188,** 393–398.
24. Spangrude, G. J., Brooks, D. M., and Tumas, D. B. (1995) Long-term repopulation of irradiated mice with limiting numbers of purified hematopoietic stem cells: *in vivo* expansion of stem cell phenotype but not function. *Blood* **85,** 1006–1016.
25. Rebel, V. I., Dragowska, W., Eaves, C. J., Humphries, R. K., and Lansdorp, P. M. (1994) Amplification of Lin⁻Sca⁺WGA⁺ cells in serum-free cultures containing Steel Factor, Interleukin-6, and Erythropoietin with maintenance of cells with long-term *in vivo* reconstituting potential. *Blood* **83,** 128–136.
26. Trevisan, M. and Iscove, N.N. (1995) Phenotypic analysis of murine long-term

hemopoietic reconstituting cells quantitated competitively *in vivo* and comparison with more advanced colony-forming progeny. *J. Exp. Med.* **181,** 93–103.

27. Yonemura, Y., Ku, H., Hirayama, F., Souza, L., and Ogawa, M. (1996) Interleukin 3 or interleukin 1 abrogates the reconstituting ability of hematopoietic stem cells. *Proc. Natl. Acad. Sci. USA* **93,** 4040–4044.

28. Yonemura, Y., Ku, H., Lyman, S., and Ogawa, M. (1997) *In vitro* expansion of hematopoietic progenitors and maintenance of stem cells: comparison between Flt3/Flk-2 ligand and kit ligand. *Blood* **89,** 1915–1921.

29. Holyoake, T., Freshney, M., McNair, L., Parker, A., McKay, P., Steward, W., et al. (1996) Ex vivo expansion with stem cell factor and interleukin-11 augments both short-term recovery posttransplant and the ability to serially transplant marrow. *Blood* **87,** 4589–4595.

30. Matsunaga, T., Kato, T., Miyazaki, H., and Ogawa, M. (1998) Thrombopoietin promotes the survival of murine hematopoietic long-term reconstituting cells: comparison with the effects of FLT3/FLK-2 ligand and interleukin-6. *Blood* **92,** 452–461.

31. Zandstra, P., E, Conneally, E., Petzer, A., Piret, J., and Eaves, C. J. (1997) Cytokine manipulation of primitive human hematopoietic cell self-renewal. *Proc. Natl. Acad. Sci. USA* **94,** 4698–4703.

32. Petzer, A., Zandstra, P., Piret, J., and Eaves, C. J. (1996) Differential cytokine effects on primitive (CD34$^+$CD38–) human hematopoietic cells: novel responses to flt3–ligand and thrombopoietin. *J. Exp. Med.* **183,** 2551–2558.

33. Piacibello, W., Sanavio, F., Garetto, L., Severino, A., Bergandi, D., Ferrario, J., et al. (1997) Extensive amplification and self-renewal of human primitive hematopoietic stem cells from cord blood. *Blood* **89,** 2644–2653.

34. Sitnicka, E., Lin, N., Priestley, G., Fox, N., Broudy, V., Wolf, N., et al. (1996) The effect of thrombopoietin on the proliferation and differentiation of murine hematopoietic stem cells. *Blood* **87,** 4998–5005.

35. Ramsfjell, V., Borge, O., Cui, L., and Jacobsen, S. (1997) Thrombopoietin directly and potently stimulates multilineage growth and progenitor cell expansion from primitive (CD34$^+$CD38$^-$) human bone marrow progenitor cells: distinct and key interactions with the ligands for c-kit and flt3, and inhibitory effects of TGF-b and TNF-a. *J. Immunol.* **158,** 5169–5177.

36. Fischer, M., Goldschmitt, J., Peschel, C., Brakenhoff, J., Kallen, K.-J., Wollmer, A., et al. (1997) A bioactive designer cytokine for human hematopoietic progenitor cell expansion. *Nat. Biotechnol.* **15,** 142–145.

37. Audet, J., Miller, C., Rose-John, S., Piret, J., and Eaves, C. (1998) *In vitro* expansion of *in vivo* repopulating hematopoietic stem cells from adult mouse bone marrow using hyperIL-6, an engineered hybrid cytokine of human interleukin-6 and its soluble receptor. *Exp. Hematol.* **26,** 700.

38. Zandstra, P. W., Conneally, E., Piret, J. M., and Eaves, C. J. (1998) Ontogeny-associated changes in the cytokine responses of primitive human haemopoietic cells. *Br. J. Haematol.* **101,** 770–778.

39. Rebel, V.I. and Lansdorp, P.M. (1996) Culture of purified stem cells from fetal liver results in loss of *in vivo* repopulating potential. *J. Hematother.* **5,** 25–37.

40. Koller, M., Bradley, M., and Palsson, B. (1995) Growth factor consumption and production in perfusion cultures of human bone marrow correlate with specific cell production. *Exp. Hematol.* **23,** 1275–1283.

41. Zandstra, P., Petzer, A., Eaves, C., and Piret, M. (1997) Cellular determinants affecting the rate of cytokine depletion in cultures of human hematopoietic cells. *Biotechnol. Bioeng.* **54,** 58–66.

42. Audet, J., Zandstra, P. W., Eaves, C. J., and Piret, J. M. (1998) Advances in hematopoietic stem cell culture. *Curr. Opin. Biotechnol.* **9,** 146–151.

43. Zandstra, P. W., Eaves, C. J., and Piret, J. M. (1999) Environmental requirements of hematopoietic progenitor cells in ex vivo expansion systems, in *Ex Vivo Cell Therapy,* (Schindhelm, K. and Norton, R., eds.), Academic Press, San Diego, CA, pp. 245–272.

44. Williams, S. F., Lee, W. J., Bender, J. G., Zimmerman, T., Swinney, P., Blake, M., et al. (1996) Selection and expansion of peripheral blood CD34+ cells in autologous stem cell transplantation for breast cancer. *Blood* **87,** 1687–1691.

45. Reiffers, J., Cailliot, C., Dazey, B., Duchez, I., Pigneux, A., Cousin, T., et al. (1998) Infusion of expanded CD34+ selected cells can abrogate post myeloablative chemotherapy neutropenia in patients with hematologic malignancies. *Blood* **92,** 126a.

46. McNiece, I., Hami, L., Jones, R., Bearman, S., Cagnoni, P., Nieto, Y., et al. (1998) Transplantation of ex vivo expanded PBPC after high dose chemotherapy results in decreased neutropenia. *Blood* **92,** 126a.

47. Shpall, E. J., Quinones, R., Hami, L., Jones, R., Bearman, S., Cagnoni, P., et al. (1998) Transplantation of cancer patients receiving high dose chemotherapy with ex vivo expanded cord blood cells. *Blood* **92,** 646a.

48. Moore, M. and Hoskins, I. (1994) Ex vivo expansion of cord blood-derived stem cells and progenitors. *Blood Cells* **20,** 468–481.

49. Bhatia, R., McGlave, P., Miller, J., Wissink, S., Lin, W.-N., and Verfaillie, C. (1997) A clinically suitable ex vivo expansion culture system for LTC-IC and CFC using stroma-conditioned medium. *Exp. Hematol.* **25,** 980–991.

50. Brugger, W., Heimfeld, S., Berenson, R. J., Mertelsmann, R., and Kanz, L. (1995) Reconstitution of hematopoiesis after high-dose chemotherapy by autologous progenitor cells generated ex vivo. *N. Engl. J. Med.* **333,** 283–287.

51. Koller, M., Bradley, M., and Palsson, B. (1993) Large-scale expansion of human stem and progenitor cells from bone marrow mononuclear cells in continuous perfusion cultures. *Blood* **82,** 378–384.

52. Pecora, A. L., Preti, R., Jennis, A., Goldberg, S., Stiff, P., Bachier, C., et al. (1998) Aastrom Replicell System expanded bone marrow enhances hematopoietic recovery in patients receiving low doses of G-CSF primed blood stem cells. *Blood* **92,** 126a.

53. Jaroscak, J., Martin, P. L., Waters-Pick, B., Armstrong, R. D., Driscoll, T., Howrey, R. P., et al. (1998) A phase I trial of augmentation of unrelated umbilical cord blood transplantation with ex-vivo expanded cells. *Blood* **92,** 646a.

54. Stiff, P., Pecora, A., Parthasarathy, M., Preti, R., Chen, B., Douville, J., et al. (1998) Umbilical cord blood transplants in adult using a combination of

unexpanded and ex vivo expanded cells: preliminary clinical observations. *Blood* **92,** 646a.

55. Bachier, C. R., Gokmen, E., Teale, J., Lanzkron, S., Childs, C., Franklin, W., et al. (1999) Ex-vivo expansion of bone marrow progenitor cells for hematopoietic reconstitution following high-dose chemotherapy for breast cancer. *Exp. Hematol.* **27,** 615–623.

56. Zandstra, P., Eaves, C. J., and Piret, J. (1994) Expansion of hematopoietic progenitor cell populations in stirred suspension bioreactors of normal human bone marrow cells. *Bio/Technol.* **12,** 909–914.

57. Kogler, G., Callejas, J., Miggliaccio, A., and al., e. (1996) The effects of different growth factor combinations and medium on the ex vivo expansion of umbilical cord blood committed and primitive progenitors in "steady-state" or stirred suspension cultures. *Blood* **88,** 603a.

58. Iscove, N. N., Guilbert, L. J., and Weyman, C. (1980) Complete replacement of serum in primary cultures of erythropoietin-dependent red cell precursors (CFU-E) by albumin, transferrin, iron, unsaturated fatty acids, lecithins and cholesterol. *Exp. Cell. Res.* **126,** 121–126.

59. Worton, R.G., McCulloch, E.A., and Till, J.E. (1969) Physical separation of hematopoietic stem cells from colony forming cells in culture. *J. Cell Physiol.* **74,** 171–182.

60. Thomas, T. E., Miller, C. L., and Eaves, C. J. (1999) Purification of hematopoietic stem cells for further biological study, in *Methods: A Companion to Methods in Enzymology*, Academic Press, 17, pp. 202–218.

61. Baum, C. M., Weisman, I. L., Tsukamoto, A. S., Buckle, A. M., and Peault, B. (1992) Isolation of a candidate human hematopoietic stem-cell population. *Proc. Natl. Acad. Sci. USA* **89,** 2804–2808.

62. Craig, W., Kay, R., Cutler, R. L., and Lansdorp, P. M. (1993) Expression of Thy-1 on human hematopoietic progenitor cells. *J. Exp. Med.* **177,** 1331–1342.

63. Yin, A. H., Miraglia, S., Zanjani, E. D., Almeida-Porada, G., Ogawa, M., Leary, A. G., et al. (1997) AC133, a novel marker for human hematopoietic stem and progenitor cells. *Blood* **90,** 5002–5012.

64. de Wynter, E. A., Buck, D., Hart, C., Heywood, R., Coutinho, L. H., Clayton, A., et al. (1998) CD34+AC133+ cells isolated from cord blood are highly enriched in long-term culture initiating cells, NOD/SCID-repopulating cells and dendritic cell progenitors. *Stem Cells* **16,** 387–396.

65. Zanjani, E. D., Almeida-Porada, G., Livingston, A. G., Flake, A. W., and Ogawa, M. (1998) Human bone marrow CD34− cells engraft *in vivo* and undergo multilineage expression that includes giving rise to CD34+ cells. *Exp. Hematol.* **26,** 353.

66. Bhatia, M., Bonnet, D., Murdoch, B., Gan, O. I., and Dick, J. E. (1998) A newly discovered class of human hematopoietic cells with SCID-repopulating activity. *Nat. Med.* **4,** 1038–1045.

67. Spangrude, G. J., Heimfield, S., and Weissman, I. L. (1988) Purification and characterization of mouse hematopoietic stem cells. *Science* **241,** 58–62.

68. Okada, S., Nakauchi, H., Nagayoshi, K., Nishikawa, S., Nishikawa, S., Miura, Y.

et al. (1991) Enrichment and characterization of murine hematopoietic stem cells that express c-kit molecule. *Blood* **78,** 1706–1712.

69. Orlic, D., Fischer, R., Nishikawa, S., Nienhuis, A. W., and Bodine, D. M. (1993) Purification and characterization of heterogenous pluripotent hematopoietic stem cell populations expressing high levels of c-kit receptor. *Blood* **82,** 762–770.

70. Osawa, M., Hanada, K., Hamada, H., and Nakauchi, H. (1996) Long-term lymphohematopoietic reconstitution by a single CD34⁻low/negative hematopoietic stem cell. *Science* **273,** 242–245.

71. Morel, F., Galy, A., Chen, B., and Szilvassy, S. J. (1998) Equal distribution of competitive long-term repopulating stem cells in the CD34⁺ and CD34⁻ fractions of Thy-1^{low} Lin$^{-/low}$ Sca-1$^+$ bone marrow cells. *Exp. Hematol.* **26,** 440–448.

14

Hematopoietic Development of ES Cells in Culture

Gordon M. Keller, Saiphone Webb, and Marion Kennedy

1. Introduction

Under appropriate culture conditions, ES cells will spontaneously differentiate and generate colonies known as embryoid bodies (EBs) that contain precursors of multiple lineages, including those of the hematopoietic system *(1–7)*. Previous studies have demonstrated that the molecular events leading to hematopoietic commitment, as well as the kinetics of lineage development within the EBs, parallel that found in the normal mouse embryo *(5)*. More recent studies *(8–11)* have supported these earlier findings and have provided evidence that hematopoietic development within EBs can be divided into the following distinct stages: hemangioblast, primitive and early definitive, and multilineage definitive. These stages most closely correspond to the preblood island, the early-mid yolk sac, and the late yolk sac-early fetal-liver hematopoietic programs within the mouse embryo.

Given these well-characterized patterns of development, the in vitro differentiation of ES cells provides a powerful model for studying embryonic hematopoiesis, using a number of experimental approaches. EBs provide easy access to multiple stages of development, enabling the identification, isolation, and characterization of the earliest committed hematopoietic precursors *(8,10)*. Differentiation of genetically altered ES cells provides a good assay for defining the role of a specific gene in the development of the embryonic hematopoietic system. With respect to loss of function studies, in vitro differentiation of gene-targeted ES cells offers a complementary approach to the analysis of knock-out mice, as it is quick, inexpensive, and can be used for the analysis of genes that are essential for embryonic and fetal development *(12–15)*. The ES/EB system is also well-suited to gain-of-function studies, as the consequences

From: *Methods in Molecular Medicine, vol. 63: Hematopoietic Stem Cell Protocols*
Edited by: C. A. Klug and C. T. Jordan © Humana Press Inc., Totowa, NJ

of overexpression of specific genes on hematopoietic commitment can be determined *(16,17)*. The protocols in this Chapter cover all aspects of ES differentiation and the generation of specific hematopoietic lineages from the developing EBs.

2. Materials
2.1. Media

1. Dulbecco's Modified Eagle Medium (DMEM): (for 1 L)
   DMEM powder: Gibco-BRL #12100–046: package for 1 L.
   Penicillin/streptomycin (100X): Gibco-BRL #15070–063: 10 ml/L.
   HEPES buffer 1 M: Gibco-BRL #15630–080: 25 ml/L.
   $NaHCO_3$: 3.025g/L*.
   Tissue-culture grade H_2O (TC-H_2O): make up to 1 L.
   Filter-sterilize.
   *The amount of $NaHCO_3$ has been adjusted to that of IMDM.
2. Iscove's Modified Dulbecco's Medium (IMDM): (for 1 L)
   IMDM powder: Gibco-BRL #12200-036: package for 1 L.
   Penicillin/streptomycin (100X): Gibco-BRL #15070–063: 10 mL/L.
   $NaHCO_3$: 3.025 g/L.
   TC-H_2O: make up to 1 L.
   Filter-sterilize.
   IMDM can also be purchased ready-made from a number of different suppliers.
3. 10X Phosphate-Buffered Saline (PBS): (for 1-L stock).
   Dissolve the following in approx 800 mL of TC-H_2O: NaCl (80 g), KCl (2 g), Na_2HPO_4 (14.4 g), KH_2PO_4 (2.4 g).
   Adjust pH to 7.4.
   Adjust final volume to 1 L with TC-H_2O and filter-sterilize.
   Dilute stock 1:10 with sterile TC-H_2O for use.
4. DMEM-ES and IMDM-ES Medium:
   DMEM or IMDM (85%).
   Fetal bovine serum (FCS) pretested for maintenance of ES cells (15%).
   Monothioglycerol ($1.5 \times 10^{-4}M$).
   Leukemia inhibitory factor (LIF) (10 ng/mL mouse recombinant or conditioned medium [CM]).
5. IMDM-FCS Medium: IMDM (95%), fetal calf serum (FCS) (5%), monothioglycerol ($1.5 \times 10^{-4}M$).
6. Macrophage Medium I: IMDM + $1.5 \times 10^{-4}M$ monothioglycerol (80%), FCS (10%), L-cell CM (10%), IL-3 (1 ng/mL mouse recombinant or CM).
7. Macrophage Medium II: IMDM + $1.5 \times 10^{-4}M$ monothioglycerol (80%), FCS (10%), L-cell CM (10%).
8. Mast-Cell Medium: IMDM + $1.5 \times 10^{-4}M$ monothioglycerol (90%), FCS (10%), IL-3 (1 ng/mL mouse recombinant or CM), c-kit ligand (KL) (100 ng/mL mouse recombinant or CM).

9. Hemangioblast Medium: This medium is used to expand both hematopoietic and endothelial cells from the blast-cell colonies, and contains the following serum and cytokines that have been selected to stimulate the growth of these lineages: FCS (10%), horse serum (HS)(10%), vascular endothelial growth factor (VEGF) (5 ng/mL), insulin-like growth factor (IGF-1) (10 ng/mL), basic fibroblast growth factor (bFGF) (10ng/mL), Epo (2 U/mL), KL (100 ng/mL mouse recombinant or CM), IL-3 (1 ng/mL mouse recombinant or CM), endothelial cell- growth supplement (ECGS) (100 μg/mL), IMDM + MTG ($1.5 \times 10^4 M$); make to 100%.

10. Methylcellulose Stock (2.0%):

   a. Weigh a sterile 2-L Erlenmeyer flask, add 450 mL autoclaved TC-H$_2$O, and bring to a boil on a hotplate.

   b. Add 20 g of methylcellulose powder and bring to a boil for 3 min. The mixture must be swirled repeatedly during this step, as it will rise and flow over the flask as it boils. Swirling the mixture as it begins to rise will prevent this.

   c. Allow this mixture to cool to room temperature.

   d. While the mixture is cooling, make 500 mL of 2X IMDM with 2X MTG ($3.0 \times 10^4 M$) using the above IMDM recipe with one-half the amount of water. Filter-sterilize prior to use.

   e. When the methylcellulose mixture has cooled to room temperature, add the 2X IMDM and swirl to mix.

   f. Weigh the flask and adjust the weight with sterile water. The final weight of the methylcellulose mix minus the flask should be 1000 g.

   g. Allow the methylcellulose to thicken at 4°C overnight, aliquot, and store at –20°C. Swirl the mixture two times during the first hour of this cooling period to prevent separation. The methylcellulose must be frozen before it can be used.

2.2. Conditioned Media (CM)

L-Cell CM: Medium conditioned by L929 cells provides a good source of M-CSF for the growth of large numbers of EB-derived macrophages. CM is prepared as follows:

   a. Seed L929 cells into a flask containing IMDM with 10% FCS. We routinely use NUNC triple flasks (NUNC #132867) that hold 150 mL of medium.

   b. Harvest the supernatant shortly after the cells have reached confluence, and add fresh medium to the cells.

   c. Harvest supernatant again following 72–96 h of conditioning, and repeat procedure 3–4 times, as long as the cells remain healthy.

   d. Pool, filter (0.2 μm), and test CM. The CM should be tested for its ability to stimulate EB-derived macrophage colonies in methylcellulose assays. A good CM should have maximal activity at 10% or less. When tested, CM should be aliquoted and stored frozen at –20°C.

IL-3 Conditioned Medium: For many experiments CM from cell lines engineered to express IL-3 can be used. We routinely use CM from X63 AG8–653 myeloma cells transfected with a vector expressing IL-3 *(18)*. IL-3 CM from these cells is generated as follows:

a. Cells are initially grown in IMDM-FCS and G418 (1 mg/mL) for 3–4 d to select and maintain those containing the expression vector. Following this selection step, cell numbers are expanded in IMDM-FCS without G418 in T75 flasks. When the cells have reached sufficient density (1×10^5/mL-2×10^5/mL), the contents of three T75 flasks are pooled and passaged to a NUNC triple flask with 150 mL IMDM-FCS for the generation of the CM.
b. CM is harvested as it acidifies, prior to significant cell death. The contents of the NUNC triple flasks are poured into 200-mL (NUNC conical) tubes, and the cells are pelleted by low-speed centrifugation. Because many of the cells are slightly adherent, they will remain in the flask and can be used for conditioning the next batch of medium. Following centrifugation, harvest and filter-sterilize the supernatant. One-half of the cell pellet is returned to the original triple flask with 150 mL of new medium, and the conditioning step is repeated. At this stage, conditioning takes approx 48–72 h.
c. Medium can be changed 5–6 times using the same cell population.
d. When conditioning is complete, test the pooled harvests for activity. Testing should include the stimulation of proliferation of an IL-3-dependent cell line, as well as the growth of colonies in methylcellulose. Most batches of X63 AG8–653 CM show maximum activity in these assays below a final concentration of 1%. When tested, CM should be aliquoted and stored frozen at –20°C.

KL and LIF-CM: We use medium conditioned by Chinese hamster ovary (CHO) cells transfected with either a KL or LIF expression vector (provided by Genetics Institute, Cambridge MA) as a source of KL and LIF for most experiments. This CM is produced by the same protocol used for the generation of L-cell CM. KL-CM can be tested for its ability to stimulate the growth of mast cells in liquid culture or mast cell colonies in methylcellulose cultures. LIF-CM is tested for its ability to maintain feeder-independent ES cells in an undifferentiated state through 4–5 passages. Most batches of CHO-KL and CHO-LIF-CM show optimal activity at a final concentration of 1%. When tested, CM should be aliquoted and stored frozen at –20°C.

D4T Endothelial-Cell-CM: Medium conditioned by the embryonic endothelial cell line D4T is used together with VEGF to support the growth of EB-derived hemangioblast colonies *(8,10)*. D4T-CM is produced as follows:

a. D4T cells are grown on gelatinized flasks in IMDM with 10% FCS (selected for hemangioblast growth) and ECGS (50 mg/mL).

b. When the cells reach confluency, replace medium and allow new medium to condition for 72 h.

c. Conditioning can be repeated 4–5 times with the same cell population.

d. Filter and test conditioned medium. D4T-CM should be tested for its ability to stimulate EB-derived blast-cell colonies in cultures containing VEGF. Most batches of D4T-CM are used between 15–25%. When tested, CM should be aliquoted and stored frozen at –20°C.

2.3. Reagents and Cytokines

1. Trypsin-EDTA: Trypsin (1.25 g, trypsin 1:250: Sigma T-4799).
   0.5 *M* ethylenediaminetetraacetic acid (EDTA) (1.08 mL).
   PBS (500 mL).
   Warm to dissolve, filter-sterilize, aliquot, and store at –20°C.
2. Collagenase: Dissolve 1.0 g of collagenase (Sigma C0130) in 320 mL PBS.
   Filter-sterilize (use prefilter; may need to use more than one filtration apparatus).
   Add 80 mL FCS.
   Aliquot and store frozen at –20°C. One cycle of freeze-thaw is acceptable.
3. DNase: Make a stock of 1 mg/mL (DNase I: Calbiochem #260912) in TC-H$_2$O.
   Aliquot in 1-mL amounts and store frozen at –20°C.
   Use aliquots once and discard excess.
4. Collagenase/DNase: Add DNase at a final concentration of 10 μg/mL to collagenase just prior to EB dissociation.
5. Gelatin: Prepare a 0.1% solution of gelatin (Sigma #G 1890) in 1X PBS, dissolve, and sterilize by autoclaving.
6. Gelatinized flasks and dishes: Gelatinization is accomplished by covering the surface of a dish or flask (e.g., 2.0 mL for a T25 flask) with the gelatin solution for 20 min at room temperature. Dishes and flasks can be prepared in advance and stored with the gelatin solution at 4°C for up to 1 wk. Remove excess gelatin solution prior to use.
7. Ascorbic Acid (AA): Prepare a stock solution of 5 mg/mL (L-ascorbic acid: Sigma A-4544) in cold TC-H$_2$O, filter-sterilize, aliquot and store at –20°C. Use once and discard excess.
8. Monothioglycerol (MTG): The amounts of MTG (SIGMA #M6145) indicated are the recommended concentrations. However, it is important to test each new batch of MTG, as there is variability between them. MTG should be aliquoted (1.0 mL) and stored frozen (–20°C). When aliquots are thawed, they can be used for several experiments and then discarded. Aliquoting of MTG is strongly recommended, as it minimizes the amount of oxidation caused by repeated opening of the stock bottle.
9. L-Glutamine: Gibco-BRL #25030–081.
10. Transferrin (TRANS): Boehringer Mannheim #652202.
11. Protein-Free Hybridoma Medium (PFHM-II): Gibco-BRL #12040–093.
12. Methylcellulose (MeC): It is important to test different batches of methylcellulose (FLUKA #64630) for their ability to support the growth of hematopoietic cells.

13. Fetal Bovine Plasma-Derived Serum; Platelet-Poor (PDS): Antech, Tyler, TX: Request Keller lab protocol serum.
14. Penicillin/Streptomycin (Pen/Strep): Gibco-BRL #15070–063.
15. Matrigel: Becton Dickinson #40230 (growth factor reduced). The stock bottle of Matrigel is thawed slowly on ice, diluted 1:1 with IMDM, aliquoted (0.5 mL) and stored frozen (–20°C).
16. Endothelial Cell Growth Supplement (ECGS): Collaborative Biomedical Products, Becton Dickinson #40006B.
17. Recommended Culture Dishes:
    a. For EB generation: 60×15mm Petri dish (5 mL) VWR#25384-060.
    b. For hematopoietic colony assays: 35×10 mm Petri dish: FALCON #1008.
18. Cytokines: Cytokines can be purchased from a number of different suppliers. We use the following from R&D Systems:

    G-CSF: #414-CS   TPO: #488-TO
    GM-CSF: #415-ML   EPO: #287-TC
    M-CSF: #416-ML   KL: #455-MC
    VEGF: #293-VE   LIF: #449-L
    IL-3: #403-ML   bFGF: #233-FB
    IL-6: #406-ML   IGF-1: #291-G1
    IL-11: #418-ML

3. Methods

The method used for ES differentiation in our lab, outlined in **Fig. 1**, involves three different stages: preparation of ES cells for differentiation, the generation of EBs from ES cells, and the isolation of hematopoietic cells from EBs. For ES cell differentiation to be efficient and reproducible, it is important to begin with healthy, well-maintained ES cells and to accumulate a set of tested proven reagents. Each aspect of the ES cell-differentiation protocol is discussed in **Subheading 3.1.** In addition to the differentiation protocols, we have also provided some standard protocols for the growth and maintenance of undifferentiated ES cells. More detailed information on different aspects of ES cells—including growth, maintenance, and derivation—can be found elsewhere *(19)*.

3.1. Growth and Maintenance of ES Cells

ES cells are routinely maintained on irradiated or mitomycin C-treated primary mouse embryonic or STO fibroblasts in medium containing LIF (DMEM-ES) *(19)*. Although LIF is not necessary for maintaining ES cells on feeder cells, it is essential for the growth of feeder-independent ES cells *(20,21)*. For the sake of convenience, we use the same media for the growth of all ES cells. Maintenance of ES cells on feeder cells is important for preserving their potential to contribute to the germ line following injection into host blastocysts. ES cells used only for in vitro differentiation can be maintained in the absence of feeders in medium supplemented with LIF, although prolonged growth (>3 wk) in these conditions is not recommended. ES cells divide rapidly, and therefore cultures should be monitored daily and the cells passaged frequently, usually every 2 d. When passaging ES cells, it is important to dissociate cell clusters well with trypsin to ensure a good single-cell suspension. Passaging of undissociated cell clusters results in the development of large aggregates of ES cells that can begin to undergo spontaneous differentiation.

1. To passage cells from a confluent T25 flask, remove the DMEM-ES medium, add 1.5 mL trypsin-EDTA, and incubate at 37°C for 3 min. It is important to use high-strength trypsin to ensure that the dissociation is complete in less than 5 min. Long periods of trypsinization can be detrimental to the cells.
2. Following this short incubation, the cells can be easily dissociated by gently shaking the flask and/or by pipetting. In some instances, relatively dense cultures require an additional minute of incubation.
3. When the cells have been dissociated, add 3.5 mL of DMEM-ES medium to dilute and inactivate the trypsin. For normal maintenance, approx 10% of these cells are passaged to a new flask with DMEM-ES medium and fresh feeder cells. During this dilution, aliquots of the trypsinized suspension can be passaged directly to the new flask without centrifugation. If a significantly larger volume is passaged to the new flask, it is advisable to first pellet the cells by low-speed centrifugation to remove the trypsin.

3.2. Preparation of ES Cells for In Vitro Differentiation

Prior to differentiation, it is advisable to remove the ES cells from the feeder cells—which, when present in excess numbers—can affect the development of EBs. Feeders can be removed either by selective adhesion to tissue-culture plastic or by subcloning the ES cells directly onto a gelatinized culture vessel. Because the adhesion procedure is fast and easy, it is the recommended first approach for most ES cell lines.

3.2.1. Depletion of Feeder Cells by Adherence

1. Trypsinize the ES cells and feeder cells, centrifuge the suspension, and resuspend the pellet in an appropriate volume for cell counting.
2. Seed the ES and feeder cells into a 100×15 mm tissue-culture-grade dish in DMEM-ES medium at an approximate concentration of 1×10^6 cells/mL in a total of 7–10 mL.
3. Culture at 37°C for 1.5–2.0 h, during which time the feeders, but not the ES cells, will adhere to the dish.
4. Remove the nonadherent ES cell-enriched fraction and transfer it to a gelatinized flask in DMEM-ES medium.

5. The adherence procedure is successful if greater than 75% of the cells in the culture have the morphology of ES cells. Further passaging can usually eliminate the remaining feeder cells. However, excessive passaging in the absence of feeder cells is not recommended. If significant numbers of feeder cells are present in the culture following the first adherence step, it should be repeated. The entire process of depleting feeder cells should not require more than five passages. When the ES population is relatively free of feeder cells, large numbers of aliquots should be frozen for the differentiation experiments. Additional vials of ES cells can be frozen from the first few passages in the absence of feeder cells. It is important to accumulate an adequate stock of gelatin-adapted cells for a particular ES cell line so that the feeder-cell depletion step does not have to be constantly repeated. Feeder-independent ES cells should not be carried longer than 2–3 wk in culture. At this stage, they should be discarded, and a new vial thawed.

Some ES cells undergo some spontaneous differentiation when removed from feeder cells and maintained on gelatinized flasks. This is not of concern if the number of differentiated cells is less that 10% of the population. However, if significant numbers of differentiated cells persist with repeated passaging, the ES line should be subcloned.

3.2.2. Subcloning of ES Cells

Subcloning can be used to separate ES cells from differentiating progeny or to remove ES cells from feeder cells.

1. Dissociate the cells with trypsin as in **Subheading 3.2.1., step 1** and culture in a gelatinized 100×15 mm tissue-culture-grade dish in DMEM-ES medium at concentrations ranging from 3×10^3 to 1×10^5 per dish. The goal of this step is to achieve a cell density in which single, well-dispersed ES-cell colonies will develop over a 2–3 d culture period.
2. When colonies have reached a reasonable size (200–500 cells), they can be picked directly from the liquid culture with a finely drawn 10-µL glass micropipet (VWR #53432–728). Choose clones with a three-dimensional appearance, free of surrounding differentiating cells or feeder cells.
3. Individual clones are placed in microtiter wells containing 50 µL of PBS. Add 100 µL of prewarmed trypsin-EDTA to each well and incubate for 3 min at 37°C. Stop the reaction by adding 50 µL of FCS to the well, and disperse the colony by gentle pipetting.
4. Transfer the cells from each clone into one well of a gelatinized 24–well plate containing DMEM-ES medium. It is not necessary to wash the cells during this passage. The medium should be changed frequently, and the growth of clones monitored daily. When the cells have reached 75% confluence, the contents of a well can be passaged to a gelatinized T25 flask. Most clones will reach this stage within 3–4 d. An aliquot of the T25 flask can be frozen at the time of passaging.

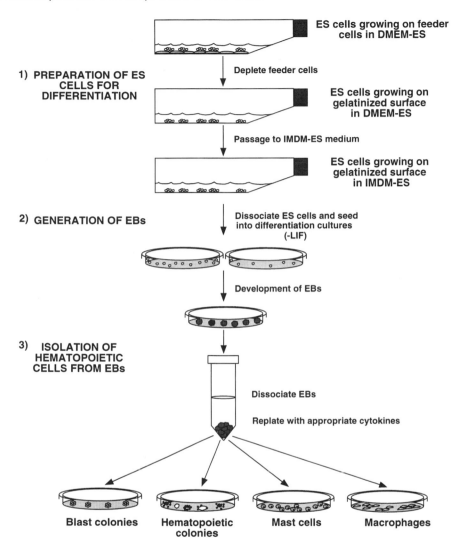

Fig. 1. Protocol for ES cell differentiation.

To ensure that the subcloning is successful, select approx 24–48 clones per ES cell line. When the clones have been expanded and aliquots frozen, each should be tested for its capacity to generate EBs.

3.3. Generation of EB from ES Cells

The generation of healthy, robust embryoid bodies (EBs) is an important first step in the differentiation of ES cells to the hematopoietic lineage. The two variables that impact EB development most dramatically are the state of the ES cells and the lot of FCS used for differentiation. Selection of appropriate FCS for differentiation is discussed in **Subheading 3.5.**

1. Twenty-four to 48 h prior to the initiation of EB generation, passage ES cells into IMDM-ES media in a T25 gelatinized flask. This step is designed to reduce possible stress from moving cells directly from DMEM-ES medium to IMDM medium, which is used in all differentiation cultures. ES cells are not maintained for extended periods of time in IMDM-ES medium, as they grow faster and the resulting clusters are considerably flatter then those maintained in DMEM-ES medium.

2. Following 1–2 d of culture in IMDM-ES medium, harvest the ES cells by trypsinization, wash 2 times in IMDM-FCS, and do a viable cell count. You should expect to recover between 2×10^6 and 8×10^6 cells from a single T25 flask, and cell viability should be near 100%.

3. To generate EBs, ES cells are cultured in the absence of LIF and under conditions that prevent them from adhering to the surface of the culture dish. This can be achieved by culturing the cells either in methylcellulose-containing medium or in liquid cultures in Petri-grade dishes. Testing different brands of Petri-grade dishes is sometimes required to select those which display the least adhesiveness for the developing EBs. Methylcellulose is recommended for long-term cultures (>9 d), as EBs tend to become more adherent with time. Liquid is more convenient for shorter-term cultures (2–9 d), because it is easier to harvest the EBs from these conditions.

4. The components of the differentiation culture will vary depending upon the stage of hematopoietic development to be studied. **Table 1** summarizes the culture conditions used to generate EBs representative of the three stages of hematopoietic development; hemangioblast, primitive, and early-definitive and multilineage definitive.

5. Liquid cultures are usually carried out in a volume of 5 mL per 60×15mm Petri-grade dishes or in a vol of 10 mL per 100×15 mm dish. Methylcellulose cultures can be done in 100×15 mm, 60×15 mm or 35×15 mm Petri-grade dishes, using vol of 10, 5, and 1.5 mL of culture mix respectively. **Table 1** provides an estimate of the number of CCE ES cells that should be plated to obtain reasonable numbers of EB-derived cells at different time-points. When differentiated in methylcellulose cultures, the efficiency of EB formation for CCE cells is 20–50%.

The number of input CCE ES cells recommended in **Table 1** should yield 2.5×10^6 to 5×10^6 per 5-mL plated. It is important to titrate the number of input cells for each ES cell line to be used in the differentiation assay, as the efficiency of EB formation varies considerably between cell lines. If the efficiency of EB formation is very low (<1% EB formation in methylcellulose or a recovery of less than 1×10^6 cells per 1×10^5 input ES cells in liquid), the ES cell line should be subcloned (*see* **Subheading 3.2.2.**). Cytokines (KL, IL-3, and IL-11) are added to late-stage cultures (9–14 d) to maintain the precursor content of the EBs (*see* **Table 1**). In addition, long-term differentiation cultures should be fed as indicated in **Table 1**. Cytokines are not required for the initiation of hematopoiesis in EBs during the first 6 d of differentiation.

3.4. Isolation of Hematopoietic Cells from EB

Developing hematopoietic precursors within the EBs can be identified and studied using several different approaches. Standard colony-forming cell (CFC) assays can be used for a quantitative assessment of precursor development. For this type of analysis, EB-derived cells are cultured in methylcellulose-containing medium supplemented with hematopoietic cytokines. Precursor numbers and developmental potential are determined from the number and type of hematopoietic colonies that develop. Colony assays are useful for quantification and characterization of precursors, but do not provide large numbers of lineage-specific hematopoietic cells for further molecular and biochemical studies. Large numbers of cells for such studies can be generated from the mast cell and macrophage lineages.

3.4.1. Harvesting EBs

1. EBs generated in liquid cultures are transferred to a 50-mL tube and allowed to settle by gravity for approx 10 min. This step separates the EBs from the dead cells that did not participate in EB formation. A maximum of eight 60×15 dishes (40 mL) can be harvested into each tube. When the majority of EBs have settled into a pellet, the supernatant can be removed and the EBs dissociated (*see* **Subheading 3.4.2.**). It is not necessary to wash the EBs prior to dissociation.
2. EBs grown in methylcellulose cultures should be loosened with a cell scraper, as some adhesive cells can develop over a period of time. The methylcellulose is next diluted with an equal volume of IMDM-FCS to convert the entire culture to a liquid consistency that can be removed with a pipet. The contents of the differentiation cultures are transferred to a 50-mL tube with additional IMDM-FCS to further dilute the methylcellulose. A maximum of four dishes can be harvested into a 50-mL tube. Older EBs (10 or more days) are less compact than younger ones, and often have hematopoietic cell populations growing out of them. To prevent loss of these maturing populations, the cells and EBs are collected by centrifugation.

3.4.2. Dissociation of EBs

EBs differentiated for 7 d or less can be easily dissociated with trypsin, whereas those differentiated 9 d or longer require collagenase treatment.

3.4.2.1. TRYPSIN TREATMENT OF EBS (2–7 DAYS)

1. Add 3 mL of trypsin to the EB pellet, incubate for 3–5 min in a 37°C-water bath, and then stop the reaction with the addition of 1 mL of FCS. Dissociate the EBs by passaging them 2 times through a 5-mL syringe with a 20-gauge needle.
2. Following the dissociation procedure, add 5–6 mL of IMDM-FCS, centrifuge at 1000–1400 rpm, and resuspend the pellet in an appropriate volume for cell counting and distribution. Using the CCE ES cell line, EB cell yields should range between 5×10^5–1×10^6 cells per mL from a 60×15 mm dish. Cells should be >95% viable after this treatment.

3.4.2.2. COLLAGENASE TREATMENT OF EBS (>9 DAYS)

1. Resuspend the EB pellet collected from one or two 60×15 mm dishes in 5 mL of collagenase-DNase solution and incubate at 37°C for 1–2 h. The suspension should be vortexed every 30 min.
2. Dissociate the EBs by passing them through a 20-gauge needle 4 times. Centrifuge the dissociated cells, and resuspend the pellet in IMDM-FCS. A 60×15-mm culture of d 12 CCE-derived EBs should yield between 4.0×10^5 and 8.0×10^5 cells per mL with >90% viability.

3.4.3. Methylcellulose Colony-Forming Assay

The procedure for assaying EB-derived precursors in methylcellulose is identical to that used for precursors from fetal liver and adult bone marrow. Cells are mixed into the methylcellulose-containing medium with specific hematopoietic cytokines, and aliquots are plated into 35×10 mm Petri-grade dishes, which are incubated at 37°C for various periods of time. Colonies that develop from the hematopoietic precursors are scored between 5–10 d following the initiation of culture. The types of precursors present will depend on the age of the EBs. The changing precursor populations provide the basis for defining the three different stages of EB hematopoietic development. The earliest stage, the hemangioblast stage, contains the VEGF-responsive blast-CFC able to generate both endothelial and hematopoietic progeny (**Table 2**). EBs at the next stage, the primitive and early-definitive stage, contain primitive erythroid (E^p), definitive erythroid (E^d), macrophage (Mac), bipotential E^d/Mac bipotential E^d/megakaryocyte (E^d/Mega), and multipotential precursors. The multilineage definitive stage EBs contain E^d, bipotential E^d/mast cell (mast), Mast, bipotential E^d/Mega, Mega, bipotential E^d/Mac, Mac, neutrophil (Neut), bipotential Mac/Neut (GM), and multipotential precursors. Few, if any, E^p pre-

Table 1
Conditions for the Generation of EBs with Different Populations of Hematopoietic Precursors

	Hemangioblast stage	Primitive and early definitive stage	Multilineage definitive stage[b]
Culture Components	d 3.0–3.5	d 5–7	d 9–d 14
MeC Stock (50%) [a]	+/–[a]	+/–[a]	+
FCS 15%	+	+	+
Glutamine (2 mM)	+	+	+
TRANS (300 ug/mL)	+	+	+
MTG ($4 \times 10^{-4}M$ final)	+	+	+
AA (50 ug/mL)	+	+	+
PFHM-II (5%)	–	+	+
Cytokines	–	–	+
KL (100 ng/mL or CM)	–	–	+
IL–3 (1 ng/mLor CM)	–	–	+
IL–11 (5 ng/mL)	–	–	+
IMDM (to 100%)	+	+	+
Cell Input and Yield			
Input for CCE ES cells/mL	7500–10,000	500–1500	300–500
Yield/ml	0.5×10^6–1.0×10^6	0.5×10^6–1.0×10^6	0.5×10^6–1.0×10^6

[a]Day 3–7 EBs can be generated in either methylcellulose or liquid cultures. Methylcellulose is recommended for later-stage cultures.

[b]For the generation of d 12–14 EBs, the methylcellulose cultures should be fed with 2 mL of fresh methylcellulose mix on d 9 or 10. Add the feeding mix in small amounts over the surface of the existing culture.

cursors are found in the multilineage definitive stage of development. These various populations are representative of populations that develop in the embryonic yolk sac and fetal liver of the normal mouse embryo. Conditions that support the growth of specific lineage-restricted precursors as well as those that support the growth of all precursors from EBs at these various stages of development are outlined in **Table 2**.

3.4.3.1. THE HEMANGIOBLAST

Recent studies have demonstrated that precursors with the potential to generate both hematopoietic and endothelial lineages develop within the EBs prior to the onset of any other hematopoietic programs *(10)*. These bipotential precursors, also referred to as hemangioblasts, represent a transient population

that develops between d 3.0 and d 3.25 of differentiation, and persists for 12–
18 h. These times can vary by 3–6 h, depending on the batch of FCS and on the
ES cell line used. The EB-derived hemangioblasts grow in response to VEGF
and generate colonies consisting of cells with undifferentiated blast-cell morphology. Consequently, we have referred to these hemangioblast-derived colonies as blast-cell colonies. Growth of blast-cell colonies is enhanced by the
addition of CM from an embryonic endothelial-cell line, D4T *(8)*. Although
this effect is most pronounced in sparse cultures, growth-promoting effects can
be observed at most cell densities, and therefore we routinely include D4T-CM
in all of our hemangioblast assays. It is possible that CM from other endothelial or stromal-cell lines can be used in place of D4T-CM, although we have
not carried out extensive comparisons.

1. To generate colonies from hemangioblasts, plate varying numbers of cells
   (3.0×10^4/mL to 1.5×10^5/mL) from d 3.0–3.5 EBs in the appropriate methylcellulose mixture (**Table 2**).
2. Colonies develop from the hemangioblasts within 3–4 d of culture and can be
   recognized as loose clusters of cells that are easily distinguished from the compact secondary embryoid bodies (*see* **ref. 8**). Blast-cell colonies and secondary
   EBs are the only colonies present in these replated cultures.
3. The potential of the hemangioblast-derived colonies is best assayed by plating
   them in microtiter wells precoated with a thin layer of Matrigel, and in medium
   containing cytokines that support the growth of both the hematopoietic and endothelial lineages (hemangioblast medium). To coat the wells with Matrigel, add
   5 uL to each and spread it over the surface with the tip of an Eppendorf pipet.
   This step should be carried out on ice. When the required number of wells have
   been treated, allow the microtiter plate to incubate on ice for 10–15 min. Following this step, aspirate the excess Matrigel from each well and incubate the plate at
   37°C for an additional 15 min. The plate is now ready to use. Under these culture
   conditions, individual blast-cell colonies will generate both adherent and
   nonadherent cell populations which can distinguished within 24 h of culture. The
   nonadherent cells contain hematopoietic precursors that can easily be harvested
   by pipetting and assayed in methylcellulose cultures for colony-forming potential, using the cytokine mix designated for the growth of all precursors (*see* **Table
   2**). The adherent population contains cells that express endothelial markers *(10)*,
   including PECAM-1 *(22)*, flk-1 *(23,24)*, flt-1 *(25)*, and TIE-2 *(26)*.

3.4.3.2. Primitive Erythroid Precursors

Primitive erythroid precursors develop within EBs shortly after the
hemangioblasts, and can be detected as early as d 4.0 of differentiation. Their
number increases dramatically over the next 2–3 d and can represent 1–2% of
the total EB population by d 6–7 of differentiation *(5)*. Beyond this stage, their

number declines sharply to almost undetectable levels by d 10–12 of differentiation. E^p precursors require only Epo for growth and generate relatively small (<100 cells) brilliant red colonies (*see* **ref. *15***). We have not identified any other cytokines that will stimulate the growth of these colonies. E^p colonies have several specific growth requirements that differ from other types of hematopoietic colonies. First, they require platelet-poor plasma-derived serum (PDS) for growth, as they do not develop well in most batches of normal FCS. Second, their growth and development is enhanced significantly by the addition of PFMH-II (5%) to the methylcellulose cultures. The active component within PFMH-II is currently unknown. The identification of a colony as primitive erythroid can be confirmed by morphological assessment of the cells and by analysis of the globin expression patterns. Primitive erythrocytes are large and nucleated, and express embryonic globins *(27–29)*. We have found $\beta H1$ expression to be the best molecular marker for primitive erythrocytes *(8)*.

3.4.3.3. Definitive Hematopoietic Precursors

All precursors, other than primitive erythroid, are considered members of the definitive hematopoietic system. Precursors of the macrophage and definitive erythroid lineages develop shortly after the onset of primitive erythropoiesis, and persist within EBs for several weeks.

The earliest definitive erythroid precursors that develop within the EBs (d 5–6 of differentiation) are the equivalent of BFU-E and require both c-kit ligand (KL) and Epo for growth *(5)*. The colonies that develop from these precursors are easily distinguished from E^p colonies, because they are considerably larger and contain small cells that express β major but no $\beta H1$ globin *(8,15)*. If Tpo is included in the cultures, many of these definitive colonies will also develop megakaryocytes. Precursors that generate these bilineage colonies are more frequent in d 6 EBs than in those differentiated for longer periods of time.

Macrophage colonies develop best in response to a combination of M-CSF and IL-3. These colonies are easily identified based on growth characteristics, cell morphology, and expression of macrophage-specific genes such as c-fms. A subpopulation of macrophage colonies also contain a definitive erythroid component (E^d/MAC colonies). Mast cell precursors develop within the EBs between d 6–8, whereas those of the neutrophil lineage are delayed and are not consistently detectable until d 12–14 of differentiation. As with the megakaryocyte lineage, the earliest mast cells often develop in colonies together with E^d cells. Mast-cell restricted precursors that generate pure mast-cell colonies are not found in high numbers until d 10–12 of differentiation. Megakaryocyte, mast-cell, and neutrophil colonies are easily identified by their size and shape, and by the morphology of the cells within them. Standard histochemical analysis can be used to confirm that the cells within the colonies represent the respective lineages.

The development of bilineage E^d/Mac, E^d/Mega, and E^d/Mast colonies suggests that precursors with these restricted potentials exist. Although we have not formally demonstrated the clonal origin of these bilineage colonies, we have indicated the presence of these restricted precursors in **Table 2**. The patterns of lineage development described here are highly reproducible for a given ES cell line and set of reagents. Although there can be some difference in the onset of hematopoiesis within the EBs, there is little variation in kinetics of lineage development.

3.4.4. Liquid Expansion Cultures

Large numbers of ES cell-derived mast cells and macrophages can be easily generated in liquid cultures for molecular biology and biochemical analysis.

3.4.4.1. MAST CELLS

1. Harvest d 6 EBs as described in **Subheading 3.4.**
2. Pellet the cells by centrifugation, wash once with IMDM-FCS, and then culture in 6-well dishes in mast-cell medium at a concentration of 1.0×10^6–2.0×10^6 cells per mL in a final vol of 3–4 mL. Both adherent fibroblasts/endothelial cells and nonadherent hematopoietic precursors will develop rapidly in these cultures.
3. 24 h following the initiation of the cultures, transfer the nonadherent cells to new plates with fresh mast-cell medium. For this initial transfer, move the contents of one well to a new well without diluting the number of cells. Adherent cells will likely develop in these secondary cultures as well, and when significant numbers are present (>50% confluent), passage the nonadherent population again. The extent of adherent cell growth should diminish significantly by the third passage.
4. The cultures will undergo a crisis over the next 4–7 d as many of the hematopoietic lineages begin to die. Mast cells will persist and continue to expand during this phase of the culture.
5. Replace approx one half of the media every 2–3 d. This is done by carefully aspirating old medium from the side of the well and replacing with new medium.
6. When the mast cells begin to grow and dominate the cultures, they can be passaged and their numbers expanded. Mast cells grow best at a reasonably high density, and therefore a dilution of approx 1:3 is recommended when passaging. Mast cells can be maintained in culture for 6–8 weeks with media changes every 2–3 d.

3.4.4.2. MACROPHAGES

1. Harvest d 6 EB cells as described in **Subheading 3.4.**
2. Pellet the cells by centrifugation, wash once with IMDM-FCS and culture at 1×10^6 per mL in 100×15 mm tissue-culture-grade dish in a final vol of 10 mL of

Table 2
Growth of Hematopoietic Precursors from Different Stages of EB Development

EB age	D 3.0–3.5	D 5–7					D 9.0–14	
Precursor content	Hemangio-blast ES cells	E^P, E^D, E^D/Mega, Mega, E^D/Mac, Mac, Multipotential					E^D, Mac, Mega, Mega, E^D/Mega, Mast, E^D/Mast, Neut/Mac, Neut, Multipotential	
Growth of defined lineage-specific precursors	Hemangio-blast	EryP	EryD	Mac	Mega	All precursors	Mast	All precursors
Culture components								
MeC Stock (50%)	+	+	+	+	+	+	+	Same as d 5–7 mix
PDS (10%)[a] or	+	+	+	+	+	+	+	
FCS (10%)[a]	+	–	+	+	+	+	+	
Glutamine (1%)	+	+	+	+	+	+	+	
PFHM-II (5%)	–	+	+	+	+	+	+	
TRANS (300 ug/mL)	+	–	–	–	–	–	–	
MTG ($4 \times 10^{-4} M$)[b]	+	–	–	–	–	–	–	
AA (25 ug/mL)[b]	+	–	–	–	–	–	–	
VEGF (5 ng/mL)	+	–	–	–	–	–	–	
D4T CM (20%)	+	–	–	–	–	–	–	
Epo (2 u/mL)	–	+	+	–	+	+	–	
KL (100 ng/mL)[c]	–	–	+	+	+	+	+	
IL-3 (1 ng/mL)[c]	–	–	–	+	+	+	+	
M-CSF (5 ng/mL)	–	–	–	+	–	+	–	
Tpo (5 ng/mL)	–	–	+	–	+	+	–	
IL-11 (5 ng/mL)	–	–	–	–	+	+	–	
G-CSF (30 ng/mL)	–	–	–	–	–	+	–	
GM-CSF (3 ng/mL)	–	–	–	–	–	+	–	
IL-6 (5 ng/mL)	–	–	–	–	–	+	–	
Approx # of EB cells plated per mL	$3 \times 10^4 - 1.5 \times 10^5$	$3 \times 10^4 - 1.5 \times 10^5$					$7.5 \times 10^4 - 1.5 \times 10^5$	

[a]Either PDS or FCS can be used for the growth of colonies from most hematopoietic precursors. PDS is required for the growth of colonies from primitive erythroid precursors. [b]Add ascorbic acid to the mix last. [c]Conditioned medium can be used in place of these recombinant cytokines.

macrophage medium 1. Macrophage precursors develop initially as nonadherent cell clusters in these cultures.

3. Forty-eight h later, harvest the nonadherent clusters and pellet by centrifugation.
4. Resuspend the pellet in macrophage medium 2, and culture in 100 × 15 mm tissue-culture-grade dishes. Culture the contents of one dish in each new dish
5. Macrophages will grow and begin to adhere to the dish within the next 2–3 d. Cultures should be fed every 2–3 d and can be harvested 5–7 d later. As mature macrophages are very adherent, combinations of trypsinization and cell scraping are often required to harvest them from the culture dishes. More than 90% of the cells should be of the macrophage lineage as determined morphology and by the expression of lineage-specific markers such as F4/80 *(30)*.

3.5. Serum Selection

Serum is the most critical component of the differentiation culture, and therefore considerable time and effort is required to select appropriate batches.

3.5.1. Growth of ES Cells

Pretested serum for ES cell growth is available from several different companies. Alternatively, various lots can be tested for their ability to maintain ES growth. To select an appropriate serum, passage the ES cells 4–5 times in the various test lots and monitor the cultures for cell viability, growth, and maintenance of cells with an undifferentiated morphology. It is easiest to test serum on feeder-cell-depleted ES-cell populations.

3.5.2. Generation of EBs

The lot of serum selected for growth of ES cells is often not the best for EB generation. Serum for differentiation should be selected based on its ability to support the efficient development of EBs and on the hematopoietic potential of the EBs that develop. To assess efficiency of EB development, EB numbers can be counted if tested in methylcellulose, or total cell numbers from the differentiation cultures can be evaluated if tested in liquid. Hematopoietic potential is determined by assaying EBs at different stages of development for the desired precursor populations. Serum selection for the hemangioblast stage is most difficult, given the highly sensitive and transient nature of this population. In our experience, a given lot of serum that supports the efficient development of the hemangioblast will often support the development of primitive and definitive precursors in later-stage EBs. However, the reverse is not always true, as some sera will support the efficient development of hematopoietic precursors in d 5–14 Ebs, but are not optimal for the early stages of development. Therefore, the serum test should be set-up based on the types of precursors to be studied.

Table 3
Troubleshooting

Problem	Cause	Solution
Large cell aggregates in ES cell maintenance culture	Incomplete cell dissociation during trypsinization	Trypsinize for a longer period of time and/or replace trypsin
Persistence of differentiated cells in feeder-cell-depleted cultures	Unstable ES cell line Insufficient amount of LIF in media	Subclone ES cell line Titrate LIF concentration
Low numbers of EBs in differentiation cultures	Suboptimal serum Suboptimal ES cells Suboptimal ES cell concentration	Select new lot of serum Subclone ES cell line Titrate ES cell number
Adherent EBs	Adherent petri dishes Suboptimal serum Overcrowded cultures	Select a new brand of Petri dishes Select a new lot of serum Titrate ES cell number
Low numbers of hematopoietic precursors in EBs	Suboptimal serum for EB differentiation	Select a new lot of serum

3.5.3. Generation of Hematopoietic Cells from EBs

For the methylcellulose colony assay, serum should be selected based on two criteria: the ability to support the growth of large numbers of colonies, and the ability to support the growth and maturation of cells within the colonies. With respect to maturation, the most sensitive cells are those of the primitive erythroid lineage. As indicated above, we have found that PDS best supports the development of these colonies *(5)*. PDS will also support the growth of other colonies and therefore we use it routinely for all our colony assays. Selected lots of normal FCS will support the development of colonies from all definitive lineages, and may be used in place of PDS. Hemangioblast-derived colonies will grow in either pretested lots of PDS or FCS. This serum should be selected based on numbers of blast-cell colonies that develop and on the potential of the colonies to generate both hematopoietic and endothelial progeny.

Acknowledgments

We wish to thank Dr. Scott Robertson, Dr. Chris Hogan, and Dr. Lia Gore for their critical review of this manuscript, and Kelly Bakke for help in the preparation. This work was supported in part by NIH grant HL48834-06.

References

1. Doetschman, T. C., Eistetter, H., Katz, M., Schmidt, W., and Kemler, R. (1985) The in vitro development of blastocyst-derived embryonic stem cell lines: formation of visceral yolk sac, blood islands and myocardium. *J. Embryol. Exp. Morphol.* **87,** 27–45.
2. Wiles, M. and Keller, G. (1991) Multiple hematopoietic lineages develop from embryonic stem (ES) cells in culture. *Development* **111,** 259–267.
3. Schmitt, R., Bruyns, E., and Snodgrass, H. (1991) Hematopoietic development of embryonic stem cells in vitro: cytokine and receptor gene expression. *Genes Dev.* **5,** 728–740.
4. Burkert, U., von Ruden, T., and Wagner, E. F. (1991) Early fetal hematopoietic development from in vitro differentiated embryonic stem cells. *New Biol.* **3,** 698–708.
5. Keller, G., Kennedy, M., Papayannopoulou, T., and Wiles, M. (1993) Hematopoietic commitment during embryonic stem cell differentiation in culture. *Mol. Cell. Biol.* **13,** 473–486.
6. Nakano, T., Kodama, H., and Honjo, T. (1994) Generation of lymphohematopoietic cells from embryonic stem cells in culture. *Science* **265,** 1098–1101.
7. Keller, G. (1995) In vitro differentiation of embryonic stem cells. *Curr. Opin. Cell Biol.* **7,** 862–869.
8. Kennedy, M., Firpo, M., Choi, K., Wall, C., Robertson, S., Kabrun, N., et al.

(1997) A common precursor for primitive erythropoiesis and definitive haematopoiesis. *Nature* **386,** 488–493.

9. Kabrun, N., Buhring, H. J., Choi, K., Ullrich, A., Risau, W., and Keller, G. (1997) Flk-1 expression defines a population of early embryonic hematopoietic precursors. *Development* **124,** 2039–2048.

10. Choi, K., Kennedy, M., Kazarov, A., Papadimitriou, J. C., and Keller, G. (1998) A common precursor for hematopoietic and endothelial cells. *Development* **125,** 725–732.

11. Nishikawa, S. I., Nishikawa, S., Hirashima, M., Matsuyoshi, N., and Kodama, H. (1998) Progressive lineage analysis by cell sorting and culture identifies FLK1+VE-cadherin+ cells at a diverging point of endothelial and hemopoietic lineages. *Development* **125,** 1747–1757.

12. Weiss, M., Keller, G., and Orkin, S. (1994) Novel insights into erythroid development revealed through in vitro differentiation of GATA-1⁻ embryonic stem cells. *Genes Devel.* **8,** 1184–1197.

13. Tsai, F. Y., Keller, G., Kuo, F. C., Weiss, M., Chen, J., Rosenblatt, M., et al. (1994) An early haematopoietic defect in mice lacking the transcription factor GATA-2. *Nature* **371,** 221–226.

14. Porcher, C., Swat, W., Rockwell, K., Fujiwara, Y., Alt, F. W., and Orkin, S. H. (1996) The T cell leukemia oncoprotein SCL/tal-1 is essential for development of all hematopoietic lineages. *Cell* **86,** 47–57.

15. Epner, E., Reik, A., Cimbora, D., Telling, A., Bender, M. A., Fiering, S., et al. (1998) The beta-globin LCR is not necessary for an open chromatin structure or developmentally regulated transcription of the native mouse beta-globin locus. *Molecular Cell* **2,** 447–455.

16. Helgason, C. D., Sauvageau, G., Lawrence, H. J., Largman, C., and Humphries, R. K. (1996) Overexpression of HOXB4 enhances the hematopoietic potential of embryonic stem cell differentiated in vitro. *Blood* **87,** 2740–2749.

17. Keller, G., Wall, C., Fong, A., Hawley, T., and Hawley, R. (1998) Overexpression of HOX11 leads to the immortalization of embryonic precursors with both primitive and definitive hematopoietic potential. *Blood* **92,** 877–887.

18. Karasuyama, H. and Melchers, F. (1988) Establishment of mouse cell lines which constitutively secrete large quantitites of interleukin 2, 3, 4, or 5 using modified cDNA expression vectors. *Eur. J. Immunol.* **18,** 97–104 .

19. Robertson, E. J., ed., (1987) *Teratocarcinomas and embryonic stem cells: a practical approach.* (D. Rickwood and B. Hames, eds. Hames.) IRL Press, Oxford, Washington, DC.

20. Williams, R. L., Hilton, D. J., Pease, S., Willson, T. A., Stewart, C. L., Gearing, D. P., Wagner, E. F., Metcalf, D., Nicola, N. A., and Gough, N. M. (1988) Myeloid leukaemia inhibitory factor maintains the developmental potential of embryonic stem cells. *Nature* **336,** 684–687.

21. Smith, A. G., Heath, J. K., Donaldson, D. D., Wong, G. G., Moreau, J., Stahl, M., et al. (1988) Inhibition of pluripotential embryonic stem cell differentiation by purified polypeptides. *Nature* **336,** 688–690.

22. Newman, P. J. (1994) The role of PECAM-1 in vascular cell biology. *Ann. NY Acad. Sci.* **714,** 165–174.
23. Millauer, B., Wizigmann-Voos, S., Schnurch, H., Martinez, R., Moller, N. P., Risau, W., et al. (1993) High affinity VEGF binding and developmental expression suggest Flk-1 as a major regulator of vasculogenesis and angiogenesis. *Cell* **72,** 835–846.
24. Yamaguchi, T. P., Dumont, D. J., Conlon, R. A., Breitman, M. L., and Rossant, J. (1993) flk-1, an flt-related receptor tyrosine kinase is an early marker for endothelial cell precursors. *Development* **118,** 489–498.
25. Fong, G. H., Klingensmith, J., Wood, C. R., Rossant, J., and Breitman, M. L. (1996) Regulation of flt-1 expression during mouse embryogenesis suggests a role in the establishment of vascular endothelium. *Dev. Dyn.* **207,** 1–10.
26. Dumont, D. J., Yamaguchi, T. P., Conlon, R. A., Rossant, J., and Breitman, M. L. (1992) tek, a novel tyrosine kinase gene located on mouse chromosome 4, is expressed in endothelial cells and their presumptive precursors. *Oncogene* **7,** 1471–1480.
27. Russel, E. (1979) Heriditary anemias of the mouse: a review for geneticists. *Adv. Genet.* **2,** 357–459.
28. Barker, J. (1968) Development of the mouse hematopoietic system I. Types of hemoglobin produced in embryonic yolk sac and liver. *Dev. Biol.* **18,** 14–29.
29. Brotherton, T., Chui, D., Gauldie, J., Patterson, M. (1979) Hemoglobin ontogeny during normal mouse fetal development. *Proc. Natl. Acad. Sci. USA* **76,** 2853–2857.
30. Hume, D. A., Robinson, A. P., Macpherson, G. G., and Gordon, S. (1983) The mononuclear phagocyte system of the mouse defined by immunohistochemical localization of antigen F4/80. *J. Exp. Med.* **158,** 1522–1536.

15

Genetic Modification of Murine Hematopoietic Stem Cells by Retroviruses

Christian P. Kalberer, Jennifer Antonchuk, and R. Keith Humphries

1. Introduction

Among the currently available methods for gene transfer, recombinant murine retroviruses remain the best established method for achieving stable integration of a transgene with high efficiency. Pioneering work by a number of groups has demonstrated the feasibility of using this method for gene transfer to primitive, multipotential long-term repopulating hematopoietic stem cells (HSC) *(1–4)*. In the case of the hematopoietic system, it is required that the introduced gene integrates into the genome of HSC in order to be expressed in multiple lineages over an extended period of time. However, HSC are found at low frequency, and are normally in a quiescent or slow cycling state. Both factors represent challenges to successful retroviral gene transfer. The former places a premium on high titer, and the latter dictates methods to trigger HSC cycling during the infection, since stable integration of murine retroviruses requires cell division of the target cell and breakdown of the nuclear membrane *(5,6)*. In general, titers greater than 1×10^5 U/mL allow some degree of gene transfer for HSC, but 1×10^6 or higher are a reasonable goal for achieving useful efficiencies of at least 20%. For activation of HSC, most protocols invoke a combination of in vivo and in vitro stimulation. The former is most easily and routinely achieved by administration of cytotoxic agents like 5-fluorouracil (5-FU) 4 d prior to bone-marrow harvest. This procedure removes a large proportion of actively cycling, more differentiated cells, thus achieving a degree of enrichment of HSC and CFU-S. It also triggers cycling of these cells *(7,8)*. Many groups have established the importance of cytokine stimulation in

From: *Methods in Molecular Medicine, vol. 63: Hematopoietic Stem Cell Protocols*
Edited by: C. A. Klug and C. T. Jordan © Humana Press Inc., Totowa, NJ

vitro, usually involving a combination of exposure to growth factors for 24–48 h prior to virus exposure (prestimulation period) and throughout the subsequent period of virus infection *(9,10)*. These cytokines are critical to both maintain/trigger cycling and promote survival of HSC during the infection procedure.

The protocol described in this Chapter represents a robust approach for retroviral gene transfer to HSC. Numerous variations can be successfully employed, including alternatives to in vivo treatment with 5-FU such as in vivo administration of growth factors *(11)*, various growth-factor combinations for HSC stimulations, various viral packaging systems, and other methods to increase cell-virus encounters, including flowthrough systems *(12)*. This protocol should provide a framework for initial forays into the use of this powerful method for genetic manipulation of hematopoietic cells.

2. Materials

2.1. Generation of Retroviral Producer Cells

1. Retroviral vector: The marker gene that is incorporated into the retroviral vector influences the way that retroviral producer cells are generated. Numerous genes whose expression can be identified by fluorescence-activated cell-sorting (FACS) analysis, such as CD24 *(13)*, CD8 *(14)*, or the low-affinity nerve-growth-factor *(15)* have been used. More recently, green fluorescent protein (GFP) has been used as an intracellular marker gene *(16,17)*. All these markers are expressed by the infected cells as early as 24–48 h postretroviral infection, and the transduction efficiency can be determined by FACS. This short selection period is crucial to minimize the loss of HSC during the in vitro culture period. Alternatively, the Neo^R gene conferring resistance to the cytotoxic drug G418 (or any other resistance marker gene, such as for puromycin or hygromycin) is a useful marker in retroviral vectors that are primarily used for in vitro experiments in which drug selection can be readily employed.
2. $Ca_3(PO_4)_2$ transfection kit (e.g., Pharmacia).
3. Amphotropic-packaging-cell line capable of high-level transient virus production (*see* **Note 1**): Phoenix-ampho *(18)*.
4. Ecotropic-packaging-cell line for long-term virus production: GP+E86 *(19)*.
5. Dulbecco's modified Eagle medium (DMEM) supplemented with 10% fetal calf serum (FCS) and penicillin/streptomycin (by StemCell Technologies, or Gibco-BRL).
6. Selection medium: DMEM supplemented with:
   a. HXM: hypoxanthine (15 mg/mL, Sigma), xanthine (250 mg/mL, Sigma), mycophenolic acid (25 mg/mL, Sigma).
   b. G418 (1 mg/mL, Gibco-BRL).
7. Sterile-filter: 0.45 μm, low-protein binding (Gelman Acrodisc).

8. Protamine sulfate or polybrene (both from Sigma): prepare stock solution at 5 mg/mL, final concentration: 5 μg/mL.

2.2. Retroviral Titer Assay

1. NIH-3T3 cells.
2. Retroviral supernatant (frozen or fresh).
3. Medium supplemented with the appropriate drug for selection (e.g., G418 for vectors carrying the Neo^R gene).
4. Methylene blue staining solution: 0.2g methylene blue in 100 mL methanol.
5. FACS buffer: phosphate-buffered saline (PBS) 2% FCS, 0.5 μg/mL propidium iodide (PI) (Sigma)
6. Protamine sulfate or polybrene (both from Sigma): 5 μg/mL (final concentration).

2.3. Bone-Marrow Infection

1. Donor and recipient mice: It is convenient to employ histocompatible donor-recipient pairs that differ by readily detectable markers such as the surface antigen Ly5.1/5.2, hemoglobin variants or glucose phosphate isomerase (GPI) to enable ready determination of the degree of reconstitution with donor-derived cells.
2. For supernatant infection: retroviral supernatant (frozen or fresh).
3. For cocultivation: tissue-culture dishes with ~90 % confluent ecotropic producer cells, irradiated *in situ*.
4. Cytokines for bone-marrow culture (final concentration): m IL-3: 6 ng/mL; h IL-6: 10 ng/mL; m steel factor (SF): 100 ng/mL. Since repeated thawing and freezing of concentrated cytokine solutions is detrimental to their activity, prepare concentrated stock solution in medium without FCS, and store aliquots at – 20°C.
5. Fibronectin (Sigma) or fibronectin fragment CH-296 (Takara).
6. Methylcellulose for colony-forming cells (CFC) assays (StemCell Technologies).
7. Protamine sulfate or polybrene (both from Sigma): prepare stock solution at 5 mg/mL, final concentration: 5 μg/mL.
8. 5-fluorouracil (5-FU).

3. Methods

3.1. Retroviral Producer Cells

Generating stable retroviral producer cells is a multi-step process. For application to murine target cells, first generate amphotropic retrovirus containing supernatant by transfection of Phoenix-*Ampho* cells, which are optimized for high-level transient virus packaging *(18)*. This supernatant is used to infect an ecotropic-packaging-cell line optimized for long-term stable virus production (e.g., GP+E86) *(19)*. To increase titers expose ecotropic-packaging-cells many times with the amphotropic supernatant. Transduced cells are subsequently selected, either by drug selection or by FACS sorting. Once the integrity of the proviral copy has been confirmed by Southern blot analysis and a high-titer clone has been identified, supernatant is collected to infect the final target cells, such as bone-marrow cells.

Alternatively, if only small amounts of retroviral supernatant are needed, transient transfection of Phoenix-*Eco (18)* or BOSC cells *(20)* might yield enough supernatant to directly infect murine bone-marrow cells. However, the titer from stable producer cells are usually higher, and there are less batch-to-batch variations (*see* **Note 2**).

Clonal drift resulting in loss of packaging function may cause producer cells to give lower titers when cultured over extended periods of time. It is therefore advisable to freeze a number of aliquots of these cells, which can then be thawed in regular intervals, as soon as possible.

3.1.1. Generation of Retroviral Producer Cells

1. The retroviral vector plasmid DNA is introduced into Phoenix-*Ampho* cells by CaPO$_4$ transfection. Standard protocols as published in *Current Protocols in Molecular Biology* are used. Further useful details are described by Dr. Gary Nolan, whose lab generated the Phoenix-*Eco* and -*Ampho* packaging-cell-lines, on his web page (www-leland.stanford.edu/group/nolan).
2. The supernatant is collected 24–48 h posttransfection and filtered through 0.45 μm low-protein binding filter.
3. Ecotropic packaging cells are plated at a low density in 6-cm tissue-culture dishes 1 d prior to use (1×10^5 cells/dish).
4. The medium is removed from the ecotropic packaging cells and replaced by retroviral supernatant harvested from the transient transfection. For convenience, supernatant from Phoenix-*Ampho* transfections can be stored frozen (–80°C) prior to use, although some reduction in titer (up to 50%) can be expected.
5. Protamine sulfate is added to the dishes to a final concentration of 5 μg/mL.
6. Because of the short half-life of retroviruses of 5–8 h *(21)*, the media should be replaced after 8 h, either by fresh medium or by new retroviral supernatant.
7. The packaging cells can be infected multiple times by retroviral supernatant at 8–12 h intervals. This procedure increases the chances of multiple retroviral integrations, which in turn leads to higher titers. If necessary, the cells should be split to maintain them in exponential growth phase.
8. After 5–10 infection cycles, the retroviral producer cells are selected on the basis of the expression of the marker gene. In the case of a surface marker, FACS can be used to assess transduction efficiency and to sort transduced cells. In the case of the neo-resistance marker, G418 is added to the media (*see* **Note 3**).
9. The selected producer cells are expanded and analyzed as follows:
   a. Southern blot analysis: To demonstrate the integrity of the proviral copies. If additional rearranged forms are observed, cloning may enable the isolation of producers with only the full-length form.

b. Titer assay (*see* **Subheading 3.2.**): To determine the amount of infectious particles in the culture supernatant. The infected NIH-3T3 cells should also be analyzed by Southern blot to confirm transmission of the full-length provirus to the target cells.

3.1.2. Cloning and Selection of Retroviral Producer Clones

Once a retroviral producer-cell line has been generated, clones should be established as soon as possible, either by limiting-dilution analysis (LDA) under drug selection or by single-cell deposition of transduced cells by FACS. Cloning of retroviral producer cells serves two purposes. First, retroviral vectors may integrate not only in full-length proviral form, but also in rearranged subgenomic forms. Retroviral producer cells that carry only the full-length form can be separated by cloning from those that carry subgenomic forms. However, cloning is only advised if the full-length band is the most prominent one—otherwise, the chances to find a clone with only the full-length integration are very low. In this case, it may be faster to repeat the procedure, starting with generating fresh transient retroviral supernatant. Changes in the vector design may ultimately be the only recourse if generation of the full-length virus remains problematic.

Second, cloning allows the identification of highest-titer clones, because considerable variation occurs as a result of the integration site and number of proviral integrations. Thus, from all the clones with only the full-length provirus, viral supernatant are generated and titered, while a Southern blot analysis of the clones is simultaneously performed to determine the proviral copy number. Based on these analyses, retroviral producer-cell clones can be identified that are stable and produce high-titer supernatant.

3.1.3. Collection of Viral Supernatant

1. Expand viral producer cells and plate $5–10 \times 10^5$ cells/10-cm tissue-culture-grade dish.
2. Change medium at 90–95% confluency: 8–10 mL fresh medium.
3. Collect supernatant after 12–36 h and filter supernatant through 0.45-μm low-protein-binding filter. The optimal time at which the supernatant should be harvested must be determined for each vector. Although some groups report the collection of viral supernatant at 32°C in order to slow down cell growth and increase viral production (*22*), we have not observed significant differences in titers of supernatant collected at 32°C or 37°C.
4. Store aliquots in cryotubes at −80°C.
5. Use one aliquot to determine retroviral titer.

3.2. Retroviral Titer Assay

The marker gene of the retroviral vector defines how the titer of the viral supernatant is determined. Although any marker gene is expressed within 24–48 h of retroviral infection, transduction efficiency can only be measured immediately if the marker gene can be identified by FACS. In the case of drug-resistance markers, the selection period lasts 1–2 wk.

Accordingly, the titer assays for these two types of retroviral vectors exhibit two main differences. First, the expression/selection period lasts 2 or 14 d for FACS- or G418-selectable vectors, respectively. Second, supernatants that are titered by FACS are diluted only up to 100-fold, whereas when titered by drug selection, the supernatants are diluted from 10^3- to 10^6-fold to facilitate colony scoring.

In an attempt to increase titers, simplified retroviral vectors have been designed that have no selection marker. To determine titers of such viruses, RNA-based methods have been successfully applied *(23)*.

3.2.1. Titration by FACS Analysis (GFP-Vectors)

1. Plate 0.5–2×10^5 NIH-3T3 cells per well of a 6 well plate 1 d prior to the assay. Prepare 3–4 wells for each supernatant to be titered.
2. Obtain fresh viral supernatant or thaw a frozen aliquot.
3. Prewarm 10% FCS medium to 37°C.
4. Harvest NIH-3T3 cells from two wells and determine number of cells per well at the time of infection.
5. Prepare serial dilutions of viral supernatant (total volume: 500 μL):

neat:	500 μL supernatant	+	0 μL medium
1/3:	166 μL supernatant	+	334 μL medium
1/10:	50 μL supernatant	+	450 μL medium
1/33:	16 μL supernatant	+	486 μL medium

6. Remove medium from NIH-3T3 cells and replace by dilutions of viral supernatant.
7. Add protamine sulfate to each well: 5 μg/mL final concentration. Alternatively, polybrene (Sigma) can be used at the same concentration.
8. Add 2–3mL prewarmed medium to each well 3–4 h postinfection.
9. Incubate for 2 d at 37°C and 5% CO_2 for maximal GFP expression in infected NIH-3T3 cells.
10. Trypsinize NIH-3T3 cells and wash once with PBS 2% FCS.
11. Resuspend cell pellet in 400–500 μL FACS buffer.
12. Determine % GFP-positive NIH-3T3 cells by FACS.
13. Calculate titer as follows:
    % GFP$^+$ cells × NIH-3T3 cells/well (d 0) × 2 (only 500 μL supernatant was used in the test) × 1/dilution = U/mL.

3.2.2. Titration by Drug Selection (Neo-Vectors)

1. Plate 1×10^5 NIH-3T3 cells per 6-cm tissue-culture dish 1 d before the assay. Six dishes per viral supernatant should to be prepared.
2. Infect NIH-3T3 cells with dilutions of viral supernatants. Because viral particles are not very stable at room temperature, set all other components first, and add freshly harvested or thawed viral supernatant to the tubes as a last step:
   a. label 6-mL tubes (control = no virus, neat virus, and viral dilutions of 10^{-3}, 10^{-4}, and 10^{-5},10^{-6}). Dilutions of 10^{-3} to 10^{-5} cover the usual range of titers to be expected (10^4 to 10^6).
   b. prepare serial dilutions of viral supernatant in a total volume of 1 mL.
   c. all the dilutions should contain protamine sulfate at 5 µg/mL.
3. Remove media from NIH-3T3 cells and immediately add diluted viral supernatant.
4. Incubate for 4 h, then add 4 mL more media.
5. After 2 d, add G418 to all plates at final concentration of 1 mg/mL or as previously determined to yield no background growth of nontransfected NIH-3T3 cells.
6. Culture NIH-3T3 cells for 2 wk under G418 selection. Change media every 2–3 d, but do not split cells.
7. After 10–14 d, fix cells onto dish and stain G418-resistant colonies with methylene blue:
   a. remove media from dish.
   b. carefully rinse dish with PBS.
   c. add methylene blue solution to cover dish (2–3 mL for 6-cm dish).
   d. leave 10 min at RT.
   e. remove methylene blue solution (can be reused), and wash 2 × with dH_2O.
   f. allow dishes to dry.
8. Count colonies and calculate titer as follows: number of colonies × 1/dilution = virions/mL.

3.3. Bone-Marrow Infection

Stable integration of murine retroviral vectors requires cell division of the target cells. The HSC, however, is quiescent or cycling very slowly. Therefore, to activate HSC into cell cycling, bone-marrow donor mice are injected with 5-FU. Bone marrow harvested from 5-FU-treated mice contains a higher frequency of cycling HSC susceptible to retroviral infection, and decreased proportion of more mature cell types (*see* **Note 4**). To minimize loss of HSC function in vitro, a cytokine cocktail containing IL-3, IL-6, and SF is added to the bone-marrow culture medium during the entire culture period (*see* **Note 5**).

The infection protocol consists of a 2-d prestimulation and a 2-d infection period. If there is a FACS-selectable marker incorporated into the vector, the bone-marrow cells are cultured for an additional 2 d to allow the expression of the marker gene.

3.3.1. Infection by Cocultivation (see **Note 6**)

1. Day 0: inject donor mice intravenously, with 5-FU (150 mg/kg).
2. Day 4: flush bone marrow with 27-gauge needles and 12-mL syringe and medium containing 2% FCS. Expected cell yield: $2–5 \times 10^6$ leukocytes per mouse (2 femurs and 2 tibias), which is about 10-fold lower than a bone-marrow harvest from untreated normal mice. If bone-marrow cells are harvested earlier (2–3 d after injection of 5-FU), the cell yield is higher, and the frequency of cycling HSC is lower.
3. Prestimulate bone-marrow cells at $3–5 \times 10^5$ cells/mL (15% FCS medium plus cytokines) at 37°C/ 5% CO_2. Use Petri dishes to minimize adherence of cultured bone-marrow cells.
4. Split and plate producer cells into new tissue-culture dishes so that they are about 90% confluent at d 6.
5. Day 5: change medium of the viral producer cells.
6. Day 6: harvest bone-marrow cells (scrape plates with cell lifter), count, and resuspend cells in 15% FCS medium at $3–5 \times 10^5$ cells/mL (expect two- to fivefold reduction of cells during prestimulation period).
7. Add cytokines and protamine sulfate.
8. Irradiate culture dishes with viral producer cells with 40 Gy.
9. Remove media from viral producer plate(s) and gently add bone-marrow cells to irradiated producer cells. Do not place more than 5×10^6 bone-marrow cells into a 10-cm dish.
10. Leave a small amount of bone-marrow cells uninfected, and culture on irradiated parental packaging cells (mock control).
11. Day 8: remove bone-marrow cells from producer cells. Be careful not to disrupt adherent producers. Recover as many bone-marrow cells as possible by carefully adding medium 2% FCS dropwise to packaging cells (3–5 times). Combine all bone-marrow cells and pellet (expect one- to twofold reduction of cell number). When using drug-selectable marker (e.g., neo):
12. Inject total bone-marrow cells intravenously into recipient mice that have been lethally irradiated with 9 Gy 2–24 h earlier. Transplant $>1 \times 10^6$ cells for long-term repopulating assays (LTRA) and $5–10 \times 10^3$ cells for CFU-S assays.
13. Plate bone-marrow cells into methyl cellulose (at 10^3 to 10^4 cells/dish) +/– G418 to determine gene-transfer efficiency to progenitors. When using FACS-selectable marker (e.g., GFP):
14. Place cells back into culture (media 15% FCS plus cytokines) at $1–3 \times 10^5$ cells/ mL for 2 d more to allow expression of marker gene. Expect cell numbers to increase two- to tenfold during this culture period.
15. Day 10: determine gene-transfer efficiency by FACS analysis.
16. Sort transduced cells (if desired) prior to IV injection into recipient mice that have been lethally irradiated with 9 Gy 2–24 h earlier. Transplant $3–5 \times 10^5$ FACS-selected cells or $>1 \times 10^6$ unsorted cells for LTRA and $5–10 \times 10^3$ cells for CFU-S assays.

3.3.2. Infection by Retroviral SN (see **Note 7**)

Bone-marrow harvest and prestimulation are performed as described in **Subheading 3.3.1.** Continue the infection protocol as follows:

1. Day 6: coat Petri dishes with 3–5 µg/cm^2 fibronectin (FN), diluted in PBS (10-cm dish: 51 cm^2, 6-cm dish: 21 cm^2).
2. Dry for several hours in sterile hood.
3. Incubate fibronectin-coated Petri dishes with 3–4 mL of viral supernatant for 20min–1 h at 4°C. This process increases the number of viral particles that bind to the fibronectin and come in contact with the bone-marrow cells.
4. In the meantime, harvest bone-marrow cells with cell lifter and count (expect two- to fivefold reduction of cell number).
5. Pellet bone-marrow cells and resuspend in viral supernatant, 3–5 × 10^5 cells/mL. (*see* **Note 8**).
6. Add cytokines and protamine sulfate.
7. Remove viral supernatant from fibronectin-coated Petri dishes and replace by bone-marrow cell suspension.
8. Day 7: replace media with fresh viral supernatant and add cytokines and protamine sulfate.
9. Day 8: harvest bone-marrow cells with cell lifter, pellet, and count (expect one- to twofold reduction of cell number). Finish infection protocol as mentioned in **Subheading 3.3.1.**

4. Notes

1. The two packaging-cell-lines described here (Phoenix-*Ampho* and GP+E86) have been used in our laboratory most successfully. However, there are many more packaging-cell-lines available, such as Cre *(28)* that can be successfully employed.
2. The titers of retroviral supernatant from stable ecotropic producer clones are highly dependent on the vector. Supernatants derived from simple vectors with a cDNA driven off the proviral LTR promoter can reach titers of 1 × 10^6 U/mL or higher. More complex vectors with multiple transcription initiation sites and/or genomic form of the gene of interest usually yield lower titers. Multiple clones may need to be screened to identify those with usable titers of >1 × 10^5 U/mL.
3. The incorporation of a FACS-selectable marker into retroviral vectors allows purification of transduced cells as early as 24–48 h postinfection. We have shown that sorting eliminates the bias against HSC *(30)*. In the case of complex vectors, which can achieve only low transduction efficiencies, this allows one to conduct experiments with cells that are 100% transduced.
4. Beside 5-FU treated bone-marrow cell, alternative sources for HSC have been described. Sorted Sca-1$^+$lin$^-$ stem cells have also been used *(27)*. Although fetal liver cells have a high content of cycling stem cells, after retroviral transduction relatively high cells numbers must be transplanted.

5. The cytokines described here for the in vitro culture of 5-FU-treated mouse bone-marrow cells have been found to be highly effective for induction of cell cycle and preservation of HSC function. However, this is an evolving field of research with new combinations continuously reported (24,25). HSC from other hematopoietic sources, such as fetal liver or unmanipulated bone marrow, may require cytokine cocktails of different composition and concentrations. Alternatively, the use of stromal cells in supporting HSC maintenance is also actively investigated (26).

6. Cocultivation of bone-marrow cells and retroviral producer cells that have been irradiated or growth-arrested with mitomycin C usually leads to a higher transduction efficiency than supernatant infection, mainly because the producer cells continuously release viral particles into the culture media. However, the HSC recovery is compromised, because HSC are often strongly attach to the producer cells.

7. The advantage of supernatant infections is that the quality of different batches of retroviral supernatant can be tested in advance, which provides better control over the infection condition. Since there is no contact of the bone-marrow cells with the producer cells, all the cells can be recovered at the end of the infection period from the culture dish. However, the transduction efficiency is limited by the short half-life of retroviruses in culture of 5–7 h (12). This problem can be partially overcome by changing the viral supernatant during the infection period. The use of fibronectin in supernatant infection was pioneered by Hanenberg et al. (29). Our protocol is based on this study.

8. There is a strong correlation between the titer of the retroviral supernatant and the transduction efficiency of 5-FU-treated bone-marrow cells. The higher the titer, the higher the percentage of transduced cells. Supernatants with $\sim 2 \times 10^5$ U/mL transduce only about 10–20%, while supernatant with $> 1 \times 10^6$ U/mL should transduce >50% of the bone-marrow cells based on the percentage of GFP-positive cells 2 d postinfection. Supernatants with titers $<1 \times 105$ U/mL yield very low transduction rates, and are generally usable only for cell lines that can be selected and expanded in vitro.

References

1. Keller, G., Paige ,C., Gilboa, E., and Wagner E. F. (1985) Expression of a foreign gene in myeloid and lymphoid cells derived from multipotent haematopoietic precursors. Nature 318, 149–154.

2. Williams, D. A., Lemischka, I. R., Nathan, D. G., and Mulligan R. C. (1984) Introduction of new genetic material into pluripotent haematopoietic stem cells of the mouse. Nature 310, 476–480.

3. Dick, J. E., Magli, M. C., Huszar, D., Phillips, R. A., and Bernstein A. (1985) Introduction of a selectable gene into primitive stem cells capable of long-term reconstitution of the hemopoietic system of W/Wv mice. Cell 42, 71–79.

4. Lemischka, I. R., Raulet, D. H., and Mulligan, R. C. (1986) Developmental potential and dynamic behavior of hematopoietic stem cells. Cell 45, 917–927.

5. Miller, D. G., Adam, M. A., and Miller, A. D. (1990) Gene transfer by retrovirus vectors occurs only in cells that are actively replicating at the time of infection

(published erratum appears in *Mol. Cell. Biol.* 1992 Jan;12(1):433), *Mol. Cell. Biol.* **10,** 4239–4242.

6. Hajihosseini, M., Iavachev, L., and Price, J. (1993) Evidence that retroviruses integrate into post-replication host DNA. *EMBO. J.* **12,** 4969–4974.

7. Harrison, D. E. and Lerner, C. P. (1991) Most primitive hematopoietic stem cells are stimulated to cycle rapidly after treatment with 5-fluorouracil. *Blood* **78,** 1237–1240.

8. Bodine, D. M., McDonagh, K. T., Seidel, N. E., and Nienhuis A. W. (1991) Survival and retrovirus infection of murine hematopoietic stem cells in vitro: effects of 5-FU and method of infection. *Exp. Hematol.* **19,** 206–212.

9. Luskey, B. D., Rosenblatt, M., Zsebo, K., and Williams, D. A. (1992) Stem cell factor, interleukin-3, and interleukin-6 promote retroviral-mediated gene transfer into murine hematopoietic stem cells. *Blood* **80,** 396–402.

10. Bodine, D. M., Karlsson, S., and Nienhuis, A. W. (1989) Combination of interleukins 3 and 6 preserves stem cell function in culture and enhances retrovirus-mediated gene transfer into hematopoietic stem cells. *Proc. Natl. Acad. Sci. USA* **86,** 8897–8901.

11. Bodine, D. M., Seidel, N. E., Gale, M. S., Nienhuis, A. W., and Orlic, D. (1994) Efficient retrovirus transduction of mouse pluripotent hematopoietic stem cells mobilized into the peripheral blood by treatment with granulocyte colony-stimulating factor and stem cell factor. *Blood* **84,** 1482–1491.

12. Palsson, B. and Andreadis, S. (1997) The physico-chemical factors that govern retrovirus-mediated gene transfer. *Exp. Hematol.* **25,** 94–102.

13. Pawliuk, R., Kay, R., Lansdorp, P., and Humphries, R. K. (1994) Selection of retrovirally transduced hematopoietic cells using CD24 as a marker of gene transfer. *Blood* **84,** 2868–2877.

14. Hollander, G. A., Luskey, B. D., Williams, D. A., and Burakoff, S. J. (1992) Functional expression of human CD8 in fully reconstituted mice after retroviral-mediated gene transfer of hemopoietic stem cells. *J. Immunol.* **149,** 438–444.

15. Mavilio, F., Ferrari, G., Rossini, S., Nobili, N., Bonini, C., Casorati, G., et al. (1994) Peripheral blood lymphocytes as target cells of retroviral vector-mediated gene transfer. *Blood* **83,** 1988–1997.

16. Bierhuizen, M. F., Westerman, Y., Visser, T. P., Dimjati, W., Wognum, A. W., and Wagemaker G. (1997) Enhanced green fluorescent protein as selectable marker of retroviral- mediated gene transfer in immature hematopoietic bone marrow cells. *Blood* **90,** 3304–3315.

17. Persons, D. A., Allay, J. A., Allay, E. R., Smeyne, R. J., Ashmun, R. A., Sorrentino, B. P., et al. (1997) Retroviral-mediated transfer of the green fluorescent protein gene into murine hematopoietic cells facilitates scoring and selection of transduced progenitors in vitro and identification of genetically modified cells in vivo. *Blood* **90,** 1777–1786.

18. Kinsella, T. M. and Nolan, G. P. (1996) Episomal vectors rapidly and stably produce high-titer recombinant retrovirus. *Hum. Gene Ther.* **7,** 1405–1413.

19. Markowitz, D., Goff, S., and Bank, A. (1988) A safe packaging line for gene transfer: separating viral genes on two different plasmids. *J. Virol.* **62,** 1120–1124.
20. Pear, W. S., Nolan, G. P., Scott, M. L., and Baltimore D. (1993) Production of high-titer helper-free retroviruses by transient transfection. *Proc. Natl. Acad. Sci. USA* **90,** 8392–8396.
21. Andreadis, S. T., Brott, D., Fuller, A. O. and Palsson, B. O. (1997) Moloney murine leukemia virus-derived retroviral vectors decay intracellularly with a half-life in the range of 5.5 to 7.5 h. *J. Virol.* **71,** 7541–7548.
22. Kaptein, L. C., Greijer, A. E., Valerio, D., and van Beusechem, V. W. (1997) Optimized conditions for the production of recombinant amphotropic retroviral vector preparations. *Gene Ther.* **4,** 172–176.
23. Murdoch, B., Pereira, D. S., Wu, X., Dick, J. E., and Ellis J. (1997) A rapid screening procedure for the identification of high-titer retrovirus packaging clones. *Gene Ther.* **4,** 744–749.
24. Miller, C. L. and Eaves, C. J. (1997) Expansion in vitro of adult murine hematopoietic stem cells with transplantable lympho-myeloid reconstituting ability. *Proc. Natl. Acad. Sci. USA* **94,** 13,648-13,653.
25. Neben, S., Donaldson, D., Sieff, C., Mauch, P., Bodine, D., Ferrara, J., Yetz-Aldape, J., and Turner, K. (1994) Synergistic effects of interleukin-11 with other growth factors on the expansion of murine hematopoietic progenitors and maintenance of stem cells in liquid culture. *Exp. Hematol.* **22,** 353–359.
26. Moore, K. A., Ema, H., and Lemischka, I. R. (1997) In vitro maintenance of highly purified, transplantable hematopoietic stem cells. *Blood* **89,** 4337–4347.
27. Spain, L. M. and Mulligan, R. C. (1992) Purification and characterization of retrovirally transduced hematopoietic stem cells. *Proc. Natl. Acad. Sci. USA* **89,** 3790–3794.
28. Danos, O. and Mulligan, R. C. (1988) Safe and efficient generation of recombinant retroviruses with amphotropic and ecotropic host ranges. *Proc. Natl. Acad. Sci, USA* **85,** 6460–6464.
29. Hanenberg, H., Xiao, X. L., Dilloo, D., Hashino, K., Kato I., and Williams D. A. (1996) Colocalization of retrovirus and target cells on specific fibronectin fragments increases genetic transduction of mammalian cells. *Nat. Med.* **2,** 876–882.
30. Pawliuk, R., Eaves, C. J., and Humphries, R. K. (1997) Sustained high-level reconstitution of the hematopoietic system by preselected hematopoietic cells expressing a transduced cell-surface antigen. *Hum. Gene Ther.* **8,** 1595–1604.

16

Retroviral Transduction of FACS-Purified Hematopoietic Stem Cells

Claudiu V. Cotta, C. Scott Swindle, Irving L. Weissman, and Christopher A. Klug

1. Introduction

Since the mid-1980s, murine retroviral vectors have been used extensively by a number of investigators to clonally mark and genetically modify primitive hematopoietic stem cells (HSC) *(1,2)*. During this period, both vectors and packaging systems used to generate virus have undergone considerable modification. This has led to increased production of high-titer, replication-defective retrovirus that is more resistant to gene inactivation following integration into hematopoietic cells. Current approaches to murine HSC transduction have become increasingly more standardized, although there remain numerous variations on a theme (*see* Chapter 15). This "classical" method utilizes preconditioned bone-marrow cells (typically from 5-fluorouracil [5-FU]-treated animals) and coculture of these cells with virus-producing packaging cells in the presence of exogenous cytokines. This approach generally yields high proportions of transduced cells that can repopulate lethally irradiated recipient mice for long periods of time, indicating that self-renewal activity is maintained—at least to some extent—in conditions that promote stem-cell cycling. With this approach, it is difficult to re-isolate transduced cells from packaging cells and from nontransduced bone marrow, which would be desirable in some clinically relevant cases.

The ability to transduce pure populations of HSC that have been isolated using the fluorescence-activated cell sorter (FACS) has certain advantages that can be weighed against the disadvantage of the generally lower transduction

From: *Methods in Molecular Medicine, vol. 63: Hematopoietic Stem Cell Protocols*
Edited by: C. A. Klug and C. T. Jordan © Humana Press Inc., Totowa, NJ

rates resulting from the use of viral supernatants instead of coculture. Transduced cells can readily be repurified from nontransduced cells by using a selectable marker expressed from the integrated proviral vector *(3–5)*. These cells are then transplanted into lethally irradiated mice for analysis. This approach has the advantages of high multiplicity of infection (MOI), (generally from 10–100), the elimination of transduction of bone-marrow cells that contribute to the "noise" of a genetic assay, and the advantage of being able to immediately assay conditions that enhance stem-cell transduction. References are made to other chapters discussing retroviral transduction of HSC to avoid repetition of fully covered topics.

2. Materials

2.1. Isolation of Murine HSC from Bone Marrow

See Chapter 2 for more complete protocol.

1. Staining media (SM): *H*ank's *B*alanced *S*alt *S*olution (HBSS) (Gibco-BRL, Cat. #14025–092) supplemented with 2% heat-inactivated donor calf or fetal calf serum (FCS). Phosphate-buffered saline (PBS) supplemented with 2% serum is also acceptable.
2. 25-gauge needle and 10-cc syringe for flushing marrow.
3. 10-cm Petri dishes (Corning 25025 or comparable dish).
4. Razor blade.
5. Monoclonal antibodies (MAbs) to stem-cell antigens (E13-161-7, anti-Sca-1 conjugated to Texas red; 19XE5, anti-Thy-1.1 conjugated with fluorescein-5-isothiocyanate (FITC); 2B8, anti-c-kit conjugated to allophycocyanin (APC); 3C11, anti-c-kit conjugated with biotin) and to antigens present on more mature blood cell lineages (6B2, anti-B220; M1/70, anti-Mac-1; 8C5, anti-Gr-1; Ter-119, anti-erythrocyte-specific antigen; KT31.1, anti-CD3; 53–7.3, anti-CD5; GK-1.5, anti-CD4; and 53–6.7, anti-CD8). All of the lineage antibodies are direct conjugates with phycoerythrin and are commercially available through Pharmingen. An anti-Fc-receptor blocking antibody (2.4G2) is unconjugated and available through Pharmingen, as are the other antibodies, although the exact conjugates that are marketed may vary. Adaptation of the antibody combination described here may be required because of the available conjugates and the restraints of the flow-cytometer laser configuration that is used for the sorting (*see* Chapter 2).
6. Ammonium chloride/potassium bicarbonate (ACK) solution for red-cell lysis: 8.3 g of ammonium chloride and 1.0 g potassium bicarbonate in 1 L of ddH$_2$O. Filter or autoclave.
7. 50-mL conical tubes.
8. Nylon filters (Falcon #2350).
9. 96-well flat-bottom tissue-culture plates (Costar #3596 or equivalent).

10. Stem-cell media (DMEM, high glucose; Gibco-BRL, Cat. #11965–092). Media is supplemented with 10% heat-inactivated FCS tested for growth and maintenance of embryonic stem (ES) cells (Gibco-BRL, Cat. #16141–079), penicillin (100 IU/mL)-streptomycin (100 mg/mL), 1× nonessential amino acids, 1× sodium pyruvate (1 mM), and 50 µM beta-mercaptoethanol (B-ME). Other synthetic or serum-free media (SFM) should also work well although these have not been tested by our laboratory.

11. Streptaridin microbeads (Miltenyi Biotech, #130-048-101).

12. Minimax columns (Miltenyi Biotech, #130-042-201).

2.2. Cytokine Prestimulation of Sorted HSC

1. Cytokines: IL-6 (5 ng/mL, R&D Systems), stem cell factor (SCF) (50 ng/mL, R&D Systems), and leukemia inhibitory factor (LIF) (1×, ESGRO, Chemicon, Cat. #ESG1107). Flk-2 ligand (50 ng/mL) can also be used without detrimental effects on HSC transduction or reconstitution.

2. Stem-cell media (*see* above).

3. Tissue-culture incubator set at 5% CO_2.

2.3. Generation of Retrovirus by Transient Transfection

1. Phoenix or BOSC23 (*6*) retroviral packaging-cell-line (*see* Garry Nolan web site at Stanford University for information on Material Transfer Agreements and procurement of the cells from American Type Culture Collection (ATCC)—www.stanford.edu/group/nolan/). Other systems for retroviral packaging are also available (*see* www.imgenex.com).

2. 2 *M* $CaCl_2$ (Sigma, C-5080).

3. Sterile water.

4. 2× HBS (pH 7.05): Dissolve 8.0 g NaCl, 6.5 g HEPES (sodium salt, Sigma, H-1016), 105 mg sodium phosphate (dibasic, Sigma, S-0876) in 400 mL of water. Adjust the pH to precisely 7.05; then bring the volume to 500 mL. Filter-sterilize and aliquot to 50 mL conical tubes for freezing. Working stocks are stable for at least a few months, in our experience.

5. 6-cm tissue-culture dishes (Corning 25010).

6. 5-mL sterile polystyrene Falcon tubes (Falcon #2058).

7. Plasmid DNA purified by $CsCl_2$ gradient or kits available from a number of commercial sources, such as Qiagen or BioRad.

8. 0.1 *M* chloroquine diphosphate (2000× stock, Sigma, C-6628).

2.4. Hematopoietic Stem Cell Transduction Using Viral Supernatant

1. Filtered viral supernatant (from a frozen stock stored at –80°C) or fresh.

2. 100× stock of polybrene (hexadimethrine bromide, Sigma, H-9268). 100× polybrene is 400 µg/mL in water.

3. Retronectin (recombinant C-terminal fragment of fibronectin—CH-296, BioWhittaker Cat. #T100A).

3. Methods

3.1. Isolation of Murine HSC from Adult Bone Marrow

To facilitate the analysis of retrovirally transduced HSC following transplantation into lethally irradiated recipient mice, bone marrow should be obtained from inbred strains that are congenic at a particular locus like Ly-5, which is expressed in all hematopoietic progeny except for red blood cells (RBC)(C57B/6 strains congenic at the Ly-5 locus are available from sources such as Jackson Laboratories). Transduced cells of one Ly-5 type are then transplanted into a lethally irradiated congenic animal of the other Ly-5 type. There are commercially available MAbs for both Ly-5 alleles (Pharmingen, as well as other sources), which makes it possible to monitor donor reconstitution in the transplant recipient. As an alternative to the Ly-5 system, HSC from the bone marrow of male mice can be transduced and transplanted into female mice to differentially mark donor cells from recipient cells.

The protocol described in **steps 1–11** is a slight variation from that described by Morrison (*see* Chapter 2), and was developed in the laboratory of Dr. Irving Weissman by Dr. Sam Cheshier and Dr. Jos Domen (submitted manuscript). We have included a few additional details that are relevant for retroviral transduction of FACS-purified stem cells. One can expect to obtain from 500–2000 cells of the long-term reconstituting HSC phenotype (LT-HSC) from the four long bones of a 6–10-wk-old animal using most positive selection approaches. Other marker systems have been used to enrich or purify HSC, and would also be appropriate.

1. Flush the marrow from the tibias and femurs of 5–12-wk-old animals using cold staining media (SM) and a 25-gauge needle. Once the cells have been collected in a 10-cm tissue-culture dish, make a single-cell suspension of the marrow by repeatedly drawing and expelling the cells into the dish using the syringe. Filter the homogenous cell suspension through a nylon screen into a 15-mL or 50-mL conical tube. For all steps in the procedure, the cells should be kept on ice.
2. Spin the cells in a tabletop microfuge at 1000 rpm (about 300*g*) for 5–10 min.
3. Completely aspirate the media and add 1 mL of ACK solution per mouse equivalent of bone-marrow cells. Incubate the cells on ice for 4–5 min; then fill the remaining volume of the tube with SM and pellet the cells by centrifugation. Aspirate and repeat the wash step with SM (*see* **Note 1**). ACK will lysis RBC and leave the white blood cells (WBC) intact.
4. Resuspend the cell pellet in SM (use 500 µL of SM per mouse equivalent of bone marrow, *see* **Note 2**). Filter the resuspended cells through a nylon screen.
5. Block Fc-receptor binding of mouse antibody by staining the cells with unconjugated 2.4G2 (Pharmingen) for 20 min on ice. Wash the cells by filling the conical tube with SM, and then centrifuge at 200–300*g* for 10 min.

6. Stain the cells with anti-c-kit (biotin-conjugated 3C11) antibody for 20–25 min at 4°C. Wash as described above.

7. Resuspend the cell pellet in 100 µL of SM per mouse equivalent of bone marrow, and then add 20 µL of streptavidin microbeads (Miltenyi Biotech) per mouse equivalent of bone marrow (*see* **Note 3**). Stain for 20–25 min at 4°C. Sca-1 biotin can be used in place of c-kit. If this is done, stem cells should be isolated according to the protocol described in Chapter 2.

8. During the magnetic bead staining, begin to degas about 50 mL of SM on ice.

9. After staining with streptavidin microbeads, wash the cells with degassed SM. Repeat the wash and then resuspend the cell pellet in 500 µL of degassed SM per Miltenyi column to be used. Generally, use one MiniMACS column (Miltenyi) for every two mouse equivalents of bone marrow. The number of columns used will be determined by the total number of cells that are expected to be bound by magnetic beads (*see* manufacturer's instructions). Filter the cells through a nylon screen before adding them to the column.

10. Attach the column to the magnet. The columns should be equilibrated by adding 500 µL of degassed SM before loading the cells. After the column has ceased to drip, load the cells in a 500-µL vol to the equilibrated column. Once all of the cell suspension has entered the column, wash the column with 800 µL of SM. After washing, elute the bound fraction of cells by removing the column from the magnet and plunging 700–800 µL of SM into a new tube.

11. Spin the eluted cells, and then resuspend the pellet in the directly conjugated antibodies to lineage markers and to stem-cell surface antigens (*see* **Note 4**). Make up the antibody cocktail in 100–200 µL of SM per column used to enrich the cells (the column capacity is about 10^7 cells). Stain for 20 min at 4°C. Wash and resuspend the cells in SM containing propidium iodide (PI) to mark dead cells during cell sorting (*see* **Note 5** for details about cell sorting). If only three-color sorting is possible, the antibody combination of Sca-1 (FITC), c-kit (Apc) and Lin (PE) works well and results in greater recovery.

3.2. In Vitro Stimulation of HSC Cell Cycle Using Cytokines

A number of cytokine combinations have been used to maintain the LT-HSC phenotype in short-term liquid culture and would probably be appropriate for retroviral transduction. The cytokines used here will induce cell division of LT-HSC within 32–40 h. Cell division is necessary for nuclear entry and integration of murine retroviral vectors into the genome *(7,8)*.

1. Do the re-sort of LT-HSC directly into one well of a 96-well tissue-culture dish containing 200 µL of stem-cell media supplemented with cytokines (*see* **Subheading 2.**). Incubate the plate for 22–24 h in a humidified incubator at 37°C at 5% CO_2 (*see* **Note 6**).

3.3. Generation of Retrovirus by Transient Transfection

Retroviral production by transient transfection is useful when the retrovirus carries a gene that may have detrimental effects on the growth of the retroviral packaging cell line. This method also provides a more rapid means of producing virus that can be of sufficient titer to transduce purified stem cells (we have found that viral titers below 3×10^5 infectious units (IU)/mL are not suitable for stem-cell transduction—ideal titers are 1×10^6 IU/mL or greater). In general, stable production of retrovirus (*see* Chapter 15) can generate somewhat higher titers on a more consistent basis, although it is more time-intensive. Stable retroviral production also allows one to do co-culture experiments, which lead to higher transduction efficiencies because the stem cells are in direct contact with the viral producer cells. Additional information about retroviral packaging cells and retroviral vectors can be found on the Nolan web site (*see* **Subheading 2.3., step 1**) or in **refs. *9–11***.

1. The day before transfection, plate 2×10^6 retroviral producer cells (BOSC 23 or Phoenix-*Eco*) onto a 6-cm tissue-culture dish in a vol of 3 mL. The cells should be about 60–70% confluent the following day, just prior to transfection.
2. Prewarm stem-cell media without cytokines to 37°C. Just prior to transfection, change the media on the retroviral producer cells to stem-cell media supplemented with 50 μ*M* chloroquine diphosphate. Because the retroviral producer cells are loosely adherent on the dish, care must be taken whenever the media is changed. Incubate the dish at 37°C for 10 min.
3. To a 5-mL sterile Falcon tube, add the following in order:
   a. 430 μL of sterile water.
   b. 10–15 μg of plasmid DNA (*see* **Note 7**).
   c. 61 μL of 2 *M* CaCl$_2$ (the water and DNA should reach a total vol of 439 μL). Mix the solution by gentle vortexing.
4. Using a P1000 pipetman, vigorously expel 500 μL of 2X HEPES-buffered saline (HBS) (pH 7.05) to the solution. Gently vortex the tube for about 10 s. As an alternative to "splashing" the HBS into the tube, the HBS can be added while gently bubbling air into the mixture. The HBS should be titrated over a narrow pH range (6.95–7.1) to obtain optimal co-precipitation of DNA.
5. Add the 1 mL of DNA/Ca$_3$(PO$_4$)$_2$ precipitate dropwise to the dish containing the retroviral producer cells. Incubate the dish at 37°C for 7–8 h.
6. Gently change the media on the producer cells by aspirating the chloroquine-containing media and adding 3 mL of fresh, prewarmed stem-cell media (without cytokines) to the side of the dish; avoid dislodging the producer cells.
7. Incubate the cells for an additional 12–16 h; then replace the 3 mL of media with 2 mL of fresh media. Incubate the cells for 24 h and then harvest the retrovirus-containing supernatant (*see* **Note 8**).
8. Filter the supernatant from the retroviral producer cells through a 0.45-micron, low-protein-binding syringe filter into a 15-mL conical tube. Freeze the superna-

tant in 300–500 μL aliquots in cryotubes on dry ice. Titer an aliquot of the frozen supernatant, using NIH-3T3 cells. Titer the virus according to the procedure described in Chapter 15.

9. Check the transfection efficiency of the viral producer cells by trypsinizing the cells after the supernatant has been collected. If a GFP-containing virus (or other virus with a FACS-selectable marker) was used, assay transfection efficiency by flow cytometry. One should expect to see greater than 50% transfection efficiency. A transfection efficiency of 80–100% is not uncommon.

3.4. Retroviral Transduction of Murine LT-HSC

Optimal transduction of purified LT-HSC is obtained with a combined used of retronectin *(12)* and "spinoculation" *(13,14)*. Re-sorting of transduced cells is done about 24 h following transduction if FACS-selectable markers are incorporated into the retrovirus.

1. Prior to transducing the stem cells, coat the well of a 96-well tissue-culture dish with 50 μg/mL (in PBS) retronectin as described in Chapter 17. A similar procedure is also described in Chapter 15.
2. Carefully pipet off the media from the cultured stem-cell well so that less than 50 μL of media remains on the cells. Be careful not to disturb the stem cells at the bottom of the well.
3. Resuspend the stem cells in the remaining volume, and measure the volume using a pipetman. Transfer the cells to the retronectin-coated well along with the following:
   a) 140 μL of freshly thawed and prewarmed viral supernatant.
   b) 6 μL of cytokine cocktail (2 μL each of IL-6, Stl, and LIF from 100X stocks).
   c) 2 μL of 100X polybrene (final concentration=4 μg/mL).
   d) stem-cell media without cytokines to make up 200 μL.
4. Spin the 96-well plate at 700–800g for 1–2 h at room temperature in a tabletop centrifuge equipped with 96-well plate carriages.
5. Remove the plate and place it in a tissue-culture incubator overnight (after the spin, 150 μL of supernatant can be removed and replaced with another 150-μL aliquot of virus, polybrene, and cytokines).
6. About 8 h prior to re-sorting the transduced HSC, replace 150 μL of the media with fresh, prewarmed stem-cell media and cytokines (use 1.5 μL of each 100X stock).
7. Re-sort HSC based on green fluorescent protein (GFP) fluorescence or cell-surface marker expression, and transplant into recipient animals (*see* **Note 9**).

4. Notes

1. We and others (in the Weissman laboratory) have found no detrimental effect of ACK treatment on stem cell reconstitution or on the ability to retrovirally-transduce HSC after cell sorting. Because ACK tends to cause some of the cells to clump, filtration is necessary before proceeding to additional staining steps.

2. The number of bone-marrow cells obtained from the four long bones in one mouse should be between 5×10^7 and 1×10^8 cells, depending on the age of the animal and how extensively the bones were flushed. If cell numbers differ significantly from this, the volume of SM added to the ACK-lysed cells should be adjusted.

3. The streptavidin microbeads can be titrated using whole bone-marrow cells for optimal staining and retention of cells in the MiniMACS column (Miltenyi Biotech). We have noted some variability in the enrichment step that could be due to the antibody used for positive selection, the amount of microbeads used or the particular microbead or column lot used.

4. All antibodies should be titrated for optimal staining before use.

5. LT-HSC should be sorted once and then re-sorted for purity. Purity after the first sort depends largely on the sort mode set on the flow cytometer and the extent of column enrichment. One can typically expect the first sort purity to range between 25–75% when a four-color sort is done. Cell purity following the second sort is greater than 98%. To minimize cell losses, the first sort is done into a 96-well tissue-culture plate containing 100 µL of cold SM. The second sort is done into stem-cell media supplemented with cytokines.

6. Optimal transduction efficiencies are obtained when cells are prestimulated for 22–30 h. The timing of transduction is intended to target cells with retrovirus when they are in the G_1 phase of the cell cycle. Cells in middle to late S phase have progressed too far into the cycle to permit entry, reverse transcription, and integration of a retroviral complex before mitosis *(8)*, thus reducing transduction efficiencies. A minimal cell number for transduction would be about 3000 cells. Ideally, transduction of 10,000–20,000 LT-HSC cells per construct works best, but this number is often difficult to obtain unless large amounts of bone marrow are used for HSC isolation.

7. More DNA may need to be used if a plasmid is exceptionally large, in order to attain molar equivalents between different constructs. Use of 10 µg of plasmid works well with plasmid sizes of approx 6 kb. Using more DNA in the transfection will increase the transfection efficiency somewhat, but will not lead to significantly higher viral titers.

8. Optimal viral production occurs 18–36 h following the initiation of the transfection procedure. Titers are about 20–30% lower when collection is done between 24–48 h posttransfection, which is often more convenient.

9. Re-sorting cells after a 24-h transduction protocol does not compromise the ability to quantitatively recover nearly all of the transduced cells. Leaving cells longer before re-sorting to allow maximal reporter-gene-expression yields brighter signals, but no significant increase in the absolute number of positive cells, suggesting that most of the retroviral integration occurs early in the transduction protocol. One should expect 10–40% transduction efficiency using this approach. Significant variability resulting from the health of the cells following the original cell sort and the titer of the virus that is being used in the experiment may be observed.

Vectors that contain internal ribosome entry sites to obtain expression of the GFP reporter typically have lower titers (approx two- to threefold in our studies) than vectors without an internal ribosomal entry site (IRES) sequence.

References

1. Dick, J. E., Magli, M. C., Huszar, D., Phillips, R. A., and Bernstein, A. (1985) Introduction of a selectable gene into primitive stem cells capable of long-term reconstitution of the hemopoietic system of W/W^v mice. *Cell* **42,** 71–79.
2. Keller, G., Paige, C., Gilboa, E., and Wagner, E. F. (1985) Expression of a foreign gene in myeloid and lymphoid cells derived from multipotent haematopoietic precursors. *Nature* **318,** 149–154.
3. Ruggieri, L., Aiuti, A., Salomoni, M., Zappone, E., Ferrari, G., and Bordignon, C. (1997) Cell-surface marking of CD(34+)-restricted phenotypes of human hematopoietic progenitor cells by retrovirus-mediated gene transfer. *Hum. Gene Ther.* **8,** 1611–1623.
4. Persons, D. A., Allay, J. A., Allay, E. R., Smeyne, R. J., Ashmun, R. A., Sorrentino, B. P., et al. (1997) Retroviral-mediated transfer of the green fluorescent protein gene into murine hematopoietic cells facilitates scoring and selection of transduced progenitors in vitro and identification of genetically modified cells in vivo. *Blood* **90,** 1777–1786.
5. Pawliuk, R., Eaves, C. J., and Humphries, R. K. (1997) Sustained high-level reconstitution of the hematopoietic system by preselected hematopoietic cells expressing a transduced cell-surface antigen. *Hum. Gene Ther.* **8,** 1595–1604.
6. Pear, W. S., Nolan, G. P., Scott, M. L., and Baltimore, D. (1993) Production of high-titer helper-free retroviruses by transient transfection. *Proc. Natl. Acad. Sci. USA* **90,** 8392–8396.
7. Miller, D.G., Adam, M. A., and Miller, A. D. (1990) Gene transfer by retrovirus vectors occurs only in cells that are actively replicating at the time of infection. *Mol. Cell Biol.* **10,** 4239–4242.
8. Roe, T., Reynolds, T. C., Yu, G., and Brown, P. O. (1993) Integration of murine leukemia virus DNA depends on mitosis. *EMBO J.* **12,** 2099–2108.
9. Miller, A. D. (1992) Retroviral vectors, in *Viral Expression Vectors*. (N. Muzyczka, ed.) Springer-Verlag, New York, NY, 1–24.
10. Miller, A. D., Miller, D. G., Garcia, J. V., and Lynch, C. M. (1993) Use of retroviral vectors for gene transfer and expression. *Methods Enzymol.* **217,** 581–599.
11. Hodgson, C. P. (1996) *Retro-Vectors for Human Gene Therapy*. R. G. Landes Company, Austin, TX, 1–145.
12. Moritz, T., Patel, V. P., and Williams, D. A. (1994) Bone marrow extracellular matrix molecules improve gene transfer into human hematopoietic cells via retroviral vectors. *J. Clin. Investig.* **93,** 1451–1457.
13. Ho, W. Z., Cherukuri, R., Ge, S. D., Cutilli, J. R., Song, L., Whitko, S., and Douglas, S. D. (1993) Centrifugal enhancement of human immunodeficiency virus

type 1 infection and human cytomegalovirus gene expression in human primary monocyte/macrophages in vitro. *J. Leuk. Biol.* **53,** 208–212.

14. Bahnson, A. B., Dunigan, J. T., Baysal, B. E., Mohney, T., Atchison, R. W., Nimgaonkar, M. T., et al. (1995) Centrifugal enhancement of retroviral mediated gene transfer. *J. Virol. Methods* **54,** 131–143.

17

Retroviral-Mediated Transduction and Clonal Integration Analysis of Human Hematopoietic Stem and Progenitor Cells

Mo A. Dao and Jan A. Nolta

1. Introduction

This chapter provides information on the methods used to introduce genes into human hematopoietic stem and progenitor cells, using Moloney Murine Leukemia (MoMuLV)-based retroviral vectors. MoMuLV-based vectors have the ability to efficiently transfer genes into mammalian cells, leading to permanent integration of a single copy of the gene of interest into the cellular chromosomes. The technique of single-colony inverse [polymerase chain reaction (PCR) can be used to track individual descendants of MoMuLV-vector-transduced hematopoietic stem cells (HSC), by capitalizing upon the unique restriction patterns generated by the random integration events *(1,2)*. Methods to adapt the inverse PCR technology to the use of other vector systems, such as lentiviral or adeno-associated virus (AAV) vectors, are currently under development. These techniques will be necessary to determine the efficacy of the newer vector systems in transducing individual human HSC that have the capacity to generate both lymphoid and myeloid progeny, as has been demonstrated in rare occurrences using MoMuLV-based vectors *(2)*.

The major drawback in the use of MoMuLV-based retroviral vectors is that they require target-cell division for successful integration into the host-cell DNA *(3,4)*. The most primitive human HSC are deeply quiescent, and thus less frequently transduced than committed progenitor cells, which can be readily induced by cytokines to enter the cell cycle. Because retroviral vectors require target-cell proliferation for successful gene insertion, efforts have been directed toward identifying conditions that will induce active cycling of the hematopoi-

From: *Methods in Molecular Medicine, vol. 63: Hematopoietic Stem Cell Protocols*
Edited by: C. A. Klug and C. T. Jordan © Humana Press Inc., Totowa, NJ

etic cells (*see* **Table 1**). Following the demonstration by Suda, Suda, and Ogawa *(5)* that the combination of interleukin-3 (IL-3) and interleukin-6 (IL-6) promoted the entry of quiescent murine hematopoietic progenitor cells into the active cell cycle, we and others determined that culturing human marrow cells in IL-3 and IL-6 greatly increased the percentages of clonogenic progenitor cells (CFU-C) which can be transduced with retroviral vectors *(6,7)*. Subsequently, we and others have shown that additional cytokines—including granulocytes-colony-stimulating factor (G-CSF), IL-1 , PIXY 321, leukemia inhibitory factor (LIF), stem-cell factor (SCF), IL-11, bFGF, TPO and flt-3 ligand—can enhance the extent of transduction into hematopoietic progenitors *(8–12)*. The presence of an underlying marrow stromal-cell layer or a fragment of fibronectin greatly enhances both survival and transduction of committed and more primitive hematopoietic progenitors *(13–18)*. However, in contrast to the relative ease of transduction of committed progenitors, the more primitive, reconstituting HSC have proven to be much more difficult to transduce, a probable result of their quiescence.

The inability to efficiently transduce pluripotent stem cells has been a major barrier to successful implementation of gene therapy for the number of diseases that are potentially amenable to treatment. The major goal for gene therapy of genetic diseases involving hematopoietic cells is transduction of long-lived pluripotent stem cells, so that a permanent source of genetically corrected hematopoietic cells can be created. Currently, many groups are attempting to solve the problem of human stem-cell transduction by examining alternative cytokines, alternative vector envelopes (Gibbon Ape leukemia virus or Vesicular Stomatitis Virus G protein), and alternative vectors (adenoassociated virus or HIV-based vectors) *(19–25)*.

The presence of an irradiated stromal or fibronectin layer during retroviral-mediated transduction greatly enhances the extent of gene transfer. Stromal cells and their extracellular matrix act to bind and colocalize the hematopoietic cells and the retroviral vector particles *(26–28)*. The use of a stromal monolayer during transduction can be replaced by plates coated with the carboxyl terminal fragment of fibronectin, sold as "retronectin" by Takara Shuzo, Otsu, Japan, and marketed through BioWhittaker in the US. The retronectin-coated plates allow transduction efficiencies that are comparable to stromal support, and maintain the primitive nature of the HSC as well as stromal support *(13)*. While stem and progenitor cells from umbilical cord blood (UCB) can be maintained with good viability in suspension culture, the multipotency of human bone marrow-derived stem cells is severely compromised following 48–72 h without a stromal or fibronectin support matrix. Such cells can only sustain short-term hematopoiesis in murine xenograft assays *(11,13,17)*.

Table 1
Components of Transduction and Their Function

Component	Function
COOH terminal fragment of fibronectin (Retronectin™)	Colocalization of retroviral vector particle and target-cell *(15,16,27,28)*. Replaces the function of stromal support *(13,17)*.
IL-3, IL-6, SCF, FL	Cytokines to maintain viability, and to stimulate cell division, once stem and progenitor cells exit the G_0 phase of the cell cycle.
Serum-free medium (SFM)	Ex-vivo 15 (BioWhittaker) or others *(41,42)* are defined media that contain the constituents necessary for cell survival. SFM contain far lower levels of TGF and other inhibitory cytokines and chemokines than serum-containing media.
Anti-TGFβ antibody	Neutralizes TGFβ in the transduction medium. TGFβ is inhibitory to hematopoietic progenitor cell-cycle entry *(44–46)*.TGF increases levels of the cDK inhibitor p15 [INK4B] in human progenitors, preventing exit from quiescence *(29)*.
Anti-p27 [kip-1] oligonucleotides	Reduces levels of the CDK inhibitor p27 [kip-1], which maintains primitive hematopoietic cells in a quiescent state *(29)*.

Transduction conditions. The function of each component of the transduction system is explained in **Table 1**. The new advances in the past several years are the use of a fibronectin matrix (the recombinant retronectin™ molecule, available from Takara Shuzo, Otsu, Japan), cytokines including Flt3 ligand (FL), serum-free rather than serum-containing media, and additives to reduce levels of the CDK inhibitors p15 and p27, which prevent cell-cycle entry.

Our studies have focused on developing the methods described in this chapter, which allow transduction of a portion of the primitive human HSC while maintaining engraftment capacity. Recently, we determined that transduction in medium with low serum, antibodies to neutralize the negative regulator TGFβ, and the cytokines IL-3, IL-6, SCF, and Flt3 ligand (FL), results in good levels of transduction of primitive, reconstituting cells on fibronectin support, as measured in a long-term xenograft system *(29)*. The addition of anti-sense oligonucleotides to the negative cell-cycle regulator p27 [kip-1] further augments gene transfer by increasing the rate of induction of the primitive cells into the cycle, and allows successful transduction to be done in a 24-h ex vivo period.

Hematopoietic Progenitors from BM, PBSC, or UCB

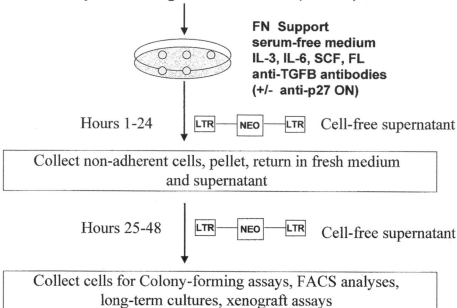

FN Support
serum-free medium
IL-3, IL-6, SCF, FL
anti-TGFB antibodies
(+/- anti-p27 ON)

Hours 1-24 | LTR—NEO—LTR | Cell-free supernatant

Collect non-adherent cells, pellet, return in fresh medium
and supernatant

Hours 25-48 | LTR—NEO—LTR | Cell-free supernatant

Collect cells for Colony-forming assays, FACS analyses,
long-term cultures, xenograft assays

Fig. 1. A sample of human hematopoietic cells is obtained from bone marrow, UCB, or M PB). The RBC are removed by ficoll-density gradient centrifugation. The CD34+ progenitors are enriched by immunomagnetic separation, and plated in medium containing the cytokines IL-3, IL-6, SCF, and FL. Plates coated with the COOH terminal domain of fibronectin (retronectin) are used to colocalize retroviral vector particles and target cells during the transduction. Sterile filtered supernatant from retroviral vector-producing fibroblasts is added at 24 h intervals for 2 d. The example shown uses the LN retroviral vector, which carries the *Neo* gene and encodes resistance to the selective agent G418. Following transduction, cells are plated in a methylcellulose-based colony-forming (CFU) assay, used to initiate long-term bone-marrow culture or transplanted into immune-deficient mice.

This decrease in the duration of ex vivo culture results in enhanced multilineage engraftment levels, with levels of transduction of the primitive, reconstituting cells ranging from 15–30% *(29)*. The techniques used to achieve this goal are fully described in this chapter.

To accomplish retroviral-mediated transduction in a 48-h period, with maintenance of engrafting cells, the steps shown in **Fig. 1** are employed. CD34+ cells are isolated from human bone marrow, mobilized peripheral blood (MPB), or UCB, using the method of choice (Dynal Dynabeads (Oslo, Norway), MiniMACS from Miltenyi Biotec (Auburn, CA), StemStep (StemCell Technologies, Inc., Vancouver, Canada), or fluorescence-activated cell-sorting (FACS) acquisition to isolate subsets of the CD34 population (*see* **refs. 30–32**). CD34$^+$ cells are plated on retronectin-coated flasks or wells at a density of 10^5 cells/mL in SFM with the cytokines IL-3, IL-6, SCF, and FL ligand present at twice the desired final concentration. Cytokines are maintained throughout transductions at concentrations of 50 ng/mL rh IL-6, 10 ng/mL rH IL-3, 50 ng/mL SCF, and 50 ng/mL Flt3 ligand. Neutralizing antibodies to TGFβ are added to a final concentration of 5 ug/mL. Anti-sense oligonucleotides to the cDK inhibitor p27 $^{kip-1}$ can be added at this stage to enhance transduction of the most primitive human hematopoietic cells *(29)*. An equal volume of filtered retroviral supernatant containing 10% fetal calf serum (FCS) is then added to each flask, bringing the final serum concentration to 5%-a level we have determined to be optimal for recruiting human hematopoietic progenitors into the S phase of the cell cycle (Dao and Nolta, Blood 92; 521a, 1998).

Approximately 24 h after addition of the first aliquot of supernatant, nonadherent cells are collected, pelleted, and resuspended in 5 mL supernatant from vector-producing fibroblasts with an equal volume of transduction medium, and returned to the original flask. The transduction medium used on d 2 is the same as that used initially. Following the second addition of supernatant, the cells are incubated for an additional 24 h, then collected for FACS or colony-forming assays (depending on the marker gene used), to initiate long-term cultures (LTC), or to transplant into immune-deficient mice.

The most important considerations for achieving adequate levels of gene transfer using the protocols provided in this chapter are the vector titer, incubation parameters and media, and the condition of the target cells. Supernatant collected from vector-producing fibroblasts must have a titer of at least 5×10^6 infectious U/mL. If the titer is lower, higher-titer clones should be rederived from the initial pool of packaging cells. The retronectin-coated plates can partially circumvent this problem, but titers of at least 1×10^6 are still required. The incubator must be at the appropriate CO$_2$ and temperature (32–37°C, never above). The CO$_2$ level is especially critical to achieving good transduction. The conformation of the retroviral receptors is easily altered by changes in pH, and CO$_2$ levels higher than 5.0% will abolish transduction. The media described in this unit are appropriate for transduction, as are commercially available media from StemCell Technologies. Many components must be screened to avoid nonspecific toxicity to hematopoietic cells. Progenitor cells must be healthy and dividing to allow integration of retroviral vectors. Processing samples as soon as possible after harvest is recommended. There is a progressive loss of the most primitive cells in stored samples. Cytokines must be present to sustain viability, either added to the media as recombinant factors, or produced by accessory cells or stroma (*see* **Table 1**).

2. Materials

2.1. Coating Flasks with Retronectin

1. Retronectin (Takara Shuzo, Otsu, Japan: marketed through BioWhittaker in the US).
2. 2% bovine serum albumin (BSA) solution in PBS (StemCell Technologies, Inc.).
3. 25-cm² culture flasks with 0.2-um vented filter cap (Costar, Cambridge, MA).
4. 1× PBS (Gibco-BRL).

2.2. Cell Preparation

1. Human bone marrow, MPB, or UCB, treated with anticoagulant (*see* **Note 1**).
2. Tabletop centrifuge; protocols require a maximal speed of 730*g* with 15 and 50-mL tube adaptors.
3. 15- and 50-mL polypropylene centrifuge tubes.
4. Ficoll-Paque, code #17-0840-03 (Pharmacia Biotech, Uppsala, Sweden).
5. Trypan blue vital dye solution (Gibco-BRL).
6. Hemocytometer with coverslip and microscope for counting cells.
7. CD34+ cell immunoselection system (Dynal Dynabeads), MiniMACS from Miltenyi Biotec, or StemSep from Stem-Cell Technologies, Inc.

2.3. Transduction

1. Retroviral vector supernatant, prepared as directed in **Subheading 3.4.**
2. 37°C, 5% CO_2 incubator-checked by fyrite weekly.
3. 37°C water bath.
4. Ex vivo 15 (BioWhittaker) or other SFM for hematopoietic cells (*see* **Note 2**) supplemented with cytokines (2× final concentration): 20 ng/mL Interleukin 3 (Biosource International, Camarillo, CA), 100 ng/mL Interleukin 6 (IL-6) (R&D Systems), 100 ng/mL SCF (R&D Systems), 100 ng/mL Flt3 ligand (R&D Systems).
5. Anti-TGFβ neutralizing antibody (R&D systems, cat. # AB-100-NA). *optional:* anti-p27^{kip-1} oligonucleotides (*see* **Note 3**).
6. Cell-dissociation buffer (Gibco-BRL).

2.4. Maintenance of Vector-Producing Fibroblasts and Collection of Cell-Free Supernatant

1. Vector-producing fibroblasts: PG13/LN (carries the *Neo* gene) is available from ATCC (CRL#10685).
2. 75-cm² culture flasks with 0.2-μm vented filter cap (Costar).
3. 10-mL syringes and syringe filters for retroviral supernatant (0.45-m pore-size filter; Uniflo-25 with calcium acetate membrane, Schleicher & Schuell, Keene, NH).
4. D10HG medium for growth of vector-producing fibroblasts: 450 mL Dulbecco's modified Eagle's medium with high glucose (Gibco-BRL), 50 mL heat-inactivated FCS (any vendor, screened for optimal growth of hematopoietic cells [*see*

Note 4], or purchased prescreened from StemCell Technologies, Inc.), 5 μL L-glutamine (200 m*M* stock, Gibco-BRL), 2.5 mL Pen/Strep (stock=10,000 U/mL penicillin and 10,000 ug/mL streptomycin, Gibco-BRL).

5. Trypsin/ethylenediaminetetraacetic acid (EDTA) (Gibco-BRL).

2.5. Immunomagnetic Selection Using Dynal Dynabeads System

1. 15-mL polypropylene centrifuge tubes.
2. Anti-CD34 antibody (anti-HPCA-1 from Becton Dickinson, Cat. #347660, or Purified anti-CD34 from Ancell, Bayport, MN, cat. # 183-020).
3. Goat-anti-mouse IgG magnetic beads and MPC-1 magnetic device for immunoselection (Dynal/Dynabeads).
4. PBS (Gibco-BRL).
5. Heat-inactivated fetal calf serum (any vendor, screened for optimal growth of hematopoietic cells [*see* **Note 4**], or purchased prescreened from StemCell Technologies, Inc).

2.6. Preparation of Individual CFU for PCR: Whole-Cell Lysates

1. Colony-forming unit (CFU) plates with growing colonies to be analyzed.
2. Microfuge tubes.
3. Tabletop microfuge.
4. plugged pipet tips: 200-μL vol.
5. 1× PBS (Gibco-BRL).
6. Red-blood-cell (RBC) lysis buffer: 0.32 *M* sucrose, 10 m*M* Tris-HCl (pH 7.5), 5 m*M* MgCl$_2$, 1% Triton-X-100 (all from Sigma). Store at room temperature.
7. Whole-cell lysis buffer: 50 m*M* KCL, 10 m*M* Tris-HCl (pH 8.3), 1.5 m*M* MgCl$_2$, 0.1 mg/mL gelatin, 0.45% NP40, 0.45% Tween-20 (all from Sigma). Store in 1-mL aliquots at –20°C.
8. 56°C water bath and hot plate for boiling water.

2.7. Individual Colony Clonal Integration Analysis by Inverse PCR

1. CFU plates with growing colonies to be analyzed.
2. Microfuge tubes.
3. Tabletop microfuge.
4. Plugged pipet tips: 200-μL volume.
5. Proteinase K (Sigma, 10 mg/mL stock in H$_2$O).
6. 56°C water bath.
7. Proteinase K buffer: 0.01 *M* Tris-HCl (pH 7.40), 0.15 *M* NaCl, 0.01 *M* EDTA (pH 8.0), 0.01% sodium dodecyl sulfate (SDS) with 10 μg proteinase K (Sigma).
8. Phenol/CHCl$_3$/isoamyl alcohol (25:24:1 mixture) (Sigma).
9. Glycogen (Boehringer Mannheim).
10. 10 *M* NH$_4$Ac (Sigma).
11. Absolute ethanol (any vendor).
12. Spermidine (0.1 *M*, Sigma).

13. React 2 buffer (Gibco-BRL, Grand Island, NY).
14. *Taq*1 restriction enzyme (Gibco-BRL).
15. T4 ligase and buffer (Gibco-BRL).
16. 12°C water bath.
17. Primers INVa: (5'AGGAACTGCTTACCACA), INVb: (5'CTGTTCCTTGGGA-GGGT), INVc: (5'TCCTGACCTTGATCTGA) and INVd: (5'CTGAGTGA-TTGACTACC).
18. PCR buffer and Mg^{++} (Perkin Elmer).
19. LE agarose (Seakem).
20. Nu-Sieve agarose (FMC).
21. Nylon membrane (Hybond-N+, Amersham, Arlington Heights, IL).
22. 32pγATP end-labeled oligonucleotide probe (5' GGCAAGCTAGCTTAAGT).
23. Hybridization buffer.
24. Spin-X column (Costar).
25. Circum Vent thermal cycle sequencing kit (New England Biolabs).

3. Methods

3.1. Coating Flasks with Retronectin

Prior to starting the cell-processing steps described in **Subheading 3.2.**, begin coating flasks with the fibronectin fragment retronectin to facilitate transduction. When planning the number of flasks to be coated in a given experiment, always include a "sham transduced" flask in addition to those that will receive supernatant containing each retroviral vector to be tested. The sham flask will receive medium alone when the other flasks receive viral supernatant, and will provide a baseline control for subsequent assays of gene expression from the transduced vectors.

1. Resuspend the lyophilized retronectin protein in PBS to a concentration of 50 µg/mL. This solution can be frozen once and stored at –20°C (avoid repeated freeze-thaws), or kept at 4°C for up to 1 mo without a significant loss of activity.
2. Add 2 mL of the fibronectin suspension to one well of a six-well plate or a 35-mm^2 Petri dish, or 5 mL to a 25 cm^2 (T-25) flask, laying flat. The transduction methods listed below in **Subheadings 3.2.** and **3.3.** are for the T-25 flasks. If smaller plates are used, adjust volumes accordingly. Tissue-culture treated plates can be used if they are fully coated with fibronectin (do not use a concentration lower than 50 µg/mL for coating). Allow the fibronectin fragments to bind to the plates for at least 1 h at room temperature. If processing cells simultaneously, leave the retronectin solution on the plates until only 30 min of the immunoselection procedure remains, then begin blocking.
3. When the cell-processing and sorting procedure detailed in **Subheading 3.2.** near the final steps (with approximately 30 min remaining), remove the fibronectin

from the plate and block with 2% BSA in PBS. Add 2 mL of the BSA solution and incubate at room temperature for 30 min.

4. Remove the BSA blocker, and rinse the plate very gently with PBS, by flushing from the edge. Immediately add the cells to be transduced, in the appropriate medium*, and the supernatant, as described in **Subheading 3.3.** Do not let the plates dry out.

3.2. Cell Preparation

1. Obtain marrow, cord blood, or MPB-cell sample. Dilute bone marrow or blood with an equal volume of PBS.
2. Gently layer 25 mL of the diluted cell suspension over an equal volume of ficoll in a 50 mL polypropylene centrifuge tube, avoiding mixture of the layers.
3. Centrifuge tubes at 730g for 15 min, with the centrifuge brake turned off.
4. Remove two-thirds of the yellow serum layer from the top and discard. The mononuclear cell fraction will be observed as an opaque layer (often referred to as the "buffy coat"), floating in the center of the tube.
5. Remove the buffy-coat layer, being careful not to collect more than 5 mL of the ficoll with it, and transfer it to a fresh 50-mL tube.
6. Add (Hank's Balanced Salt Solution (HBSS) or PBS to the mononuclear cells to fill the 50-mL tube, and mix. Centrifuge for 5 min at 1400 RPM.† This procedure washes the cells and dilutes out the ficoll that was removed with the mononuclear cell layer.
7. Discard supernatant, and tap the bottom of the tube to dislodge cells from the tight cell pellet, where they can clump together.§ If the cells are from a cord blood or MPB sample, proceed to **step 8** in this protocol. If the cells were isolated from bone marrow, they will contain live stromal elements that express the CD34 cell-surface determinant. Stromal cells must be removed by adherence prior to sorting and transduction, because if they are present in transduction flasks, they will be transduced by retroviral vectors during frequent divisions. Transduced stromal cells will then contaminate and invalidate subsequent assays. Therefore, for marrow samples, refer to **Note 5** before continuing with the next step.
8. Resuspend the cell pellet in 1 mL cold PBS. Take a cell count using Trypan blue

---

*The cytokines SCF and, to a lesser degree, IL-3, are required to activate the a4b1 and a5b1 integrins on the surface of the target hematopoietic progenitor, which bind to the FN CS-1 domain and RGD sequence, respectively *(33)*. Therefore at least SCF must be included in the transduction medium, to achieve effective colocalization of retrovirus and target cell.

†All centrifugations from this step onward are to be done at 1400 rpm for 5 min, with the centrifuge brake on.

§Following centrifugation, never leave the cells in a compact pellet, because of the enhanced potential for clumping. This occurs as a result of extruded DNA from cells that have ruptured. The inclusion of 20 U/mL RNase-free DNase during the ficoll and sorting procedures can alleviate this problem, and will not injure the intact cells. If clumps of cells do occur, they must be removed from the cell suspension prior to proceeding with any immunoselection process, as they will nonspecifically trap immunomagnetic beads.

exclusion: Dilute 20 µL of the cell suspension with an equal volume of Trypan blue solution. Apply to the hemocytometer and count the cells contained within one of the four large squares, in duplicate. Calculate the cell concentration; the count from one large square × dilution factor of 2×10^4 (factor for area under coverslip*) = cells per mL in the original solution.

9. Bring the cell suspension up to the concentration recommended by the immunoselection kit of choice, in the appropriate buffer. For detailed techniques to perform the isolation using the Dynal Dynabeads method (which works well, with >95% CD34 purity, for bone marrow and MPB samples) refer to **Subheading 3.5.**

10. After immunoselection, immediately resuspend the CD34+ cells in 1 mL of buffer or medium with serum, and take a count to obtain the percent yield. Typically, the CD34+ population will be 1% of the bone marrow, so 4×10^7 cells in the total mononuclear cell fraction should yield approx 4×10^5 CD34+ progenitors.

3.3. Transduction

1. Bring the CD34+ cell suspension up to 5 mL per retronectin-coated transduction flask in ex vivo 15 medium with IL-3 (20 ng/mL), IL-6 (100 ng/mL), SCF (100 ng/mL), Flt3 ligand (100 ng/mL), and anti-TGF neutralizing antibody (5 µg/mL)*. As few as 1×10^4 CD34+ progenitors, and as many as 2×10^6 per 25-cm^2 flask can be transduced with similar levels of gene transfer.
   *For increased levels of transduction of primitive, reconstituting human hematopoietic cells, anti-sense oligonucleotides to the cell-cycle inhibitor p27 kip-1 can be added at this step. *See* **Note 3** for details.

2. Place the flasks containing the hematopoietic cells into the incubator while thawing or filtering supernatant, so that the pH of the medium will be optimal when the retroviral vector is introduced. It is essential that medium is warm, pH is neutral, and that the CO_2 in the incubator is 4.5–5.0 (not higher!), or retroviral receptor conformation will be altered and retrovirus will not bind.

3. Thaw retroviral supernatant (which has been sterile-filtered and stored at –70°C (*see* **Subheading 3.4.**) as quickly as possible, in a 37°C water bath. Do not let the water bath water touch the top of the tube, and rinse the tube with 70% ETOH prior to taking it into the tissue-culture hood. Immediately add 5 mL of the thawed supernatant to the appropriate flask, which already contains the CD34+ progenitors on retronectin (Note: It is important that the supernatant be warmed to at least room temperature before adding to the CD34+ cells). Return the flask to the incubator as quickly as possible, and leave it there overnight.

4. After 24 h, carefully collect the supernatant from the transduction flask, and refeed the adherent layer 5 mL prewarmed (to room temperature, at least, or 37°C maximum) Ex vivo 15 with cytokines. Put the flask back into the incubator.

---

*Never use a chipped hemocytometer coverslip. Accurate weight of the coverslip is essential to obtaining an accurate count.

5. Spin down the nonadherent cells which will be floating in the removed supernatant. Discard the spent medium and supernatant. Resuspend pellet by tapping tube with finger, so cells will not clump.
6. Add 5 mL retroviral supernatant, which has just been thawed and warmed to 37°C. Resuspend cells in the supernatant and return them to the transduction flask. Return flask to the incubator immediately.
7. Incubate an additional 24 h. Cells are now ready to harvest (using cell-dissociation buffer as recommended by the manufacturer) from the transduction flask for CFU plating to determine the efficiency of transduction. The level of gene transfer into individual colony-forming cells (CFC) is accomplished by growth in Geneticin (G418, *see* **Note 6** for tips) for the *neo* gene, other selective agents (taxol or colchicine for the *mdr* gene), FACS analysis for eGFP or cell-surface markers, or single-colony PCR, as described in **Subheading 3.6.**, for vectors that lack markers.

The use of single-colony inverse PCR will allow determination of the number of different human hematopoietic progenitors that were transduced, by identifying the unique proviral integration sites. **Subheading 3.7.** has details on this procedure.

3.4. Maintenance of Vector-Producing Fibroblasts and Collection of Cell-Free Supernatant

Grow vector-producing fibroblasts (VPF) in 75-cm² flasks in 15 mL D10HG (*see* reagent list), keeping them subconfluent by trypsinization when they reach 80% confluency. Freeze down early passage vials to bank as "seed stocks." If they are grown for weeks at a time in vitro, they must be reselected to ensure that they have retained the vector and packaging plasmids. The selection methods appropriate for each cell line can be obtained from ATCC.

Trypsinize the vector-producing fibroblasts and plate at a concentration of one million cells per 75-cm² flask. Lay the flask down flat, and grow the cells in 15 mL D10HG (*see* **Subheading 2.**) at 37°C for 1–2 d, until almost confluent. Replace the medium in each flask with prewarmed D10HG*. Transfer to a 32°C incubator for production of supernatant. Retroviral particles are more stable at the lower temperature, but the VPF will not grow as quickly. Collect supernatant 48 h later. Discard confluent monolayers of VPF. Filter supernatant through a 0.45-μm pore-size syringe filter (Uniflo-25 with calcium acetate membrane, Schleicher & Schuell, Keene, NH), to remove VPF which may have lifted into the medium. Store supernatant in polypropylene tubes at −70°C in 5-mL aliquots until needed for transduction.

---

* The adhesive capacity of immortalized cell lines is diminished. Addition of cold medium, or growing in medium depleted of nutrients, causes VPF to lift from the plates.

3.5. Immunomagnetic Selection Using the Dynal Dynabeads Technique

1. After ficolling and counting (**Subheading 3.3., steps 1–8**), bring the cell suspension up to 1×10^7 cells per 1 mL cold 1× PBS, in a 15-mL polypropylene tube.* Add sterile anti-CD34 antibody at a concentration of 5 µg per mL cell suspension. (New antibodies may need to be titrated to find the optimal concentration). Incubate the cells with antibody on a slowly rotating platform in a 4°C cold room for 30 min.

2. Centrifuge the cells at 1400 rpm and remove the supernatant, containing PBS and antibody. Resuspend the pellet in 12 mL of cold PBS/5% FCS to wash and block nonspecific sites. Centrifuge again. Remove the supernatant from the pellet. Wash one more time in the same solution, to remove excess, unbound antibody. Centrifuge and remove supernatant.

3. Resuspend the cell pellet in cold 1× PBS at a concentration of 1×10^7 cells/mL. Add 10 µL of the magnetic bead suspension per mL: goat anti-mouse-conjugated magnetic beads (Dynal, Oslo, Norway). Return the tube to the rotating platform in the cold room for another 30–60 min.

4. Bring the volume up to 7 mL with cold 1× PBS. Place the tube in the magnet device (MPC-1, Dynal). Leave it there for 2 min, to allow the beads and attached CD34+ cells to line up on the side of the tube closest to the magnet. Carefully remove the PBS and transfer to a tube labeled "CD34–cells." Remove the tube from the magnetic holder and rewash the CD34+ cells and beads with 7 mL cold 1× PBS. Place the tube back into the magnetic holder for 2 min, and discard the PBS fraction, which contains very few cells, in the second wash.

If desired, the magnetic beads can be removed using chymopapain (chymodactin, Baxter), or detach-a bead (Dynal) . However, we would recommend leaving the beads on the cells, if possible, to obtain maximal yields and viability. They drop off naturally after 1–2 d of culture, and do not hamper transduction, growth of CFUs, or engraftment in immune-deficient mice (*1,2,11,13,17,34–38*). If FACS will be done to test transfer of cell-surface markers, the Dynal beads must be removed, or the MiniMACS or Stem Sep systems can be used for sorting. The latter two systems use smaller magnetic beads that do not interfere with FACS sorting.

---

*If small numbers of cells are used (less than 1×10^7 total) perform the antibody-binding and Dynabeads-binding steps in 1 mL PBS, in a 15-mL tube standing upright on ice. Tap the tube to mix gently at 10-min intervals during the binding steps. Wash steps and concentrations will remain the same.

3.6. Preparation of Individual CFU Colonies for PCR: Whole-Cell Lysates

The standard methods for plating of colony-forming assays are described in Chapter 7 in this volume. For analysis of the extent of gene transfer by PCR, single, well-isolated colonies are plucked from CFU dishes using a clean micropipet tip for each colony.* Cells are soaked 1 h at room temperature in 1 mL PBS to dissolve the methylcellulose, then divided into two portions. The first portion of each sample may be used to generate cytospin slides for immunohistochemical analyses or Wright/Giemsa staining. The second portion is used to detect the presence of integrated vector sequences by PCR. The sample may be directly lysed as described below, or DNA can be extracted as described in **Subheading 3.7.** Although the whole-cell lysis procedure is quicker and more convenient, PCR from extracted DNA gives more reproducible results. In the whole-cell lysate, ionic strength will vary depending on cell number in the original colony, and can affect the outcome of the PCR, which is highly sensitive to cation concentration.

1. Pull single colonies from the methylcellulose medium (MCM) in a vol of 20–40 µL, using a plugged pipet tip, under direct visualization with a phase-inversion microscope. Single CFU deposited by ACDU in a 96-well plate in MCM may be flushed out with PBS, and provide more convincing isolation of each colony, without the possibility of cross-contamination by neighboring CFU.† Choose colonies containing at least 200 cells for plucking. Keep a record of the colonies that contained erythrocytes: they will need a different buffer (*see* **step 4**).
2. Once the colony is in the pipet tip, flush it thoroughly into 1 mL 1 × PBS in a microfuge tube. Let the tube sit on the benchtop for 1 h to allow all of the methylcellulose to dissolve from the cells, or they will not form a firm pellet when centrifuged. This treatment does not lead to DNA degradation if cells are intact.
3. Centrifuge tubes for 5 min in a microfuge at 3,000 rpm. A tiny triangular pellet should be visible. Remove medium and PBS carefully. Spin the tubes again briefly, to bring down the residual droplets of PBS, and remove them. It is acceptable to leave up to 10 µL PBS on the pellet, to avoid the loss of cells. Pellets prepared by this method may be stored at −20°C, or may be lysed directly.
4. If colonies contained developing erythroblasts (BFU-E or CFU-MIX) they will

---

* Care must be taken to pluck well-isolated colonies, to avoid inclusion of cells from neighboring CFU. Cross-contamination between colonies could lead to overestimation of the extent of gene transfer. To verify that each CFU has arisen from a hematopoietic progenitor bearing a unique proviral integrant, use the inverse PCR technique described in **Subheading 3.7.**

† If plating individual cells in 96-well plates for isolation of individual clones from methylcellulose medium, make sure that the outer rows of wells are filled with water to provide extra humidity. The methylcellulose medium dries out easily.

need to be lysed to remove hemoglobin prior to preparation of the PCR lysate.*
RBC lysis buffer (200 uL; recipe in **Subheading 2.6.**) is added to the pellet, and
cells are mixed with the pipet tip. Spin for 2 min in a tabletop microfuge (1643*g*).
If the pellet is still red, repeat the lysis procedure. When the pellet is white, wash
once with 1× PBS and proceed to **step 5**.

5. Resuspend colony pellets in 20 µL whole-cell lysis buffer (for standard PCR) or
   200 µL proteinase K digestion buffer for DNA extraction and subsequent inverse
   PCR (*see* **Subheading 3.7.**). To the 20 µL whole-cell lysis buffer (for recipe, *see*
   Subheading 2.) add 2 µL proteinase K (Sigma, 10 mg/mL stock in H$_2$O). Incubate tubes at 56°C for 1 h. For large colonies, an additional 2 µL proteinage. K
   should be added after 30 min, and digestion continued.

6. Boil lysates for 10 min to inactivate the proteinase K. Do not forget this step!
   Proteinase K will otherwise digest the Taq polymerase in the PCR buffer. Whole-
   cell lysates may be stored at –20°C until used in PCR reactions.

7. 1–2 µL of the lysate will be adequate to detect the presence of most cDNAs
   carried in Moloney-based retroviral vectors by standard PCR methods.

3.7. Individual Colony Clonal Integration Analysis by Inverse PCR

The Inverse PCR method has been adapted from Rill and Brenner *(39)*. Cellular genomic DNA containing integrated vector provirus is digested with the
restriction enzyme *Taq*1 (Gibco, BRL) chosen because it cuts frequently (1/4^4,
or once every 256 bases on average) and does not cut within the LTR themselves, but just inside of the vector from each LTR. Each LTR is then on a
restriction fragment of unique size, determined by the distance to the nearest
Taq1 recognition site in the genomic DNA flanking the provirus. The LTR-
containing fragments are then self-ligated to form closed circles. PCR amplification using primer pairs complementary to the LTR directed in opposite
directions around the closed circle will produce a PCR product of characteristic size for each integration site. Thus, the progeny of each transduced cell,
which will contain the same clonotypic vector integrant, will show the same
pattern of PCR products with this method. Each vector integrant will yield two
PCR products, one from each LTR. The technique given in detail in **steps 1–12**
below is a modification of one that has been previously published *(1,2)*.

1. Collect individual, well-isolated CFU, and pellet cells as described in **Subheading 3.6., steps 1–3**.

2. Lyse Individual CFU samples containing 100–1,000 cells in 200 µL proteinase K
   buffer (0.01 *M* Tris-HCl (pH 7.40), 0.15 *M* NaCl, 0.01 *M* EDTA (pH 8.0), 0.01%
   SDS) with 10 µg proteinase K (Sigma) for 2 h at 56°C.

---

*The lysis of RBC must be done, and hemoglobin removed, because the porphyrin rings will
bind the magnesium in the PCR reaction buffer, and no amplification of the sample will occur.
Hemoglobin must therefore be washed out of the sample to avoid false-negative results.

3. Perform one extraction with 200 μL buffered phenol/ CHCL$_3$/IAA (25:24:1) mixture.
4. Precipitate the aqueous phase by addition of 2 μg glycogen (Boehringer Mannheim), 18 μL 10 *M* NH$_4$Ac, 500 μL absolute ethanol, and incubate at –20°C for at least 2 h, or in a dry ice/ethanol bath for 10 min.
5. Centrifuge the DNA for 5 min in a microfuge at 3650*g*. Remove the ethanol supernatant, and rinse in 70% ETOH. Dry on the benchtop* for 1–2 h.
6. Resuspend the dried DNA pellets in 25 μL 1X TE buffer. Add 10 uL of the sample to 3 μL spermidine (0.1 *M*, Sigma), 10 μL React 2 buffer (Gibco-BRL, Grand Island, NY), 2 μL (10 U) Taq1 restriction enzyme (Gibco-BRL), and 75 uL H20 for 2 h at 65°C. An additional 2 μL *Taq1* is added after the first hour of incubation.
7. Ligate an 8-μL sample of the cut DNA by addition of 2 μL 5× T4 ligase buffer and 1 μL T4 ligase (Gibco-BRL) at 12–15°C for 2 h. Prior to addition of ligase, the samples are heated to 56°C for 14 min, then cooled on the benchtop for 15 min. Ligase is added, and the samples are placed into the 12° water bath.
8. Following ligation, the first round of amplification of 2 μL of the circularized DNA uses the primers INVa: (5'AGGAACTGCTTACCACA) and INVb: (5'CTGTTCCTTGG-GAGGGT) in 0.5× Perkin Elmer PCR buffer† at a final Mg^{++} concentration of 1.25 m*M*. The first cycle is: 95° denaturation for 5 min, 50° annealing for 2 min, and 72° extension for 4 min. The subsequent 29 cycles are identical, except that the denaturation time is reduced to 1 min.
9. Perform the second round of nested PCR using 2 μL of the round 1 amplified product with primers INVc: (5'TCCTGACCTTGATCTGA) and INVd: (5'CTGAGTGATTGACTACC), using the same reaction conditions and cycles.
10. Electrophorese the resulting PCR products on a 2% gel (1% Seakem LE agarose and 1% Nu-Sieve, FMC), transfer to nylon membrane (Hybond-N+, Amersham), and hybridize with a 32p ATP end-labeled oligonucleotide probe (5' GGCAAGCTAGCTTAAGT) specific for LTR sequences.
11. To verify identity of clonal patterns (bands having the same apparent mol wt, excise the corresponding inverse PCR product bands from a 1% agarose gel, chop finely with a sterile scalpel, and recover the amplified DNA from the agarose by centrifugation through a Spin-X column (Costar) twice for 5 min.
12. Precipitate the DNA, resuspend in 8 μL 1X TE buffer, and sequence with the Circum Vent thermal cycle sequencing kit (New England Biolabs) using the inverse PCR primer INVc *(1,2)*.

4. Notes

1. Sources of hematopoietic cells for transduction: An excellent source of human marrow cells is the screens used to remove bony spicules from the bone marrow

---

* Caution: Do not use a vacuum to dry the pellets; it reduces the efficiency of cutting with the Taq1 restriction enzyme, which is the most critical parameter for this protocol. If the genomic DNA is incompletely digested, multiple bands will result.

† The use of "half-strength" PCR buffer decreases background in this reaction.

aspirate after harvest for allogeneic transplantation. The material trapped on the filters is often discarded as waste, but contains both stem cells and marrow stromal cells. In the operating room, the filters can be put into a 50-mL centrifuge tube containing sterile cell-culture medium (e.g., Iscove's modified Dulbecco's medium (IMDM) with 20% heat-inactivated FCS) and the cells released by either vigorous shaking of the closed tube or by vigorously washing the filter with medium using a 20-cc syringe. The filter washes are plated in several 75-cm^2 flasks for 2–6 h to allow adherence of stromal elements, and to permit the hematopoietic cells to dissociate from the bony fragments. The nonadherent cell fraction which contained the hematopoietic cells can then be collected and processed by centrifugation on a ficoll gradient as described in **Subheading 3.2.**

Other good sources of hematopoietic stem and progenitor cells are mobilized peripheral blood (MPB) cells or umbilical cord-blood cells (UCBC). UCBC can be obtained following delivery of neonates by gravity drainage of the placenta from the cut end of the umbilical cord. The cord blood can be collected into either sterile 50-mL centrifuge tubes or a sterile basin with either heparin (to achieve a concentration of at least 10 U/mL) or with CPD-A anticoagulant (citrate-phosphate-dextrose solution, Sigma cat. # C-7165, add 10 mL solution per 40 mL blood). Typical yields may range from 50–150 mL of UCBC. If none of these sources of hematopoietic cells are available, marrow may be obtained using the standard clinical procedure of marrow aspiration from the posterior iliac crest of volunteers, or purchased from the Northwest Tissue Center, Seattle, WA.

2. While we have exclusively used the medium Ex-Vivo 15 in our recent studies, other sources of serum-free medium have been used successfully, and are described in the literature. The main constituents to be added to a standard medium (such IMDM, which is particularly good for hematopoietic cells) are insulin, BSA, transferrin, low-density lipoproteins, glutamine, and β-ME. An excellent version of serum-free medium assembled from these ingredients was described by Lansdorp and Dragowska *(40)*, and its use was further examined by Petzer et al. *(41)*. Another good SFM for hematopoietic cells is StemSpan^{TM} serum-free expansion medium, available from StemCell Technologies, Vancouver, BC, Canada. The viability of hematopoietic progenitors is improved, and transduction is enhanced, if 50% fresh medium is added with each transduction cycle. This technique is used because the retroviral supernatant is depleted of sugars and amino acids. Although diluting the supernatant with fresh medium decreases by half the titer of virus added to the flask if high-titer supernatant ($>5 \times 10^6$ infectious particles per mL) is used, the extent of transduction of colony-forming progenitors on retronectin will be approx 30–50% using the methods in this chapter *(13,29)*.

3. We recently demonstrated that primitive hematopoietic stem and progenitor cells, induced into cell-cycle entry by the combination of anti-TGF antibody and anti-p27 oligonucleotides, were transduced by retroviral vectors in a 24–h period, and retained the ability to durably engraft immune deficient mice with multilineage

development. We determined that the optimal method for achieving entry of the oligonucleotide into primary hematopoietic progenitors was to use a concentration of 50 μM, without use of lipofectants. This method resulted in specific reduction of p27 levels without affecting other pathways, such as mitrogen activated protein kinase (MAPK) phosphorylation, in response to cytokines *(29)*. C-5 propyne modified phosphorothioate oligonucleotides (ON), synthesized by Operon (Alameda, CA) were used at a final concentration of 50 μM in SFM (Ex-Vivo 15, BioWhittaker). The sequence for the anti-sense ON (anti-p27) was 5'-qgC GUC UGC UCC AcagF-3', and the scrambled, or mis-sense ON was 5'qgC AUC CCC UGU Gca gF-3', as previously described *(42)*.

4. Many of the reagents used in human marrow culture can display nonspecific toxicity for hematopoietic cells, although they may be acceptable for growth of other cell types. Therefore, even tissue-culture-grade ingredients should be screened. Seemingly minor cell culture medium components (e.g., BSA) or environmental factors (e.g., incubator CO_2) can drastically affect cell growth and gene transduction. The screening of reagents requires a set of components which are already known to work, with each new individual component tested as single substitutions. Because of the sensitivity of marrow cells to contaminants, vendors and catalog numbers of products routinely used are provided in the reagents list. The commercial availability of media and individual cell-culture components from StemCell Technologies allows new labs to undertake hematopoietic cell culture by providing pre-tested reagents. This is accomplished by making a batch of methylcellulose medium, which lacks the component to be tested, then adding different samples to be screened into the appropriate volume of the stock solution to achieve the desired final concentration. As an example, to screen different lots of FBS, aliquots containing 7 mL of methylcellulose medium lacking serum are prepared. To each, an individual 3-mL aliquot of sterile, heat-inactivated serum to be tested is added. Samples are mixed well, then dispensed in duplicate or quadruplicate into 1-mL gridded culture dishes. The same number of purified CD34+ progenitors is added to each plate and mixed well. Following 14 d growth, CFU are enumerated, and the lot of FCS that had supported growth of the largest number of mixed lineage colonies is chosen for purchase. Similar screening procedures are done for the methylcellulose stocks, BSA, and geneticin (G418). To screen samples of G418, hematopoietic progenitors that have been transduced by a vector carrying the *neo* gene must be used, in comparison to nontransduced (Sham) cells. The lot of geneticin that permits maximal CFU formation from the transduced cell population while providing complete killing of the nontransduced cells should be chosen for purchase.

5. Stromal elements should be removed from bone-marrow aspirates, since the living stromal monolayer will be easily transduced by retroviral vectors *(35)*, and can invalidate subsequent CFU, FACS, or long-term culture (LTC) assays. Resuspend the cell pellet from **Subheading 3.2., step 7**, in IMDM with 20% FCS, at a concentration of 1×10^6 cells/mL, in 75-cm^2 flasks (tissue-culture-treated, 15 mL

cell suspension per flask). Place the flask into the incubator and allow stromal cells to adhere for 2 h. At the end of the adherence period, remove the nonadherent hematopoietic cells, and place them into a 50-mL centrifuge tube. Flush the flask several times with 1× PBS and add all flushings to the 50-mL tube. The stromal elements and mature monocyte/macrophages will adhere more strongly to the flask in 2 h than the hematopoietic stem and progenitor cells, and thus will remain with the flask, which can then be used to initiate stromal monolayers as described. Centrifuge the tubes containing the stromal-cell-depleted mononuclear cells for 5 min at 400*g*. Remove the supernatant, then tap the bottom of the tube immediately to disloge the cells from the tight pellet, to avoid clumping. Wash the mononuclear cells in 25 mL cold 1 × PBS, centrifuge at 400*g* for 5 min, and discard the supernatant. Resuspend in 1 mL cold PBS and count an aliquot by Trypan blue exclusion, as described in **Subheading 3.2., step 8**. Proceed with the cell separation steps, as described in **Subheading 3.2.**

6. Twenty-four hours after transfer of the *neo* gene into hematopoietic progenitors, the extent of transduction can be assessed by measuring the percentage of colony-forming progenitors resistant to the selective agent G418 (0.9 mg/mL: each lot should be screened for effective killing of nontransduced cells and lack of nonspecific toxicity) *(see* **Note 4**). For each sample, four replicate CFU plates are made and G418 (0.9 mg/mL active compound) is added to two of these, as described. 5×10^4 cells per plate are used when assaying unseparated bone-marrow mononuclear cell preparations and 500 and 1000 cells are used when assaying CD34+ cells (reduce to 250 and 500 cells per plate when working with UCB CD34+ cells). These plating densities were determined empirically to yield 50–100 colonies per plate, which is the upper limit that produces distinct, individual colonies. The numbers of total and G418-resistant progenitor-derived colonies are counted after 14 d. In all experiments, sham-transduced marrow, which does not contain the *neo* gene, should be plated for comparison, and should be completely inhibited from colony formation by the concentration of G418 that is used. To prepare geneticin (G418) for selection of transduced cells:

1. Dilute 1 *M* HEPES buffer (Sigma) 1:10 in H20 to generate a 100 m*M* stock.
2. Calculate the total mg of active protein purchased: the purity (mg active/g weight) will be listed in the acompanying data sheet.
3. Dilute in 100 m*M* HEPES buffer to make a 50 mg/mL stock (active concentration).
4. Adjust pH to 7.30 (use approx 1 drop 10 *N* NaOH per mL, and the pH will increase steadily).*
5. Make small aliquots and store at –20°C. Avoid repeated freeze-thaw cycles. Stable at 4°C for at least 2 mo after thawing.
6. For hematopoietic cell selection, use at a concentration of 0.9 mg/mL active drug.

* Be sure that the electrode on the pH meter has been soaked in H20 and rinsed extremely well to remove potentially toxic contaminants.

References

1. Dao, M. A., Yu, X. J., and Nolta, J. A. (1997) Clonal diversity of primitive human hematopoietic progenitors following retroviral marking and long-term engraftment in immune-deficient mice. *Exp. Hematol.* **25**, 1357–1366.
2. Nolta, J. A., Dao, M. A., Wells, S., Smogorzewska, E. M., and Kohn, D. B. (1996) Transduction of pluripotent human hematopoietic stem cells demonstrated by clonal analysis after engraftment in immune-deficient mice. *Proc. Natl. Acad. Sci. USA* **93**, 2414–2419.
3. Lewis, P. F. and Emerman, M. (1994) Passage through mitosis is required for oncoretroviruses but not for the human immunodeficiency virus. *J. Virol.* **68**, 510–516.
4. Miller, D. G., Adam, M. A., and Miller, A. D. (1990) Gene transfer by retrovirus vectors occurs only in cells that are actively replicating at the time of infection (published erratum appears in Mol Cell Biol 1992 Jan;12(1):433). *Mol. Cell Biol.* **10**, 4239–4242.
5. Suda, T., Suda, J., and Ogawa, M. (1983) Proliferative kinetics and differentiation of murine blast cell colonies in culture: evidence for variable G0 periods and constant doubling rates of early pluripotent hemopoietic progenitors. *J. Cell Physiol.* **117**, 308–318.
6. Bodine, D. M., Karlsson, S., and Nienhuis, A. W. (1989) Combination of interleukins 3 and 6 preserves stem cell function in culture and enhances retrovirus-mediated gene transfer into hematopoietic stem cells. *Proc. Natl. Acad. Sci. USA* **86**, 8897–8901.
7. Nolta, J. A. and Kohn, D. B. (1990) Comparison of the effects of growth factors on retroviral vector-mediated gene transfer and the proliferative status of human hematopoietic progenitor cells. *Hum. Gene Ther.* **1**, 257–268.
8. Luskey, B. D., Rosenblatt, M., Zsebo, K., and Williams, D. A. (1992) Stem cell factor, interleukin-3, and interleukin-6 promote retroviral- mediated gene transfer into murine hematopoietic stem cells. *Blood* **80**, 396–402.
9. Fletcher, F. A., Moore, K. A., Ashkenazi, M., De Vries, P., Overbeek, P. A., Williams, D. E., et al. (1991) Leukemia inhibitory factor improves survival of retroviral vector-infected hematopoietic stem cells in vitro, allowing efficient long-term expression of vector-encoded human adenosine deaminase in vivo. *J. Exp. Med.* **174**, 837.
10. Dilber, M. S., Bjorkstrand, B., Li, K. J., Smith, C. I., Xanthopoulos, K. G., and Gahrton, G. (1994) Basic fibroblast growth factor increases retroviral-mediated gene transfer into human hematopoietic peripheral blood progenitor cells. *Exp. Hematol.* **22**, 1129–1133.
11. Dao, M. A., Hannum, C. H., Kohn, D. B., and Nolta, J. A. (1997) FLT3 ligand preserves the ability of human CD34+ progenitors to sustain long-term hematopoiesis in immune-deficient mice after ex vivo retroviral-mediated transduction. *Blood* **89**, 446–456.
12. Nolta, J. A., Crooks, G. M., Overell, R. W., Williams, D. E., and Kohn, D. B. (1992) Retroviral vector-mediated gene transfer into primitive human hematopoi-

etc progenitor cells: effects of mast cell growth factor (MGF) combined with other cytokines. *Exp. Hematol.* **20,** 1065–1071.

13. Dao, M. A., Hashino, K., Kato, I., and Nolta, J. A. (1998) Adhesion to fibronectin maintains regenerative capacity during Ex vivo culture and transduction of human hematopoietic stem and progenitor cells (In Process Citation). *Blood* **92,** 4612–4621.

14. Moore, K. A., Deisseroth, A. B., Reading, C. L., Williams, D. E., and Belmont, J. W. (1992) Stromal support enhances cell-free retroviral vector transduction of human bone marrow long-term culture-initiating cells. *Blood* **79,** 1393–1399.

15. Moritz, T., Patel, V. P., and Williams, D. A. (1994) Bone marrow extracellular matrix molecules improve gene transfer into human hematopoietic cells via retroviral vectors. *J. Clin. Investig.* **93,** 1451–1457.

16. Moritz, T., Dutt, P., Xiao, X., Carstanjen, D., Vik, T., Hanenberg, H., et al. (1996) Fibronectin improves transduction of reconstituting hematopoietic stem cells by retroviral vectors: evidence of direct viral binding to chymotryptic carboxy-terminal fragments. *Blood* **88,** 855–862.

17. Nolta, J. A., Smogorzewska, E. M., and Kohn, D. B. (1995) Analysis of optimal conditions for retroviral-mediated transduction of primitive human hematopoietic cells. *Blood* **86,** 101–110.

18. Wells, S., Malik, P., Pensiero, M., Kohn, D. B., and Nolta, J. A. (1995) The presence of an autologous marrow stromal cell layer increases glucocerebrosidase gene transduction of long-term culture initiating cells (LTCICs) from the bone marrow of a patient with Gaucher disease. *Gene Ther.* **2,** 512–520.

19. Yang, Y., Vanin, E. F., Whitt, M. A., Fornerod, M., Zwart, R., Schneiderman, R. D., et al. (1995) Inducible, high-level production of infectious murine leukemia retroviral vector particles pseudotyped with vesicular stomatitis virus G envelope protein. *Hum. Gene Ther.* **6,** 1203–1213.

20. Burns, J. C., Friedmann, T., Driever, W., Burrascano, M., and Yee, J. K. (1993) Vesicular stomatitis virus G glycoprotein pseudotyped retroviral vectors: concentration to very high titer and efficient gene transfer into mammalian and nonmammalian cells. *Proc. Natl. Acad. Sci. USA* **90,** 8033–8037.

21. Miller, A. D., Garcia, J. V., von Suhr, N., Lynch, C. M., Wilson, C., and Eiden, M. V. (1991) Construction and properties of retrovirus packaging cells based on gibbon ape leukemia virus. *J. Virol.* **65,** 2220–2224.

22. Miller, J. L., Donahue, R. E., Sellers, S. E., Samulski, R. J., Young, N. S., and Nienhuis, A. W. (1994) Recombinant adeno-associated virus (rAAV)-mediated expression of a human gamma-globin gene in human progenitor-derived erythroid cells [published erratum appears in Proc. Natl. Acad. Sci. USA 1995 Jan 17;92(2):646]. *Proc. Natl. Acad. Sci. USA* **91,** 10,183–10,187.

23. Naldini, L., Blomer, U., Gallay, P., Ory ,D., Mulligan, R., Gage, F. H., et al. (1996) In vivo gene delivery and stable transduction of nondividing cells by a lentiviral vector (*see* comments). *Science* **272,** 263–267.

24. Podsakoff, G., Wong, Jr., K. K., and Chatterjee, S. (1994) Efficient gene transfer into nondividing cells by adeno-associated virus-based vectors. *J. Virol.* **68,** 5656–5666.

25. Walsh, C. E., Liu, J. M., Xiao, X., Young, N. S., Nienhuis, A. W., and Samulski, R. J. (1992) Regulated high level expression of a human gamma-globin gene introduced into erythroid cells by an adeno-associated virus vector. *Proc. Natl. Acad. Sci. USA* **89,** 7257–7261.

26. Dutt, P., Hanenberg, H., Vik, T., Williams, D. A., and Yoder, M. C. (1997) A recombinant human fibronectin fragment facilitates retroviral mediated gene transfer into human hematopoietic progenitor cells. *Biochem. Mol. Biol. Int.* **42,** 909–1017.

27. Hanenberg, H., Xiao, X. L., Dilloo, D., Hashino, K., Kato, I., and Williams, D. A. (1996) Colocalization of retrovirus and target cells on specific fibronectin fragments increases genetic transduction of mammalian cells. *Nat. Med.* **2,** 876-882.

28. Hanenberg, H., Hashino, K., Konishi, H., Hock, R. A., Kato, I., and Williams, D. A. (1997) Optimization of fibronectin-assisted retroviral gene transfer into human CD34+ hematopoietic cells. *Hum. Gene Ther.* **8,** 2193–2206.

29. Dao, M. A., Taylor, N., and Nolta, J. A. (1998) Reduction in levels of the cyclin-dependent kinase inhibitor p27(kip-1) coupled with transforming growth factor beta neutralization induces cell-cycle entry and increases retroviral transduction of primitive human hematopoietic cells. *Proc. Natl. Acad. Sci. USA* **95,** 13,006–13,011.

30. Olweus, J., Lund-Johansen, F., and Terstappen, L. W. (1994) Expression of cell surface markers during differentiation of CD34+, CD38-/lo fetal and adult bone marrow cells. *Immunomethods* **5,** 179–188.

31. Hao, Q. L., Thiemann, F. T., Petersen, D., Smogorzewska, E. M., and Crooks, G. M. (1996) Extended long-term culture reveals a highly quiescent and primitive human hematopoietic progenitor population. *Blood* **88,** 3306–3313.

32. Hao, Q. L., Smogorzewska, E. M., Barsky, L. W., and Crooks, G. M. (1998) In vitro identification of single CD34+CD38- cells with both lymphoid and myeloid potential. *Blood* **91,** 4145–4151.

33. Levesque, J. P., Leavesley, D. I., Niutta, S., Vadas, M., and Simmons, P. J. (1995) Cytokines increase human hemopoietic cell adhesiveness by activation of very late antigen (VLA)-4 and VLA-5 integrins. *J. Exp. Med.* **181,** 1805–1815.

34. Nolta, J. A., Hanley, M. B., and Kohn, D. B. (1994) Sustained human hematopoiesis in immunodeficient mice by cotransplantation of marrow stroma expressing human interleukin-3: analysis of gene transduction of long-lived progenitors. *Blood* **83,** 3041–3050.

35. Dao, M. A., Pepper, K. A., and Nolta, J. A. (1997) Long-term cytokine production from engineered primary human stromal cells influences human hematopoiesis in an in vivo xenograft model. *Stem Cells* **15,** 443–451.

36. Dao, M. A. and Nolta, J. A. (1997) Inclusion of IL-3 during retrovirally-mediated transduction on stromal support does not increase the extent of gene transfer into long-term engrafting human hematopoietic progenitors. *Cytokines Cell Mol. Ther.* **3,** 81–89.

37. Dao, M. A., Shah, A. J., Crooks, G. M., and Nolta, J. A. (1998) Engraftment and retroviral marking of CD34+ and CD34+CD38- human hematopoietic progenitors assessed in immune-deficient mice. *Blood* **91,** 1243–1252.

38. Dao, M. A. and Nolta, J. A. (1998) Use of the bnx/hu xenograft model of human hematopoiesis to optimize methods for retroviral-mediated stem cell transduction (Review) (In Process Citation). *Int. J. Mol. Med.* **1,** 257–264.
39. Rill, D. R., Santana, V. M., Roberts, W. M., Nilson, T., Bowman, L. C., Krance, R. A., et al. (1994) Direct demonstration that autologous bone marrow transplantation for solid tumors can return a multiplicity of tumorigenic cells. *Blood* **84,** 380–383.
40. Lansdorp, P. M. and Dragowska, W. (1992) Long-term erythropoiesis from constant numbers of CD34+ cells in serum-free cultures initiated with highly purified progenitor cells from human bone marrow. *J. Exp. Med.* **175,** 1501–1509.
41. Petzer, A. L., Hogge, D. E., Landsdorp, P. M., Reid, D. S., and Eaves, C. J. (1996) Self-renewal of primitive human hematopoietic cells (long-term-culture-initiating cells) in vitro and their expansion in defined medium. *Proc. Natl. Acad. Sci. USA* **93,** 1470–1474.
42. St. Croix, B., Florenes, V. A., Rak, J. W., Flanagan, M., Bhattacharya, N., Slingerland, J. M., et al. (1996) Impact of the cyclin-dependent kinase inhibitor p27Kip1 on resistance of tumor cells to anticancer agents. *Nat. Med.* **2,** 1204–1210.
43. Eaves, C. J., Cashman, J. D., Kay, R. J., Dougherty, G. J., Otsuka, T., Gaboury, L. A., et al. (1991) Mechanisms that regulate the cell cycle status of very primitive hematopoietic cells in long-term human marrow cultures. II. Analysis of positive and negative regulators produced by stromal cells within the adherent layer. *Blood* **78,** 110–117.
44. Li, M. L., Cardoso, A. A., Sansilvestri, P., Hatzfeld, A., Brown, E. L., Sookdeo, H., et al. 1994. Additive effects of steel factor and antisense TGF-beta 1 oligodeoxynucleotide on CD34+ hematopoietic progenitor cells. *Leukemia* **8,** 441–445.
45. Cardoso, A. A., Li, M. L., Batard, P., Hatzfeld, A., Brown, E. L., Levesque, J. P., et al. 1993. Release from quiescence of CD34+ CD38- human umbilical cord blood cells reveals their potentiality to engraft adults. *Proc. Natl. Acad. Sci. USA* **90,** 8707–8711.

18

Production of Lentiviral Vector Supernatants and Transduction of Cellular Targets

Richard E. Sutton

1. Introduction

Lentiviral vectors based upon human immunodeficiency type I (HIV) are increasingly being used to transduce nondividing or terminally differentiated cells, despite the fact HIV is a known, lethal pathogen. This is because lentiviruses contain multiple gene products that allow infection of cells independent of mitosis. Typically, plasmid DNA is transiently transfected into a producer-cell line, and viral supernatant is harvested a few days later. The supernatant can be used as is to transduce targets of choice, or it can be concentrated up to 1000-fold by ultracentrifugation and then used on difficult targets, such as hematopoietic stem cells (HSC). The ease of production permits any modern molecular biology laboratory to produce reasonable amounts of replication-defective virus for research purposes. The entire process is illustrated schematically in **Figure 1** and typically takes a week, depending upon the nature of the transgene.

2. Materials

1. Source of recombinant DNA (plasmid or appropriate *E. coli* host carrying recombinant clone).
2. Luria broth (LB) or other simple bacterial medium (e.g., terrific broth) and antibiotic stock (usually sodium salt of ampicillin at 100 mg/mL in water).
3. CsCl aqueous solutions (1.84 g/mL and 1.64 g/mL final density) and 5 mg/mL ethidium bromide (protected from light).
4. NaCl-saturated isoamyl alcohol (prepared by adding isoamyl alcohol to 5 M NaCl and enough solid NaCl to form a three-phase solution).
5. 10 mM ethylenediaminetetraacetic acid (EDTA), 25 mM Tris-HCl, pH 8.0, 40

From: *Methods in Molecular Medicine, vol. 63: Hematopoietic Stem Cell Protocols*
Edited by: C. A. Klug and C. T. Jordan © Humana Press Inc., Totowa, NJ

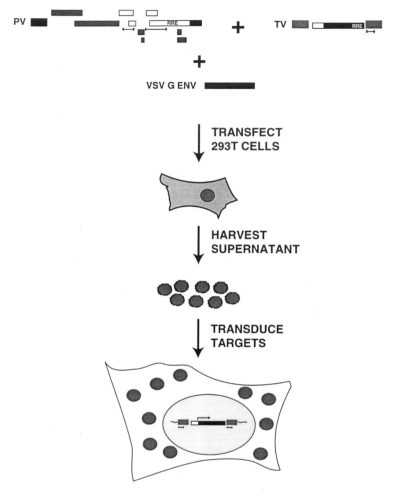

Fig. 1. Production of pseudotyped particles. At top are the three plasmids pHIV-PV, pHIV-TV, and the VSV G expression plasmid. A tri-transfection of 293T cells is performed by the calcium-phosphate technique. After 2–3 d, the supernatant is harvested (pseudotyped particles shown), and used to transduce targets. The TV becomes integrated in the host genome (note duplication of the ΔU3); and the transgene product is transcribed (*bent arrow*) and elaborated in the cytoplasm (*light gray circles*).

mM glucose (solution I); 0.2 N NaOH, 1% (w/v) sodium dodecyl sulfate (SDS) (solution II); and 3 M potassium acetate, 2M acetic acid (solution III).

6. Isopropanol and 70% ethanol.
7. 293T and HOS cells, both maintained in Dulbecco's modified Eagle's medium (DMEM) with 10% fetal calf serum (FCS) and 100 U/mL of penicillin and 100 mg/mL streptomycin (DMEM complete) at 37°C in a water-jacketed 5% CO_2

incubator. Most tissue-culture reagents are available from Gibco-BRL (Life Technologies).

8. 0.25 M CaCl$_2$, 2X HEPES-buffered saline (2X HBS; 0.28 M NaCl, 50 mM HEPES, and 1.5 mM phosphate buffer, pH 7.05), and 1 mM chloroquine.
9. 10% (v/v) dimethyl sulfoxide (DMSO) in phosphate-buffered saline (PBS), Ca^{2+} and Mg^{2+}-free.
10. X-gal. 100 mg/mL in dimethylformamide (store at –20°C in the dark).
11. X-gal staining solution: 3 mM potassium ferricyanide, 3 mM potassium ferrocyanide, and 0.8 mg/mL x-gal in PBS.
12. Fix solution: 0.3% (v/v) formaldehyde-0.4% (v/v) glutaraldehyde (prepared in PBS).
13. 0.1 M ferricyanide and 0.1 M ferrrocyanide (store at 4°C).
14. Polybrene (Sigma), 4 mg/mL in water (1000× concentrate), stored at 4°C.
15. HIV p24 antigen detection kit enzyme-linked immunosorbent assay (ELISA), from Coulter or other commercial suppliers).

3. Methods

3.1. General Safety Considerations

HIV is a known human pathogen, and infection is almost uniformly fatal. It is the etiologic agent of acquired immunodeficiency syndrome, or AIDS. Infection by HIV leads to an inexorable decline in CD4$^+$ T helper cells, although this can slowed by the use of highly active anti-retroviral therapy. Because of this, proper care must be exercised when working with HIV in the laboratory, even when it is only in vector form. Most investigators follow National Institute of Health/Centers for Disease Control (NIH/CDC) guidelines, which suggest using a BL2 facility but follow BL3 technique whenever possible (www.niehs.nih.gov/odhsb/manual/home.htm).

The following are some of the commonly accepted practices used in working with HIV vectors. All individuals should undergo bloodborne pathogen training that meets Occupational Health and Safety Administration (OSHA) standards. Prior to project initiation, personnel serum is collected and banked for future HIV serology. Periodically, serum is tested to confirm absence of HIV seroconversion. Accidental exposures to infectious material should be reported immediately to allow appropriate measures such as prophylaxis to be taken. If an investigator develops an illness that is consistent with acute HIV seroconversion, this should also be reported.

All contaminated plasticware is decontaminated with 10% bleach prior to placement in red biohazard bags. All surface spills inside the biosafety cabinet are cleansed with 70% ethanol or 10% bleach. The trap of the biosafety cabinet's aspirator apparatus should contain enough bleach so that its concentration does not fall below 10%. The only glassware used should be media

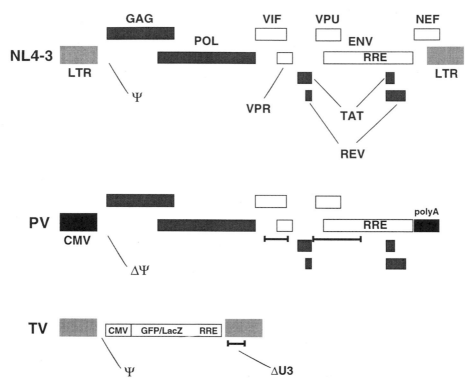

Fig. 2. HIV-based vectors. At top is a schematic of T-tropic HIV isolate NL4–3, with gene products indicated, along with the long terminal repeats (LTRs, *light gray boxes*), Rev-response-element (RRE) and packaging sequence (Ψ). Gene products required for virus production and transduction of target cells are in dark grey. The packaging vector (PV) is driven by a cytomegalovirus (CMV) immediate early enhancer/promoter, and it has deletions in *Vif, Vpr, Vpu*, and *Env (delimited lines)* and the packaging sequence (ΔΨ). The RRE is intact, and the 3' LTR has been replaced with a cellular polyadenylation signal (polyA). The transfer vector (TV) has a deletion in the 3' LTR (ΔU3) so that it is self-inactivating. Ψ and the RRE are both intact, and an internal promoter (CMV) drives the transgene reporter (*GFP* or *LacZ* indicated). Gene products are not entirely to scale.

bottles. No open aerosol solution is generated, and percutaneous exposure is minimized by absence of sharps and minimal glassware and by the use of personal protective clothing, gloves, and biosafety eyewear. After each tissue culture (TC) session, biohazard bags are autoclaved. Any viral or cell lysates are treated with nonionic or ionic detergents at a concentration of at least 0.1% prior to open handling. Sealed carriers may be used during centrifugation. Biohazard signs should be posted on the outside of the tissue-culture area, on the biosafety cabinet, and the incubator in use. Spills outside the biosafety cabinet should be cleaned up with absorbent towels and 10% bleach. Large spills or equipment contamination should be reported to the institutional biosafety officer.

3.2. Preparation of Plasmids

Currently, there are multiple HIV-based lentiviral vectors available from several different academic laboratories, including the author's *(1,3,5,8,9)*. The actual construction of these vectors is beyond the scope of this chapter. Clone construction and identity, however, can be confirmed by restriction-enzyme DNA digests and agarose-gel electrophoresis, chain-terminating (dideoxy) DNA sequencing, or Southern blotting. Many are split-coding, so that the actual transfer vector contains only long terminal repeats (LTRs), RNA packaging sequence, Rev-response-element, and transgene driven by an internal promoter (*see* **Fig. 2**). The packaging vector typically has a heterologous promoter (e.g., the cytomegalovirus immediate-early enhancer promoter) driving the structural, enzymatic, and regulatory viral genes. The accessory genes of HIV (*Vif, Vpr, Vpu,* and *Nef*) are dispensable for making high-titer pseudotyped particles. The envelope used for most studies is vesicular stomatitis virus G (VSVG) protein, expressed from a viral promoter. However, HIV appears to be remarkably flexible in terms of other envelopes that can be incorporated into infectious viral particles *(4,6)*.

1. Plasmid DNA is propagated in a non-recombinogenic *E. coli* host (e.g., HB101) and purified using standard molecular biology techniques. A suitable volume of sterile LB (500–1000 mL) is supplemented with 100 mg/mL ampicillin and inoculated with the appropriate *E. coli* recombinant clone. Bacteria are grown to saturation overnight by shaking (200–300 rpm) at 37°C.
2. Pellet bacteria by centrifugation (3000*g*) for 10 min and completely resuspend in 20 mL of solution I, using a combination of pipetting and vortexing.
3. Lyse the bacterial suspension in 40 mL of solution II and keep on ice for 4–5 min.
4. Add a total of 30 mL of solution III and keep on wet ice for 15 min. Centrifuge at 16,000*g* for 15 min.
5. Decant the supernatant through several layers of cheesecloth into 0.6 vol of isopropanol. After 15 min at room temperature, centrifuge the precipitated nucleic acid as in **step 4** and wash with 70% ethanol.
6. Resuspend the DNA (and RNA) in 1 mL of water by tilting the bottles on their side. After the nucleic acid is resuspended, add 4.5 mL of CsCl solution (1.84 g/mL) along with 0.08 mL of the ethidium-bromide solution. Load the mixture into 5-mL Beckman quick-seal ultracentrifuge tubes and seal.
7. Place the tubes in one of the vertical (Vti65.2) or near vertical (Nvti65.2) Beckman rotors and ultracentrifuge for 3.5–4 h at 400,000*g* at room temperature.
8. Collect the banded plasmid DNA in 1 mL by puncturing the tube with an 18-g. needle attached to a syringe, taking care not to disturb the gradient or remove the

RNA or other impurities. Add 4 mL of CsCl solution (1.64 g/mL, without additional ethidium bromide), and then repeat the ultracentrifugation step. Collect the banded plasmid DNA in 1 mL.

9. Remove the ethidium bromide from the DNA by extracting the DNA with the organic (top) phase of the isoamyl alcohol-NaCl three-phase solution. The number of extractions depends upon the amount of DNA and bound ethidium, but usually 20–30 vol (done repeatedly in 5–6 vol increments) is sufficient for 1 mg of DNA. At the end, no traces of ethidium in the solution should be visible to the naked eye when using a clean white sheet of paper as a backdrop.

10. Precipitate the DNA by adding 5 vol of 70% ethanol, centrifuge at 20,000*g* for 10 min, and then wash the pellet with 70% ethanol (to remove excess salt). DNA can then be dissolved in a small volume of water (to achieve a concentration of 4 mg/mL) and quantitatively precipitated in a microcentrifuge tube, using sterile technique. The resuspended DNA (at a concentration of 4 mg/mL in water) is now ready for transfection and can be stored at –20°C (*see* **Note 1**).

3.3. Preparation and Transfection of 293T Cells

293T cells are human embryonic kidney fibroblasts (293 cells) which have been stably transfected with SV40 virus large T antigen. They are resistant to G418, but do not need to be maintained in the antibiotic. They are grown in DMEM complete at 37°C in a water-jacketed 5% CO_2 incubator. The cells are very loosely adherent, and should be split 1:4 or 1:5 every 3–4 d simply by aspirating the spent medium and gently washing the cells off the plate using a small amount of fresh medium (*see* **Note 2**). Trypsin and EDTA are unnecessary, and may be harmful. During prolonged culture, the morphology of the cells change so that they become more flattened and spread out, and less clumped. In addition, the doubling time asymptotically shortens. However, the transfection efficiency and viral production of 293Ts will remain quite high, even after years of continuous culture.

1. At least 12 h prior to transfection, split the 293T cells 1:4 into 10-cm dishes (*see* **Note 4**). At the time of transfection, cells should be 40–60% confluent. Both higher and lower levels of confluency will reduce viral titers.

2. Prepare the DNA in 0.5 mL of 0.25 *M* $CaCl_2$. Usually, 40 mg of each plasmid is used in equistochiometric ratios, although some investigators reduce the amount of VSV G expression plasmid used.

3. Add an equivalent volume of 2X HBS dropwise to the DNA while bubbling the DNA-$CaCl_2$ solution. Use two automatic pipettors, one in each hand. A fine precipitate should immediately be visible. The solution will become cloudy.

4. Place the solution (1 mL) on the cells (already in DMEM complete, supplemented with 10 μ*M* chloroquine) within 20 min (*see* **Note 3**).

5. After 8–10 h, aspirate the medium and "shock" the cells using a small volume of 10% DMSO in PBS (*see* **Note 5**). Aspirate the PBS/DMSO, and then refeed the

cells using 15 mL of DMEM complete. The cells may divide once more, but by 48 h posttransfection they should show signs of cytotoxicity (from expression of VSV G), such as rounding and detachment from the plate.

6. After approx 60 h, collect the supernatant and centrifuge at 2,000g for 10 min to remove large cellular debris. Most of the cells appear nonviable at this time.

7. Titer the unconcentrated viral supernatant on a standard human adherent cell line. Although I typically use HOS cells (human osteosarcoma, available from American Type Culture Collection), other investigators use HeLa or 293 cells. Plate the target cells 1 d prior to transduction in 24-well format, at roughly 100,000 cells/well.

8. Incubate serial dilutions of virus, beginning with 0.1 mL, with the target cells. Exchange the media the next day. If a green fluorescent protein (GFP) reporter is used in the vector, transduced cells can be directly observed for expression of the transgene 48 h later, using an inverted fluorescent microscope. If the *LacZ* gene is used as a reporter, cells can be fixed for 10 min and stained overnight with an X gal solution (3 mM potassium ferricyanide, 3 mM potassium ferrocyanide, and 0.8 mg/mL x-gal in PBS). For selectable markers, targets are split into appropriate antibiotic or drug selection. Resistant colonies usually arise within 2 wk, and can be enumerated after crystal violet or giemsa staining. Titer is expressed as infectious or transducing U/mL. If 100 positive cells are observed using 0.01 mL of vector supernatant at a magnification where there are 100 microscope fields in the well, the titer is $100 \times 100 \times 100/mL = 10^6$ infectious units (IU)/mL. Most split-coding virus preparations will have a titer of between 10^5 and 10^6 IU/mL. In the case of my first-generation "proof-of-concept" vectors in which all the viral gene products are in *cis* configuration, titer is routinely 3×10^7 IU/mL, and occasionally as high as 10^8 IU/mL. At very high titer, if too much virus stock is used, the targets will demonstrate cytopathic effect, presumably because of the mutagenic nature of provirus insertion.

3.4. Concentration of Vector Supernatants and Transduction of Targets

Because of the stability of the VSV G envelope, unconcentrated vector supernatants can be concentrated using one of three methods. Virus can be concentrated by ultrafiltration, using commercially available units. I have successfully used Amicon's centriprep-10 unit, which holds up to 22 mL and has a mol wt cut-off value of 10 kd.

1. Sterilize the centriprep-10 unit by washing both the inner and outer chambers with 70% ethanol, taking care to remove most of the ethanol.

2. Load the supernatant in the outer chamber and centrifuge at 3,000g for 45–60 min at room temperature or 4°C.

3. Discard the ultrafiltrate from the inner chamber and repeat the centrifugation step. It usually takes 2.5–3 h to concentrate supernatant 10–20-fold. Recovery of

IU can be quantitated by titering material pre- and postconcentration. Losses usually do not exceed 20%.

4. Alternatively, viral supernatant can be concentrated by ultracentrifugation, using an SW28 (Beckman) rotor. Each bucket can hold up to 38 mL, so the entire rotor can accommodate up to 240 mL.

5. Wash the o-ring seals and buckets thoroughly with mild detergent and water. Rinse the rotor buckets and tubes carefully with 70% ethanol, taking care to remove most of the remaining ethanol (*see* **Note 6**), then add the supernatant.

6. Centrifuge the supernatant with the brake on at 100,000*g* for 1.5–2 h at 4°C. Remove the tubes from individual buckets using flame-sterilized forceps.

7. Aspirate the supernatant and resuspend the yellowish-brown pellet (usually a few mm in diameter) in 1/100th vol (0.4 mL) of DMEM complete by scraping and washing with a 1-mL pipet. Viral particles are fully resuspended by transferring to a sterile 15-mL polypropylene conical tube and rotating end-over-end for 3–5 h at room temperature.

8. Titer concentrated virus starting with 0.001 mL (equivalent to 0.1 mL of unconcentrated stock). Expect losses in the range of 10–20%. The 100-fold concentrated virus can be further concentrated by centrifugation in an appropriate horizontal rotor and resuspending in 1/10th the starting vol (1000-fold final concentration). This is only performed when the starting viral titer is 10^5 IU/mL and a titer of 10^8 IU/mL is required for transduction of elusive targets (*see* **Notes 7–9**). The third method is technically the easiest and involves centrifuging the vector supernatant overnight at relatively low *g* forces.

9. Centrifuge the supernatant (brake on) in a sterile 200 mL conical tube overnight (~16 h) at 4°C at 7000*g*.

10. Aspirate the supermatant carefully and resuspend the pellet as described in **step 7.**

11. Titer concentrated viral stock as described in **step 8.** Recovery of ice is typically 75–80%, with up to 25% loss in the centrifugation step.

3.5. Detection of Replication-Competent Lentivirus

Improvements in lentiviral vector design have been aimed at reducing the probability of generating a replication-competent lentivirus (RCL). RCL can arise in the producer cell by a recombination event, which can occur at the plasmid DNA level, at the level of reverse transcription during viral cDNA synthesis, or perhaps even postintegration during chromosome recombination. It is also conceivable that such a rare recombination event could arise in the transduced targets. Although these events are unlikely to produce RCL in any given cell, because of the potentially large numbers of cells involved in virus production, it is necessary to demonstrate the absence of RCL. Tests to detect RCL differ in their sensitivity and ease.

A simple but time-consuming way to determine whether RCL is present is by transducing a target adherent cell line to high efficiency (>95%), and then passaging the cells for several generations. Supernatant from the transduced targets is then serially tested for its ability to infect naïve cells, using the transgene as a readout. One may expect a few positive cells (depending upon the nature of the transfer vector), but that number should not increase over time. This method assumes that the RCL has maintained the transgene, which may not be correct.

A second way is to transduce targets to high efficiency and then serially determine capsid (CA or p24) levels in the cell-culture supernatant of the transduced targets. This can be accomplished by using a commercially available ELISA kit (Coulter). CA levels should fall exponentially over time to undetectable levels. The assumption here is that RCL will produce CA, and spreading infection by an RCL will eventually result in high levels of CA in the tissue-culture supernatant.

A third method is to transduce targets to high efficiency and then serially test tissue-culture supernatants on cells which already have an integrated HIV LTR driving a different transgene (e.g., *LacZ* or *GFP*). This type of indicator cell line is available from individual investigators *(2,5)* or the AIDS Research and Reference Reagent Program (http://www.aidsreagent.org). If RCL is present, the assumption is that it encodes *Tat*. Thus, the HIV LTR in the targets will be transactivated and positive cells will be easily detected.

The final method is probably the most sensitive, and is typically used to detect replication-competent retrovirus in Murine leukemia virus (MLV) preparations. In this marker-rescue assay, an indicator-cell line is used which has a defective HIV carrying a transgene marker (and no detectable RCL). Because such cell lines are not generally available, they may need to be created by the individual investigator. The indicator-cell line is transduced with the test supernatant and then passaged for a few weeks. Tissue culture supernatant from this transduced indicator cell line is harvested and tested for its ability to transduce a naïve-cell line with the indicator marker. Rescue (or transfer) of the marker would be consistent with the presence of RCL. This method allows for the testing of large amounts (up to 50 mL on a 15-cm plate) of unconcentrated supernatant, which is ideal for increased sensitivity. In the case of the current third-generation HIV-based vectors, RCL is undetectable using any of these methods *(1,3,9)*.

I anticipate that over the next 5–10 yr, lentiviral-based vectors will become more widely used to transfer genes into many types of nondividing and terminally differentiated cells. In addition, clinical trials will likely begin, using these vectors in select patients who have failed or are unable to tolerate conventional therapies. I am confident that as more investigators use this vector system, improvements in technique and safety and refinements in methodology will occur.

4. Notes

1. DNA prepared by double banding in CsCl is consistently of the highest purity and results in the highest-titer vector supernatant. Alternatively, DNA can be prepared by ion-exchange chromatography using any of a number of commercial kits (e.g., Qiagen). In our experience, viral titers using DNA prepared by the latter methods are reduced by several-fold.

2. It is important to maintain the 293T cells in mid-log phase. If the cells become confluent, they become contact-inhibited and go into stationary phase. For most cell types, the medium becomes more acidic, but paradoxically, in the case of 293Ts, the medium becomes more basic. 293T cells can be split 1:100, but their initial recovery and growth becomes somewhat erratic and unpredictable. Routinely, cells can be passaged every 3–4 d to maintain good growth kinetics.

3. Even fine calcium-phosphate precipitates end up clumping after a prolonged period of time, so the precipitate should be added to the cells in a timely manner. The quality of precipitate is crucial; if it is too fine it will not settle upon the cells, and if it is too clumpy the cells cannot take up the particles by endocytosis. I typically test the precipitate in a mock transfection (without DNA) to determine its suitability.

4. I have described the transfection procedure for 10-cm plates. The transfection can be scaled down to 6-well (35-mm) format or up to 15-cm or large square plates. Below the 6-well size, it becomes difficult to obtain high-quality precipitates because of the small volumes used. On the other end, it is relatively easy for a single investigator to transfect up to ten 15-cm plates. Handling more than that number of large plates at any one time becomes logistically difficult, and should be avoided if possible. Thirty large (15 cm) plates can be transfected in groups of 10 each.

5. After the DMSO shock procedure, I refeed the cells with a large volume of DMEM complete and harvest the virus 60 h later. Other investigators use a smaller, almost minimal volume, hoping that the viral titer will be higher. However, larger volumes do not appreciably reduce viral titer, perhaps because the medium is not spent as quickly. It is also possible to harvest the supernatant multiple times after transfection to increase virus yield.

6. When preparing the buckets and tubes for ultracentrifugation, care should be taken to rinse both the buckets and tubes with 70% ethanol. I do this separately, in two steps. Ethanol is first added to the empty buckets, the caps are screwed tightly, the buckets are inverted several times, and the ethanol is removed. These steps are then repeated with the tubes in place. A short centrifugation (1 min at 1,000g) will collect all the ethanol at the bottom to permit complete aspiration (done in the biosafety cabinet).

7. The actual details of the transduction process are highly dependent upon the nature of the targets. I usually perform transductions in multiwell format so that the cell concentration does not exceed 1×10^7 cells/mL. Freshly isolated or actively cycling primary cells may be used. It should be kept in mind that truly quiescent (G0 or non-cycling) cells are poorly transduced, even with lentiviral vectors *(7)*.

Transductions should be performed in the smallest volume possible to avoid reducing viral titer unnecessarily. As an example, 10^6 cells can be transduced overnight (12–16 h) in 0.5 mL medium, using 2.5×10^8 IU of previously concentrated and titered viral stock, in the presence of 4–8 µg/mL polybrene. The following day, spent medium is exchanged for fresh medium, and 2–4 d later, cells are examined for transgene expression as described above. Performing PCR-based assays to measure transduction is slightly more complicated, because there is a large amount of carryover DNA from the original transfection. Even femtogram amounts of DNA can yield a positive result, depending upon the PCR conditions used. If PCR is necessary, the target cells can be washed extensively after transduction, using large amounts of complete medium. In addition, after the final wash, medium can be supplemented with 100 µg/mL DNase I and 10 mM MgCl$_2$ so that the leftover extracellular DNA will be digested to completion. Cells remain viable, because they are impermeable to the enzyme. Unfortunately, this process sometimes fails, because the plasmid DNA appears to be relatively protected by the calcium-phosphate crystals (from the original transfection). Cells can then be directly lysed in the presence of EDTA (to inhibit DNase I) and the lysate can be heated to 95°C for 15 min to inactivate the enzyme. Samples are then ready for PCR, which can be performed using HIV vector or transgene-specific oligodeoxynucleotide primers. The details of PCR are beyond the scope of this chapter.

8. Multiplicity of infection (MOI) is a concept used in virological studies, when infection efficiency is quite high. Unfortunately, transduction of the most interesting target populations (such as HSC) is often very inefficient, and therefore MOI is not a useful parameter to consider. Viral titer (as measured on a well-characterized adherent cell line) is much more important, which suggests that transduction of each individual cell is a purely stochastic (probabilistic) process. However, any given primary cell population is likely to be heterogeneous, and thus the transduction efficiency will vary depending upon the characteristics of the target. For example, human CD34$^+$ cells require an effective viral titer of 5×10^8 IU/mL for optimal transduction efficiency. However, the maximal transduction rate is never more than 75%, which suggests that within that cell population, some cells are virtually impossible to transduce *(7)*.

9. When using ultracentrifuge-concentrated viral stocks to transduce cells, do not be alarmed by the debris observed. It is mainly of cellular origin (membranes and the like), along with the calcium phosphate crystals from the original transfection. This debris is not harmful to most cells (including HSC), and it does not impede the transduction or expression analysis (i.e., by flow cytometry). It does, however, interfere with subsequent PCR analysis (*see* **Subheading 3.4.** and **Note 7**).

References

1. Dull, T., Zufferey, R., Kelly, M., Mandel, R. J., Nguyen, M., Trono, D., et al. (1998) A third-generation lentivirus vector with a conditional packaging system. *J. Virol.* **72,** 8463–8471.

2. Kafri, T., van Praag, H., Ouyang, L., Gage, F. H., and Verma, I. M. (1999) A packaging cell line for lentivirus vectors. *J. Virol.* **73,** 576–584.
3. Miyoshi, H., Blomer, U., Takahashi, M., Gage, F. H., and Verma, I. M.. (1998) Development of a self-inactivating lentivirus vector. *J. Virol.* **72,** 8150–8157.
4. Mochizuki, H., Schwartz, J. P., Tanaka, K., Brady, R. O., and Reiser, J. (1998) High-titer human immunodeficiency virus type 1–based vector systems for gene delivery into nondividing cells. *J. Virol.* **72,** 8873–8883.
5. Naldini, L., Blomer, U., Gallay, P., Ory, D., Mulligan, R., Gage, F. H., et al.. (1996) In Vivo delivery and stable transduction of nondividing cells by a lentiviral vector. *Science* **272,** 263–267.
6. Sutton, R. E. and Littman, D. R. (1996) Broad host range of human T-cell leukemia virus type 1 demonstrated with an improved pseudotyping system. *J. Virol.* **70,** 7322–7326.
7. Sutton, R. E., Reitsma, M. J., Uchida, N. and Brown, P. O. (1999) Transduction of human progenitor hematopoietic stem cells by human immunodeficiency virus type 1 vectors is cell-cycle dependent. *J. Virol.***73,** 3649–3660.
8. Sutton, R. E., Wu, H. T., Rigg, R., Bohnlein, E., and Brown, P. O. (1998) Human immunodeficiency virus type 1 vectors efficiently transduce human hematopoietic stem cells. *J. Virol.* **72,** 5781–5788.
9. Zufferey, R., Dull, T., Mandel, R. J., Bukovsky, A., Quiroz, D., Naldini, L., et al. (1998) Self-inactivating lentivirus vector for safe and efficient In vivo gene delivery. *J. Virol.* **72,** 9873–9880.

19

Reverse Transcriptase-PCR Analysis of Gene Expression in Hematopoietic Stem Cells

Donald Orlic

1. Introduction

The events that determine whether hematopoietic stem cells (HSC) divide in the course of self-renewal or differentiate and become committed progenitor cells are regulated by specific gene expression. Although little is known of the molecular controls for these diverse events, the activation of a single gene may determine which developmental event will occur in an individual HSC. New and more precise information on the controls for gene expression in HSC may provide relevant clues to the regulation of hematopoiesis. Yet investigations of gene expression in HSC have been difficult to perform, primarily because it has been difficult to purify the large numbers of HSC needed to obtain sufficient RNA for Northern analysis or RNase protection assays. These rare cells occur in a ratio of approx 1:10,000 to 1:100,000 bone-marrow cells. Their enrichment is accomplished by coupling several procedures that include the use of lineage-specific monoclonal antibodies (MAbs) and immunomagnetic bead depletion of unfractionated bone marrow followed by fluorescence-activated cell sorting (FACS). The HSC in lineage-negative cell populations from mouse bone marrow are then sorted for HSC using MAbs specific for surface markers such as Sca-1 or c-kit (**Fig. 1**). Human HSC are lineage negative, CD34-positive and CD38-negative.

To overcome the problems associated with the low levels of mRNA obtained from enriched populations of HSC, we and others have modified (**Fig. 2**) the early reverse transcriptase-polymerase chain reaction (RT-PCR) protocols *(1–8)* and made them suitable for analysis of HSC mRNA *(9–22)*.

From: *Methods in Molecular Medicine, vol. 63: Hematopoietic Stem Cell Protocols*
Edited by: C. A. Klug and C. T. Jordan © Humana Press Inc., Totowa, NJ

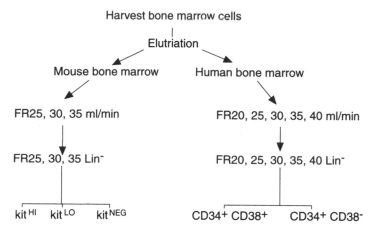

Fig. 1. This scheme shows the method we use for the purification of mouse and human HSC from elutriated bone marrow. The cells in the elutriated cell fractions (FR = flow rate in mL/min) are labeled with MAbs specific for each hematopoietic lineage. These cell populations are then depleted of lineage-positive cells using immunomagnetic beads. Finally, the lineage-negative cells from mouse bone marrow are incubated with anti c-kit MAb and the lineage-negative cells from human bone marrow are incubated with anti-CD34 and anti-CD38 MAb. With a starting population of $2–4 \times 10e8$ unfractionated mouse bone-marrow cells, a typical isolation procedure yields approx $2 \times 10e4$ FR25 lin⁻ c-kit^{HI} cells. This is the most highly enriched HSC population we have been able to obtain to date. As few as 50–100 of these cells can completely repopulate the hematopoietic tissue of an adult W/W^v mouse. However, $2 \times 10e4$ cells from this highly enriched HSC population do not provide sufficient mRNA for Northern blots or RNase protection assays, but do provide sufficient mRNA for the RT-PCR assay.

Using RT-PCR, one can analyze gene expression in as few as 10–20 HSC because of the enormous capacity of PCR to amplify rare cDNA copies. We were able to detect the expression of mRNA-encoding growth-factor receptors and transcription factors in several distinctly different populations of hematopoietic cells *(14)*. Because HSCs, progenitor cells, and maturing cells all expressed mRNA transcripts for several of the genes investigated, it was necessary to derive a formula for quantitative evaluation of the RT-PCR reaction (for the formula, *see* **Subheading 3.2., step 6**). Quantitative data on mRNA levels in these diverse populations of hematopoietic cells can provide a basis for understanding biological function in HSC, because a threshold level of protein may be required for the onset of function.

A second obstacle to accurate analysis of HSC mRNA by RT-PCR is the purity of the HSC population. Generally, it is not possible to sort HSC populations at greater than 85–95% purity, as seen by FACS reanalysis. The small

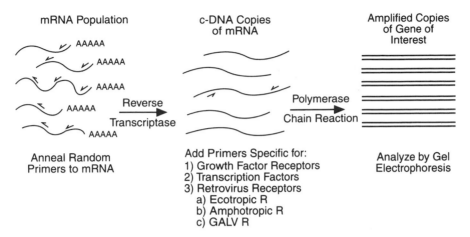

Fig. 2. The detection of specific mRNA molecules by RT-PCR is initiated with the annealing of random primers to total cellular RNA from an enriched HSC population. Reverse transcriptase is used to generate cDNA copies of the mRNA transcripts. Subsequently, growth-factor receptor, transcription factor, and retrovirus receptor cDNA or cDNA from any early acting gene in HSC can be amplified using primers specific for these cDNAs. The amplified fragments are then analyzed by gel electrophoresis.

number of contaminating cells within the HSC sample may contribute mRNA transcripts that will be amplified during RT-PCR, and thus give a false-positive result. To overcome this problem, we recommend obtaining quantitative data with the use of an internal standard such as the RT-PCR product of a constitutively expressed gene. Either β-actin or β2-microglobulin can be used as the internal standard. By limiting-dilution analysis (LDA), the product of the internal standard can be used to determine the log phase of the PCR reaction and to indicate uniform loading of the samples on the agarose gel (**Fig. 3**). The relative expression of mRNA for the gene of interest can be calculated based on the level of ß2-microglobulin mRNA in the sample. With this calculated ratio, it is possible to compare the level of mRNA for the gene of interest in multiple experimental samples. This quantitative data is especially useful for determining the level of mRNA expression when dealing with a widely expressed gene (**Fig. 4**). Whereas relative differences in mRNA expression can suggest biological function, the RT-PCR assay is also valid when no reaction product is generated for a specific mRNA transcript. From negative results, it can be concluded that the highly enriched HSC population and contaminating cells do not express the mRNA of interest.

The PCR amplification of a cDNA copy is achieved using primers designed to recognize sequences in two different exons of the genomic DNA (*see* **Note 1**) that will generate fragments from 200–600 nucleotides in length. By spanning

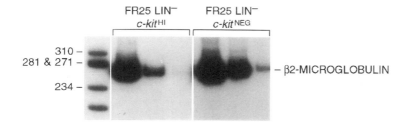

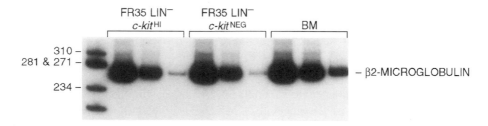

Fig. 3. Quantitative estimates of the level of mRNA in unfractionated mouse bone marrow and in purified HSC-enriched (FR25 lin⁻ c-kit^HI and FR35 lin⁻ c-kit^HI) and HSC-depleted (FR25 lin⁻ c-kit^NEG and FR35 lin⁻ c-kit^NEG) populations can be obtained by LDA. ß2–microglobulin mRNA can be used as an internal standard for RT-PCR assays because it is a constitutively expressed gene. The primers used to detect ß2–microglobulin define a fragment consisting of 258 nucleotides. To quantitate the level of ß2–microglobulin mRNA in the sample, we use a series of 10–fold dilutions to establish a value at which the level of the PCR product approaches zero. With these results, one can select a quantity of mRNA from the linear phase of the reaction curve.

an intron and calculating the expected length of the fragment, one can eliminate the possibility of error resulting from amplification of genomic DNA. Also, by amplifying a cDNA fragment that has a restriction enzyme site, one can prepare digests of the PCR product and demonstrate that the sum of the resulting fragments equals the predicted size of the original cDNA (**Fig. 5**) (*see* **Notes 2** and **3**). This further reduces the possibility that an incorrect mRNA sequence has been analyzed.

In order to demonstrate that the specificity and efficiency of RT-PCR can compare with that of Northern blot analysis, we quantified the mRNA encoding amphotropic and ecotropic retrovirus receptors using RT-PCR and conventional Northern blot analysis *(15)*. We assayed mRNA from NIH-3T3, MEL, and 32D cell lines and unfractionated mouse bone-marrow cells. The values obtained for NIH-3T3 cells by RT-PCR and Northern blot were arbitrarily set at 1.0, and the values for MEL and 32D cells and unfractionated

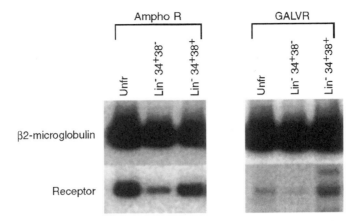

Fig. 4. This figure illustrates how ß2–microglobulin can be used as an internal standard for estimating the relative level of test gene mRNA expression and equivalent loading of each lane. In this instance, comparisons are made between ß2–microglobulin mRNA and mRNA encoding the amphotropic and Gibbon Ape Leukemia Virus receptors (amphoR and GALVR) in fresh human cord blood. By comparing the ratio of receptor mRNA with ß2–microglobulin mRNA, one can calculate the relative difference in receptor mRNA expression in HSC (lin⁻ CD34⁺ CD38–) and progenitor cells (lin⁻ CD34⁺ CD38⁺). In this example, the level of mRNA encoding both receptors is low in HSC and higher in progenitor cells. The calculation is done using the formula in **Subheading 3.2., step 6.**

bone marrow were adjusted to these standards. The relative levels of mRNA were similar when assayed by these two methods, thus demonstrating that RT-PCR provides an accurate method for the quantification of mRNA in small numbers of HSC.

New technology for the RT-PCR analysis of mRNA in single HSC is emerging. This assay, referred to as "Real-Time" PCR, requires the use of flow cytometry for sorting single HSC and TaqMan-PCR, ABI Prism 7700 Sequence Detection System, Perkin Elmer Applied Biosystems equipment. "Real-Time" PCR is based on the use of a double-labeled hybridization probe specific for a sequence within the cDNA amplicon. The probe is labeled with a 5' fluorescent reporter dye and a 3' fluorescent quencher dye. The reporter fluorescent dye emission is quenched when the probe is intact. During PCR extension, Taq polymerase displays 5' nuclease activity, and as the cDNA copy is generated the probe is cleaved. Reporter fluorescent dye emission is recorded in "Real-Time," and the fluorescence intensity in the reaction is directly proportional to the number of cDNA copies generated. Although this protocol requires equipment and expertise that many laboratories do not have, in the future "Real-

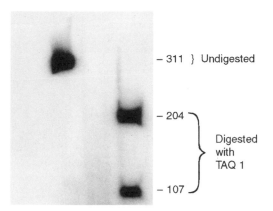

Fig. 5. The specificity of the PCR product can be established using a number of assays. The one seen here involves the digestion of the PCR product IL-2R alpha with the restriction enzyme *Taq*1. mRNA isolated from –/– thymocytes was amplified by RT-PCR using primers that predicted a 311 nucleotide fragment. The *Taq*1 digested products were 204 and 107 nucleotides in length, thus confirming the identity of the PCR product.

Time" PCR may become a powerful tool for the quantitative analysis of mRNA expression in single HSC. When this protocol *(23–25)* is eventually adapted for analysis of mRNA expression in individual HSC we may learn to distinguish quiescent, self-renewing and differentiating HSC on the basis of gene expression.

2. Materials

2.1. Purification of Total Cellular RNA

1. TRIzol (Life Technologies, Grand Island, NY).
2. Yeast tRNA (10 mg/mL, Sigma, St. Louis, MO).
3. Chloroform (Mallinckrodt Chemicals Co., Paris, KY).
4. 2-propanol (J.T. Baker, Phillipsburg, NJ).
5. 75% ethyl alcohol (Warner-Graham Co., Cockeysville, MD).
6. Diethylpyrocarbonate (DEPC) (ICN Biomedicals Inc., Aurora, IL)-dH$_2$O.

2.2. Reverse Transcriptase Reaction

1. Capped 0.5 mL polypropylene microcentrifuge tubes (GeneAmp reaction tubes, Perkin Elmer, Norwalk, CT).
2. DNA Thermal Cycler 480 (Perkin Elmer, Norwalk, CT).
3. MgCl$_2$ solution (25 mM).
4. 10X PCR buffer II.
5. Deoxyadenosine 5'-triphosphate (dATP), deoxycytidine 5'-triphosphate (dCTP), deoxyguanosine 5'-triphosphate (dGTP), and deoxythymidine 5'-triphosphate (dTTP) (10 μM each).

6. Sterile DEPC-dH$_2$O.
7. Random hexamers (50 μ*M*) or Oligo dT (50 μ*M*).
8. RNase Inhibitor (20 U/μL).
9. MuLV reverse transcriptase (50 U/μL).
10. Positive control RNA (<1 μg) (Perkin Elmer, Norwalk, CT).

2.3. PCR Reaction

1. Thin-walled 0.5-mL-capped tubes.
2. MgCl$_2$.
3. 10X PCR buffer II.
4. Forward-strand primer for mouse β-2 microglobulin 5' TGC TAT CCA GAA AAC CCC TC 3' (400 ng or 0.15 μ*M*).
5. Reverse-strand primer for mouse β-2 microglobulin 5' GTC ATG CTT AAC TCT GCA GG 3' (400 ng or 0.15 μ*M*).
6. Primers specific for the gene of interest.
7. ^{32}PdCTP, 800 Ci/mmol (Amersham Pharmacia Biotech, Piscataway, NJ).
8. Ampli*Taq* DNA Polymerase (Perkin Elmer, Norwalk, CT).
9. Mineral oil (ICN Biomedicals Inc., Aurora, IL).
10. DNA thermal cycler.

2.4. Separation of PCR Generated cDNA Fragments

1. 5% Polyacrylamide gel (National Diagnostics, Atlanta, GA).
2. Bromophenol blue solution (Sigma, St. Louis, MO).
3. Power supply, electrophoresis apparatus, gel dryer.

2.5. Quantification of cDNA Bands

1. PhosphorImager and ImageQuant Program (Molecular Dynamics Densitometer System, Sunnyvale, CA).
2. PhosphorImager cassette.

3. Methods
3.1. RNA Extraction

1. Harvest a highly purified population of HSC by flow cytometry and transfer the cells to an Eppendorf tube. Spin the cells at 300g for 5 min at 4°C.
2. Suspend the cells in 200 μL TRIzol for up to 10^6 cells and add 40 β*L* of chloroform and 1 μL tRNA (this will later help to precipitate the small number of mRNA molecules).
3. Shake the tubes gently by hand for 15 s and place at room temperature for 2–3 min. Spin the samples at 1,3600g for 15 min at 4°C.
4. Transfer the aqueous phase (approx 120 μL) to a new tube and add 2-propanol in a 1:1 ratio with the aqueous solution. Place the samples at room temperature for 10 min and spin at 13,600g for 10 min at 4°C.

5. Remove the supernatant and suspend the RNA in 200 μL of 75% ethanol and vortex gently (the sample can be stored at this stage at –20°C). Spin at 5000g for 5 min at 4°C.

6. Remove the supernatant and air-dry the pellet for 10 min or more and then resuspend the pellet in 10–40 μL DEPC-dH$_2$O. In an effort to obtain similar RNA concentrations in all samples we use the following resuspension volumes of DEPC-H2O. Fewer than 3,000 cells are resuspended in 10 μL, (*see* **Note 4**) 3,000–10,000 cells are resuspended in 20 μL, 10,000–20,000 cells are resuspended in 30 μL, and 20,000–50,000 cells are resuspended in 40 μL. The limiting-dilution assay (LDA) described in **Subheading 3.2.** below provides the final working estimate of the RNA concentration in each sample prior to the RT-PCR assay involving target gene-specific primers.

Incubate the sample at 55°C to 60°C for 10 min in a water bath. The samples can then be stored at –20°C for a period of 6 mo or more and can be at thawed several times without apparent RNA degradation (*see* **Note 5**).

3.2. Limiting-Dilution RT-PCR

The small quantity of RNA derived from highly purified HSC populations does not permit measurements by spectrophotometry for estimating RNA concentration. To circumvent this problem, one can perform a LDA based on a series of 10-fold decreases in RNA content per reaction. In the initial step the total mRNA is reverse-transcribed to cDNA, which is then amplified by PCR.

1. Label four PCR tubes for each sample: 1X dilution, 10X dilution, 100X dilution, 1000X dilution and dispense aliquots of 18 μL of RT master mix to each dilution tube. Prepare sufficient RT master mix using the following reagents in the volumes given for each reaction tube: MgCl$_2$ (*see* **Note 6**)(4 μL), 10X PCR buffer II (2 μL), dATP, dCTP, dGTP and dTTP (2 μL each), DEPC-dH$_2$O (1 μL), random hexamers (*see* **Note 7**)(1 μL), RNase Inhibitor (1 μL, recombinant enzyme from Perkin Elmer, Part No. N808-0017) and reverse transcriptase (1 μL) for a total of 18 mL per reaction.

2. Serial dilutions are prepared as follows:
   a. For the 1X dilution tubes, add 1 μL RNA and 1 μL DEPC-dH$_2$O, vortex, and spin briefly.
   b. For the 10X dilution tubes, add 2 μL of the 1X dilution RNA solution, vortex, and spin briefly.
   c. Repeat this procedure for the 100X dilution tubes and the 1000X dilution tubes.
   d. Run the RT reaction 1 cycle using the following conditions: segment 1 at 20°C for 10 min, segment 2 at 42°C for 15 min, segment 3 at 99°C for 5 min, and segment 4 at 4°C for 5 min.

3. In the PCR reaction, the quantity of cDNA can be estimated in each sample by using primers specific for a constitutively expressed mRNA species such as β-

actin or β2-microglobulin. In the event the highest concentration of RNA yields a maximum or plateau phase reaction, the diluted RNA samples will eventually fall in the linear phase of the reaction. The quantity of RNA per reaction for each sample can then be normalized, thus making it possible to obtain quantitative data that can be usefully compared from sample to sample. (*see* **step 6** in **Subheading 3.2.** for details of this analysis).

4. The PCR master mix for each reaction tube is as follows: $MgCl_2$ (2 μL), 10X PCR buffer II (4 μL), primers for mouse β-2 microglobulin (400 ng or 0.15 μ*M*), ^{32}PdCTP (0.1 μL), AmpliTaq DNA polymerase (0.25 μL) and DEPC-dH_2O (to a final volume of 40 μL per reaction). For each sample, add 40 μL PCR master mix to 10 μL cDNA, vortex gently, and add mineral oil (1 or 2 drops). The PCR reaction involves the following conditions: step-cycle 94°C for 1 min for melting, step-cycle 58°C for 1 min for annealing (this annealing temperature will vary depending upon the specific annealing conditions required for the primers for the different test genes), and step-cycle 72°C for 2 min for extension. After the completion of 35 cycles, hold the samples at 72°C for 7 min to complete the extension when dealing with long fragments, and hold at 4°C until ready to separate by polyacrylamide gel electrophoresis.

5. Load 25 μL of sample together with the loading dye (2% bromophenol blue) onto a 5% polyacrylamide gel. Run the gel at 150 V (maximum) for approx 2.5 h and dry the gel at 80°C for approx 1 h. Expose the plate of a Molecular Dynamics PhosphorImager cassette for 1 h, and quantify the appropriate bands using an ImageQuant program.

6. Calculation of the mRNA concentration in each sample is determined by assaying the level of expression of a constitutively expressed gene. We routinely use the expression of β-2 microglobulin mRNA as the internal standard. By inspecting the bands obtained using the four mRNA dilutions for each sample, one can select a representative band that is in the linear range of the amplification curve. Use the numerical value of this band as the standard to which the other samples will be adjusted. For each sample, choose the dilution that provides a band nearest the intensity of the standard band and calculate the volume required for equivalent loading of each sample per reaction. An example of this calculation follows: if the standard band has a count of 600000 and the 10X dilution of a representative band of another sample has 400000 counts, then:

$$\frac{600\,000}{400\,000} \times 0.1 = 0.15 \ \mu L/rx$$

predicts equivalent concentration in the two sample dilutions

In some studies it may be important to determine the relative level of specific gene mRNA in the HSC population with the level in a standard cell population. This can be accomplished if the mRNA in the HSC population is normalized to the level of mRNA in HeLa (human) or NIH-3T3 (mouse) cells using the following formula:

$$\frac{\text{Test gene mRNA in HSC}}{\beta 2\text{-m mRNA in HSC}} \times \frac{\beta 2\text{-m mRNA in HeLa / NIH-3T3 cells}}{\text{Test gene mRNA in HeLa / NIH-3T3 cells}} =$$

Relative level of test gene mRNA in Human/Mouse HSC

7. Using the numerical values obtained for each RNA sample, the level of mRNA expression for any gene of interest can be assayed using primers specific for that cDNA. For each sample, assay β2-microglobulin mRNA as well as the test gene mRNA. With these results, one can compare the mRNA level for the test gene with the mRNA level for β2-microglobulin. The number of reactions, or samples, multiplied by the number of primer pairs that will be used in the PCR reaction will determine the volume of the RT master mix that will be needed. For example, if there are 5 samples and 3 primer pairs, prepare sufficient master mix for 6 samples × 4 primer pairs, for a total of 24 reactions. This will ensure an adequate volume of master mix for all samples (*see* **Note 10**). The total of 10 μL of cDNA that will be used for each PCR reaction will consist of the following reagents and volumes. MgCl$_2$ (2 μL), 10X PCR buffer II (1 μL), dATP, dCTP, dGTP, and dTTP (1 μL each), DEPC·dH$_2$O (0.5 μL), Random hexamers (0.5 μL), RNase Inhibitor (0.5 μL), RT (0.5 μL), and RNA+DEPC-dH$_2$O (1 μL).

4. Notes

1. For the PCR, select a pair of primers that span an intron. Each primer may be 20–25 bases in length, and should not include long spans of the same base. It is also useful to select primers with approx 50% "C" and "G" that begin and terminate in "C" or "G," since these bases will form a stronger linkage with the cDNA strand. This is caused by the three hydrogen bonds that form with "C" and "G" compared to two with "T" and "A." As a result, the primer/cDNA complex is more stable during the changes in temperature required for PCR. Primer concentration in the range of 0.15 μM to 0.25 μM (approx 400 ng) is recommended. At higher concentrations of primers, amplification of other than the target sites may occur.
2. Calculate the predicted size of the amplified cDNA fragment.
3. Select an enzyme that has a restriction site within the fragment, and digest the reaction product and assay for the predicted size fragments.
4. When working with a small number of cells, suspend the final RNA pellet in a small volume such as 10 μL of DEPC-H2O. The final RNA solution may be added up to 2 μL for each RT reaction. Greater than 2 μL of RNA in 20 μL total volume of RT master mix will alter the buffer concentration.
5. The purified RNA can be frozen at –20°C in 75% ethanol and stored overnight if additional samples are to be obtained the following day. At that time, the RNA in each sample can be precipitated and centrifuged to form a pellet prior to final suspending in DEPC-dH$_2$O. Long-term storage of the RNA can be achieved at –80°C. However, we have not detected any loss of RNA content, even after repeated freeze/thaw cycles when stored at –20°C.
6. For the RT reaction, Oligo dT may be used in place of Random Hexamers if the target site is short and near the 3' end of the mRNA.

7. Adjust the MgCl₂ concentration to provide optimal conditions for the PCR. With each set of primers, we test 1–10 μM concentrations. This is done to optimize the annealing of primers and cDNA.
8. DNase digestion is required if the sample is positive in the RT⁻ control assay.
9. Use tRNA as a negative control reaction against contamination in the PCR master mix.
10. If there are several test genes to be assayed at the same time using different primer pairs, it may be easiest to prepare a PCR master mix, minus the primers, for the total number of samples. In turn, prepare separate tubes with the proper amounts of primers. To these tubes, add the correct amount of PCR master mix. This method allows you to make several master mixes simultaneously rather than several separate master mixes.

Acknowledgments

I would like to express my thanks to David M. Bodine and Laurie J. Girard, who participated throughout the planning and development of this RT-PCR assay.

References

1. Klotman, M. E., Kim, S., Buchbinder, A., DeRosse, A., Baltimore, D., and Wong-Staal, F. (1991) Kinetics of expression of multiply spliced RNA in early human immunodeficiency virus type 1 infection of lymphocytes and monocytes. *Proc. Natl. Acad. Sci.USA* **88,** 5011–5015.
2. Eldadah, Z. A., Asher, D. M., Godec, M. S., Pomeroy, K. L., Goldfarb, L. G., Feinstone, et al. (1991) Detection of flaviviruses by reverse-transcriptase polymererase-chain reaction. *J. Med. Virol.* **33,** 260–267.
3. Kashanchi, F., Liu, Z. Q., Atkinson, B., and Wood, C. (1991) Comparative-evaluation of bovine immunodeficiency-like virus-infection by reverse-transcriptase and polymerase chain-reaction. *J. Virol. Methods* **31,** 197–210.
4. Henderson, A. J., Narayanan, R., Collins L., and Dorshkind, K. (1992) Status of kL chain gene rearrangements and c-kit and IL-7 receptor expression in stromal cell-dependent pre-B cells. *J. Immunol.* **149,** 1973–1979.
5. Miller, W. H., Kakizuka, A., Frankel, S. R., Warrell, R. P., Deblasio, A., Levine, K., et al. (1992) Reverse transcription polymerase chain-reaction for the rearranged retinoic acid receptor-alpha clarifies diagnosis and detects minimal residual disease in acute promyelocytic leukemia. *Proc. Natl. Acad. Sci. USA* **89,** 2694–2698
6. Koralnik, I. J., Lemp, J. F., Gallo, R. C., and Franchini G. (1992) In vitro infection of human macrophages by human T-cell leukemia lymphotropic virus type-1 (HTLV-1). *AIDS Res. Hum. Retrovir.* **8,** 1845–1849.
7. Odriscoll, L., Daly, C., Saleh, M., and Clynes, M. (1993). The use of reverse transcriptase-polymerase chain reaction (RT-PCR) to investigate specific gene-expression in multi-drug resistant cells. *Cytotechnology* **12,** 289–314.
8. Gaudette, M. F., Cao, Q. P., and Crain, W. R. (1993) Quantitative analysis of

specific messenger RNAs in small numbers of preimplantation embryos, in *Methods in Enzymology* (Wassarman, P.M. and DePamphilis, M.L., eds.), Academic Press, San Diego, CA, vol. **225,** 328–344.

9. Orlic, D., Fischer, R., Nishikawa, S.-I., Neinhuis, A., and Bodine, D. M. (1993) Purification and characterization of heterogeneous pluripotent hematopoietic stem cell populations expressing high levels of c-*kit* receptor. *Blood* **82,** 762–770.

10. Yamaguchi, Y., Gunji, Y., Nakamura, M., Hayakawa, K., Maeda, M., Osawa, H., et al. (1993) Expression of c-kit messenger-RNA and protein during the differentiation of human hematopoietic progenitor cells. *Exp. Hematol.* **21,** 1233–1238.

11. Visser, J. W. M., Rozemuller, H., Dejong, M. O., and Belyavsky, A. (1993) The expression of cytokine receptors by purified hematopoietic stem-cells. *Stem Cells* **11,** 49–55.

12. Sorrentino, B. P., McDonagh, K. T., Woods, D., and Orlic, D. (1995) Expression of retroviral vectors containing the human multidrug-resistance-1 cDNA in hematopoietic cells of transplanted mice. *Blood* **86,** 491–501.

13. Ziegler, B. L., Lamping, C. P., Thoma, S. J., and Fliedner, T. M. (1995) Analysis of gene expression in small numbers of purified hematopoietic progenitor cells by RT-PCR. *Stem Cells* **13,** 106–116.

14. Orlic, D., Anderson, S., Biesecker, L. G., Sorrentino, B. P., and Bodine, D. M. (1995) Pluripotent hematopoietic stem cells contain high levels of mRNA for c-*kit*, GATA-2, p45 NF-E2 and c-*myb*, and low levels or no mRNA for c-*fms*, and the receptors for granulocyte-colony stimulating factor, and interleukin-5 and 7. *Proc. Natl. Acad. Sci. USA* **92,** 4601–4605.

15. Orlic, D., Girard, L. J., Jordan, C. T., Anderson, S. M., Cline, A. P., and Bodine, D. M. (1996) The level of mRNA encoding the amphotropic retrovirus receptor in mouse and human hematopoietic stem cells is low and correlates with the efficiency of retrovirus transduction. *Proc. Natl. Acad. Sci. USA* **93,** 11,097–11,102.

16. Yoder, M. C., Hiatt, K., Dutt, P., Mukherjee, P., Bodine, D. M., and Orlic, D. (1997) Characterization of definitive hematopoietic stem cells in the day 9 murine yolk sac. *Immunity* **7,** 335–344.

17. Orlic, D., Girard, L. J., Lee, D., Anderson, S. M., Puck, J. M., and Bodine, D. M. (1997) Interleukin-7Rα mRNA expression increases as stem cells differentiate into T and B lymphocyte progenitors. *Exp. Hematol.* **25,** 217–222.

18. Ashihara, E., Vannucchi, A. M., Migliaccio, G., Migliaccio, A. R. (1997) Growth factor receptor expression during in vitro differentiation of partially purified populations containing murine stem cells. *J. Cell. Physiol.* **171,** 343–356.

19. Orlic, D., Girard, L. J., Anderson, S. M., Yoder, M. C., Broxmeyer, H. E., and Bodine, D. M. (1998) Identification of human and mouse hematopoietic stem cell (HSC) populations with high levels of mRNA encoding retrovirus receptors. *Blood* **91,** 3247–3254.

20. Mohle, R., Bautz, F., Rafii, S., Moore, M. A. S., Brugger, W., and Kanz, L. (1998) The chemokine receptor CXCR-4 is expressed on CD34(+) hematopoietic progenitors and leukemic cells and mediates transendothelial migration induced by stromal cell-derived factor-1. *Blood* **91,** 4523–4530.

21. Persons, D. A., Allay, J. A., Allay, E. R., Ashmun, R. A., Orlic, D., Jane, S. M., et al. (1999) Enforced expression of the GATA-2 transcription factor blocks normal hematopoiesis. *Blood* **93,** 488–499.
22. Horwitz, M. E., Malech, H. L., Anderson, S. M., Girard, L. J., Bodine, D. M., and Orlic, D. (1999) G-CSF mobilized peripheral blood stem cells enter into G1 of the cell cycle and express higher levels of amphotropic retrovirus receptor mRNA. *Exp. Hematol.* **27,** 1160–1167.
23. Heid, C.A., Stevens, J., Livak, K.J., and Williams, P.M. (1996) Real time quantitative PCR. *Genome Res.* **6,** 986–994.
24. Gibson, U. E. M., Heid, C. A., and Williams, P. M. (1996) A novel method for real time quantitative RT-PCR. *Genome Research* **6,** 995–1001.
25. Fink, L., Seeger ,W., Ermert, L., Hanze, J., Stahl, U., Grimminger, F., et al. (1998) Real-time quantitative RT-PCR after laser assisted cell picking. *Nat. Med.* **4,** 1329–1333.

20

Identification of Differentially Expressed Genes in Sorted Cell Populations by Two-Dimensional Gene-Expression Fingerprinting

Alexander V. Belyavsky, Sergey V. Shmelkov, and Jan W.M. Visser

1. Introduction

Differential activity of genes is one of the major mechanisms underlying a vast array of biological phenomena. Classical genetic approaches (from phenotypes to genes) have proven their exquisite potential for dissection of complex signaling pathways regulating the development of organisms and the functioning of individual cells. In recent years, with the advent of a number of techniques for studying gene function, the reverse genetics approach (from genes to phenotypes) has received broad acceptance. One of the advantages of this strategy is that it makes genes, whose dysfunction either does not produce an evident phenotype or is lethal, amenable to analysis. Reverse genetics has spearheaded the development of procedures for identification of candidate genes for this type of analysis by detecting spatial or temporal changes in gene-expression patterns. A significant range of methods have been proposed (1–7); in particular, the advent of microarray hybridization techniques promises to increase gene-expression analysis throughput by two or more orders of magnitude (8,9). Some of these procedures have been used to identify genes expressed differentially during hematopoiesis (10,11).

Despite the plethora of techniques, it seems that the goal to develop a protocol that could be accessible for laboratories with moderate budgets, yet would provide systematic and reproducible analysis of gene-expression patterns in small cell populations, as well as discovery of new genes, has not been reached so far. A few years ago, we developed the Gene-Expression Fingerprinting

From: *Methods in Molecular Medicine, vol. 63: Hematopoietic Stem Cell Protocols*
Edited by: C. A. Klug and C. T. Jordan © Humana Press Inc., Totowa, NJ

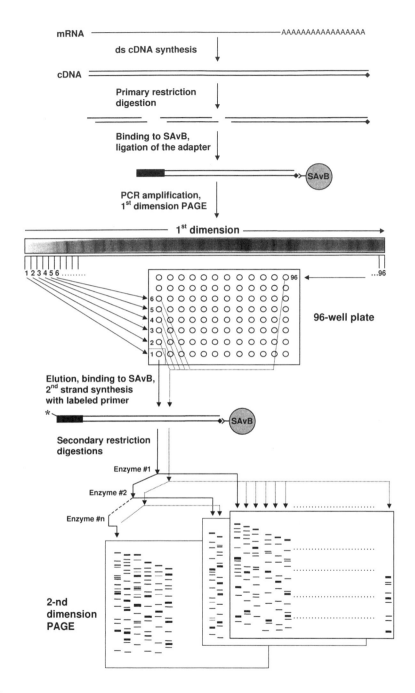

Fig. 1. Scheme of two-dimensional GEF protocol. Diamonds indicate biotin groups. SAvB: streptavidin beads.

(GEF) procedure, a gel-display technique that might satisfy at least some of the conditions cited here *(12)*.

In this chapter, we describe a two-dimensional variant of the GEF protocol that provides a much higher resolution and sensitivity than the previously proposed GEF schemes *(12,13)*. Certain amendments in the cDNA synthesis protocol have also permitted us to substantially increase the reproducibility of the procedure. The protocol was rigorously tested using the human primitive hematopoietic cell line KG-1, and its derivative KG-1a. The results demonstrate that differentially expressed sequences can be identified with high precision with the proportion of false-positives not exceeding 20% *(13a)*.

The protocol exploits the basic principle of GEF analysis, namely generation of discrete restriction endonuclease fragments of cDNA followed by their display on acrylamide gels to visualize mRNA "expression patterns." However, for separation of the cDNA fragments, a two-dimensional electrophoresis was introduced that dramatically increased the resolving power of the technique. The procedure is shown schematically in **Fig. 1**. cDNA synthesis is initiated using biotinylated anchored oligo (dT)-containing primer; second-strand synthesis is performed using the RNaseH-DNA polymerase I protocol *(14)*. After digestion with a frequently cutting restriction enzyme 3'-terminal cDNA fragments containing biotin label are isolated by binding to streptavidin beads. Following ligation of a double-stranded adapter, the 3' terminal cDNA fragments are amplified by PCR using adapter primer and the above mentioned biotinylated primer. This primary cDNA fragment population is resolved according to size on a denaturing polyacrylamide gel. Resolved fragments are subdivided into many size fractions by cutting the first-dimension lane into slices. Individual size fractions are recovered from the gel, immobilized on streptavidin beads, and end-labeled during the second strand synthesis. Beads with immobilized fragments are then treated sequentially with a set of restriction enzymes, so that every treatment liberates a subset of fragments containing restriction sites for a given enzyme. Fragment subsets liberated by one enzyme from the entire range of size fractions can be loaded on one gel to produce a two-dimensional separation picture. Alternatively, if the identification of differentially expressed mRNAs is the major objective, fragments from equivalent size fractions corresponding to two or more different cell samples can be loaded side-by-side to facilitate the comparison of the expression patterns. The latter variant is described in this chapter. The protocol was shown to work with small numbers of cells. We were able to produce high-quality GEF patterns from as little as two thousand sorted murine hematopoietic stem cells (HSC) (*see* **Fig. 2**), and our preliminary data indicate successful identification of genes expressed differentially between different subpopulations of early murine hematopoietic cells (*see* **Fig. 3**).

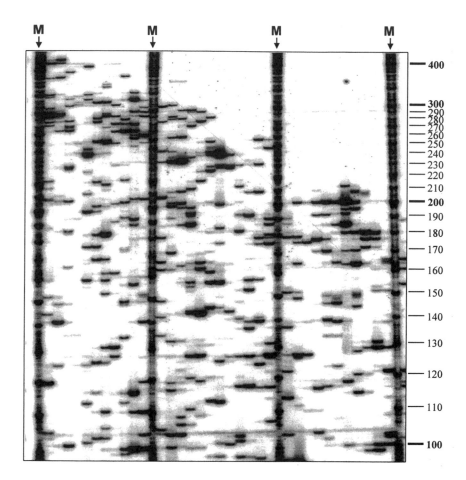

Fig. 2. Example of a two-dimensional GEF separation of the cDNA fragments. Approx 2×10^3 murine bone-marrow cells of the phenotype Rho⁻/Rho(VP)⁻ sorted according to the procedure described by Zijlmans et al. *(16)* were used for the cDNA synthesis. The picture shown was produced by the *Sty*I restriction endonuclease treatment. Prior to *Sty*I, the cDNA fragments immobilized on beads were treated sequentially with *Eco*RI, *Pst*I, *Ban*I, and *Stu*I. **M** indicate the SequaMark marker lanes. Positions of the brightest marker bands are shown on the right side. It should be noted that SequaMark provides 1 base resolution in the range of lengths of 40–400 bases.